A Pattern-Based Approach
Atlas of Lymph Node Pathology

AMY S. DUFFIELD, MD, PHD
Associate Professor
Department of Pathology
Johns Hopkins Hospital
Baltimore, Maryland

JOO Y. SONG, MD
Associate Clinical Professor
Department of Pathology
City of Hope National Medical Center
Duarte, California

GIRISH VENKATARAMAN, MD
Assistant Professor
Medical Director, Immunohistochemistry
Department of Pathology, Section of Hematopathology
University of Chicago Medicine
Chicago, Illinois

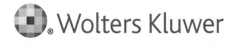 Wolters Kluwer

Philadelphia • Baltimore • New York • London
Buenos Aires • Hong Kong • Sydney • Tokyo

Acquisitions Editor: Nicole Dernoski
Development Editor: Ariel S. Winter
Editorial Coordinator: Tim Rinehart
Marketing Manager: Phyllis Hitner
Production Project Manager: Barton Dudlick
Design Coordinator: Stephen Druding
Manufacturing Coordinator: Beth Welsh
Prepress Vendor: TNQ Technologies

9 8 7 6 5 4 3 2 1

Printed in China

Library of Congress Cataloging-in-Publication Data

ISBN-13: 978-1-4963-7554-4

Cataloging in Publication data available on request from publisher.

shop.lww.com

To my mentors, trainees, and family.
Amy Duffield, MD

To Elaine and Stefania, for their tireless mentoring in teaching me the art of looking at lymph nodes under the microscope.
Girish Venkataraman, MD

To SS, my family, and mentors, for all your love and support
Joo Song, MD

PREFACE

Many traditional textbooks on lymph node pathology are arranged by diagnostic entity. This is most helpful when the pathologist already essentially knows the diagnosis, with the book serving to confirm an experienced pathologist's original hunch. As a trainee confronted with a lymph node specimen, however, it is often difficult to even begin formulate a differential diagnosis. This can lead to chaotic flipping through books in a futile attempt to "picture match."

In order to address this issue, we have structured this book to describe both normal findings and abnormalities in the different functional compartments of the node, namely the capsule, sinuses, paracortex, and cortex. In our experience, a complete understanding of normal lymph node structure—and variations on the normal structure—is limited in traditional textbooks. However, once the histology and the immunophenotypic findings in a normal lymph node are understood, abnormalities within the different compartments of the lymph node can be more readily identified. This sort of structured "march" through the parts of node can be used as an organizational guide when evaluating lymph nodes, making the process less daunting.

Another area of frustration for trainees is that many textbooks on lymph node pathology focus on neoplastic processes. However, in general practice, we are also frequently confronted by nonneoplastic findings in lymph nodes, some of which can mimic lymphoma. This book includes both neoplastic and nonneoplastic findings in lymph nodes that are encountered in everyday practice. We believe that the hematopathologists' role is not just to confirm or exclude lymphoma, but rather to establish a coherent explanation for enlarged nodes regardless of the presence of malignancy. Some of these diagnoses can be made in isolation, whereas others require clinical correlation.

Microscopic evaluation is the mainstay of lymph node pathology; however, ancillary testing is becoming increasingly more critical in the diagnosis of lymph node disorders. The appropriate use and interpretation of immunohistochemical stains is essential for lymph node evaluation. To this end, we have included an entire chapter focused on immunostains. This chapter addresses the use of internal controls and discusses best practices for the interpretation and reporting of immunostains. Flow cytometry, routine molecular studies, and fluorescence in situ hybridization (FISH) are also utilized in the pathologic evaluation of lymph nodes. While this textbook is not an exhaustive exploration of these ancillary tests, it does discuss when they should be deployed and also notes of some of their critical limitations. Additionally, there is discussion of the need for judicious use of ancillary testing when trying to be mindful of costs.

We hope that the structure of this book as well as the extensive images provide the reader with a useful framework for approaching a lymph node specimen.

Features of this textbook are described below.

- "Checklists" systematically organize complex topics.
- A chapter on the normal lymph node is included, as the morphologic and immunophenotypic findings are somewhat complex and are not always fully understood by trainees.
- "Pearls and Pitfalls" includes lessons from real-life sign-out experience with an emphasis on important diagnostic clues, mimics, and hazards.
- The "Frequently Asked Questions" section includes questions that we are often asked by both trainees as well as our colleagues who are not hematopathologists.
- "Key Features" summarizes the essential elements of an entity.
- "Sample Notes" are provided for infrequent or complex diagnoses.
- "Near Misses" are included to alert the reader to close calls and tips for avoiding pitfalls in difficult diagnoses.
- References included in each chapter are provided for further reading and may also be included in pathology reports.
- Each chapter is accompanied by an online "Quiz" section, which emphasizes important points and can be used for board review.

CONTRIBUTORS

REVA C. GOLDBERG, BS
Visiting Research Student
Department of Pathology
The University of Chicago Medicine
Chicago, Illinois

KYLE KISSICK, MD
Resident Pathologist
Department of Pathology
The University of Chicago Medicine
Chicago, Illinois

HA L. NGUYEN, MD
Staff Pathologist
Dekalb Pathology
Decatur, Georgia

LAURA WAKE, MD
Assistant Professor
Division of Hematologic Pathology
Department of Pathology
Johns Hopkins Medical Institutions
Baltimore, Maryland

ALISHA WARE, MD
Assistant Professor
Division of Hematologic Pathology
Department of Pathology
Johns Hopkins Medical Institutions
Baltimore, Maryland

CONTENTS

CHAPTER OUTLINE

Histologic evaluation of lymph nodes is not always straightforward: abnormal findings can be subtle and may require additional workup, including immunohistochemical stains, ancillary studies, and expert consultation. On the other hand, benign reactive lymph nodes may occasionally look atypical, even to the experienced eye, and may also require further evaluation. Given the breadth and depth of diagnostic categories of lymphoproliferative disorders as well as numerous reactive conditions that involve lymphoid tissue, the examination of lymph node specimens can be challenging even for experienced pathologists.

In order to facilitate the pathologic evaluation of lymph nodes, it is important to understand the structural and functional compartments of the lymph node and to interpret morphologic findings in parallel with ancillary tests. Adequate specimen preparation is also critical, as is knowledge of the patient's medical history and appreciation of the clinical context leading to the biopsy.

LYMPH NODE STRUCTURE

Normal lymph nodes are small, subcentimeter structures with several functional compartments.[1-5] Systematically identifying and evaluating each of these compartments provides a framework for the pathologist to identify a lymph node as benign, atypical, or malignant, and helps guide the appropriate diagnostic workup.

CAPSULE

A normal lymph node is surrounded by a thin rim of fibrous tissue which forms the **capsule** (Figures 1.1 and 1.2). The presence of a capsule defines the border of the lymph node and helps to differentiate between a true lymph node and a lymphoid infiltrate. The diagnostic line should reflect the classification of the tissue, which is, in part, defined by the presence or absence of a capsule.

SAMPLE SIGN OUT

(*If capsule is present*): **Lymph node** with reactive lymphoid hyperplasia.

(*If no capsule*): **Lymphoid tissue** with reactive lymphoid hyperplasia.

SINUSES

The **sinuses** are located beneath the capsule (subcapsular sinuses) and distributed throughout the lymph node (cortical and medullary sinuses). The sinuses function as a mingling area for immune cells to interact with antigen-presenting cells. In benign lymph nodes, the sinuses are open, or "patent," and contain lymphatic fluid, which enters the lymph node via the afferent lymphatic vessels at the periphery of the lymph node, traverses the subcapsular sinus, circulates through the medullary sinuses, and exits the lymph node via the efferent lymphatic vessel at the hilum.[6]

Sinuses may be difficult to visualize on an H&E-stained slide (Figure 1.3) but will often contain small lymphocytes, immunoblasts, histiocytes, and/or neutrophils (Figure 1.4). In lymph nodes involved by lymphoma, the sinuses are often filled by the neoplastic cells and are no longer patent or may be compressed to slitlike spaces by the infiltrating neoplastic cells. In other disorders, the sinuses may be distended (see Chapter 3).

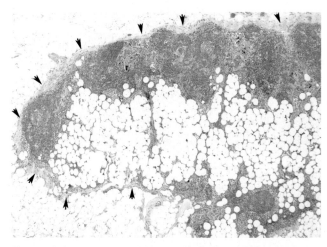

Figure 1.1. A thin rim of fibrovascular tissue surrounds lymph nodes, forming a capsule (arrowheads) that delineates the lymph node from the surrounding tissue.

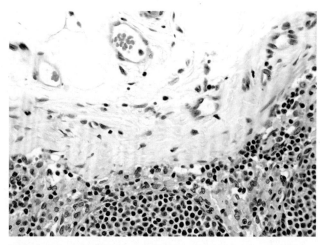

Figure 1.2. A high-power view of the capsule illustrates the presence of small vessels.

CORTEX

The peripheral zone of the lymph node subjacent to the subcapsular sinus is designated as the **cortex**. The normal lymph node cortex is composed of aggregates of cells that form follicles of various sizes and shapes (Figure 1.5). The follicles are mostly composed of B-cells (Figure 1.6), and the lymphocytes in the interfollicular areas are predominantly T-cells (Figure 1.7). The follicles are typically arrayed in the cortical area at the periphery of the node; however, histologic sections may not be taken along the central axis of the lymph node; and therefore, the normal architectural structure of the lymph node may not be apparent on all sections (Figure 1.8).

Primary follicles are present in inactive lymph nodes and are composed of small, mature B-cells (Figures 1.9-1.12). The B-cells in primary follicles express the typical mature B-cell markers, including CD20 and Pax-5, and are also positive for the anti-apoptotic protein, Bcl-2. The B-cells in primary follicles express dim CD5, but this can be difficult to visualize with the CD5 immunohistochemical stain performed in many labs. The expression of Bcl-2 on B-cells is of great functional significance, as this anti-apoptotic protein supports the survival of the B-cells in the primary follicles. The primary follicles have well-organized underlying follicular dendritic cell (FDC) meshworks.

In a simplified model, primary follicles transition into **secondary follicles** when B-cells encounter an antigen, and this process incites an immune response. Secondary follicles (Figure 1.13) contain centers of immune activity called **germinal centers** where B-cell selection occurs.[7] The primary function of a germinal center is to produce competent B-cells that will generate effective antibodies to foreign antigens but will tolerate self-antigens. In order to achieve that goal, ineffective or overeffective B-cells are destroyed via programmed cell death, and the cellular debris is engulfed by phagocytic histiocytes that are known as **tingible-body macrophages**. To allow for the apoptosis and elimination of the B-cells that generate ineffective antibodies, the anti-apoptotic protein Bcl-2 is downregulated in normal germinal center B-cells.

The germinal center B-cells are separated into zones corresponding to their stage in the selection process, and this zonation imparts a characteristic **polarized** appearance to the germinal center, consisting of a **dark zone** and a **light zone** (Figure 1.14). The dark zone is rich in large B-cells with open chromatin and several small nucleoli, known as **centroblasts**, whereas the light zone contains admixed small B-cells with mature chromatin, known as **centrocytes**. Mitotic figures and tingible-body macrophages are common in the germinal centers. FDCs are present to help B-cell selection and expansion, and—as with primary follicles—FCDs provide structural support for the secondary follicle cells.[8] FDCs are identifiable in follicles as binucleated cells with small eosinophilic nucleoli (Figures 1.15-1.18).

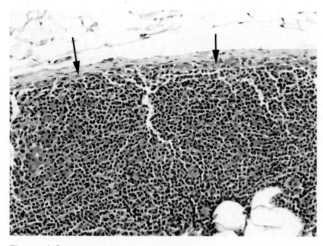

Figure 1.3. The sinuses may be difficult to visualize in some lymph nodes. Arrows point to the thin subcapsular sinus in this lymph node.

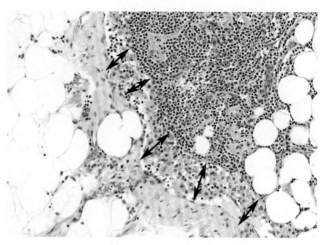

Figure 1.4. In other lymph nodes, the sinuses are relatively easy to identify. The subcapsular sinus in this node contains numerous histiocytes and small lymphocytes, and the arrows indicate the width of the sinus.

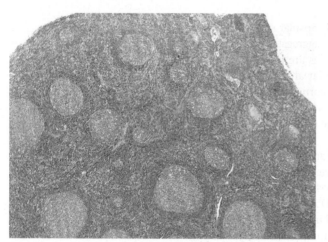

Figure 1.5. The cortex of a lymph node with follicular hypertrophy.

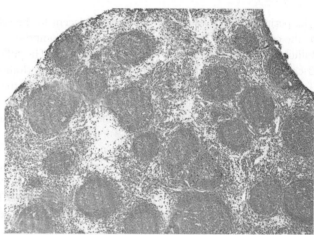

Figure 1.6. CD20 stains the B-cells, which are concentrated in follicles.

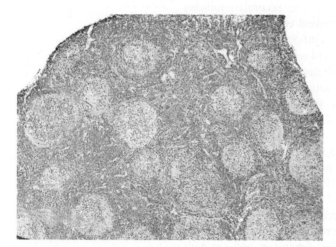

Figure 1.7. CD3-positive T-cells predominate in the paracortex, but there are also infrequent T-cells in the follicles (follicular helper T-cells).

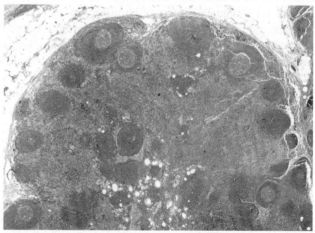

Figure 1.8. The reactive follicles are arrayed around the periphery of the node in this section, illustrating the characteristic nodal architecture.

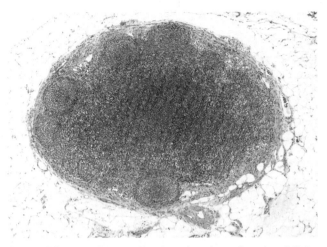

Figure 1.9. A small (2 mm) lymph node with small primary follicles arrayed around in the cortex.

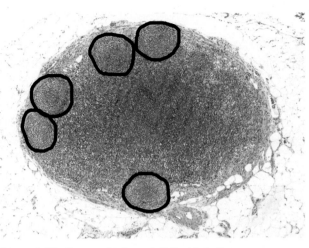

Figure 1.10. Scattered primary follicles (circled).

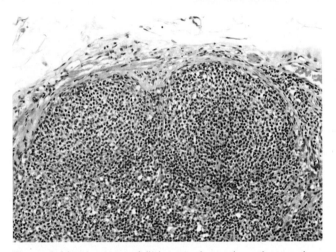

Figure 1.11. The primary follicles are subcapsular and are predominantly composed of small, mature B-cells.

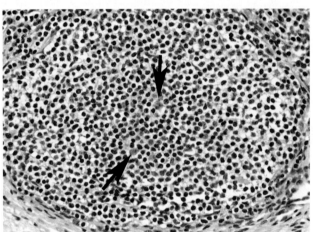

Figure 1.12. The B-cells in primary follicles are small with condensed (mature) chromatin. Most of the rare larger cells present are the follicular dendritic cells with long cellular processes that provide follicular structure (arrows).

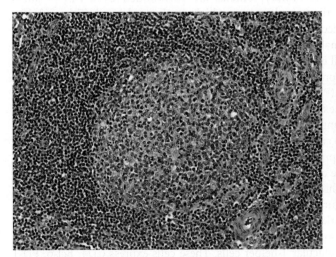

Figure 1.13. High-power view of a secondary follicle. Both the mantle zone and germinal center are polarized.

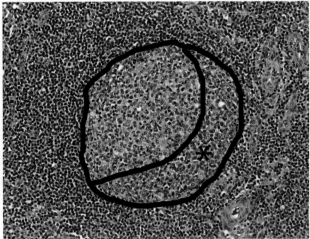

Figure 1.14. The germinal center is circled, and the dark zone is indicated with an asterisk.

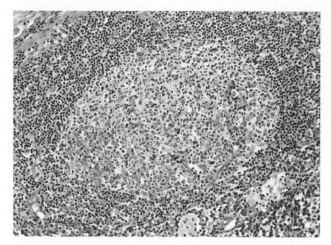

Figure 1.15. A characteristic germinal center with a polarized mantle zone. The germinal center is also polarized and contains scattered tingible-body macrophages.

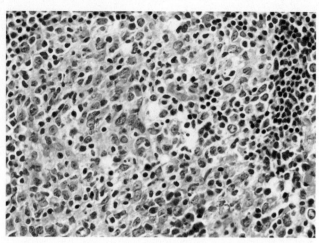

Figure 1.16. The germinal center contains a mixture of centroblasts, centrocytes, small lymphocytes, tingible-body macrophages, and follicular dendritic cells.

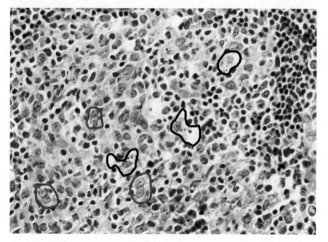

Figure 1.17. Tingible-body macrophages are outlined in black, and follicular dendritic cells are outlined in blue.

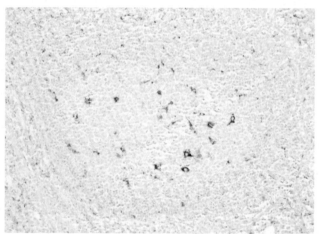

Figure 1.18. CD68 marks scattered tingible-body macrophages in the germinal center.

The germinal centers of secondary follicles are surrounded by a rim of small B-lymphocytes, known as the **mantle zone**, which is also polarized (Figure 1.19). Secondary follicles have a second thin rim of small lymphoid cells surrounding the mantle zone, comprising the **marginal zone**. However, the marginal zone is typically not visualized in H&E sections of a normal lymph node.

The immunophenotypic profile of secondary follicles is very characteristic. The germinal center B-cells express CD20 (Figure 1.20) and Pax-5 (Figure 1.21). The expression of CD20 tends to be brighter and the expression of Pax-5 tends to be dimmer on the germinal center cells as compared to the mantle zone B-cells. The centroblasts in the germinal center also express CD10 (Figure 1.22) and Bcl-6 (Figure 1.23). As noted previously, B-cells in a normal germinal center lack expression of Bcl-2 (Figure 1.24). The dark zone of the germinal centers has a relatively dense concentration of centroblasts, with a high Ki-67 proliferation index as compared to the light zone (Figure 1.25). The surrounding polarized mantle zones are highlighted by IgD (Figure 1.26), Bcl-2, and CD23 (Figure 1.27). In addition to the mantle zone cells, CD23 marks the underlying FDC meshworks, which also express CD21 (Figure 1.28). The follicle also contains scattered T-cells, which assist in the B-cell selection process and are known as follicular T-helper cells. These cells express CD4, Bcl-6, PD-1 (Figure 1.29), and Bcl-2 (Figure 1.24), and a subset are brightly CD10-positive (Figure 1.22).

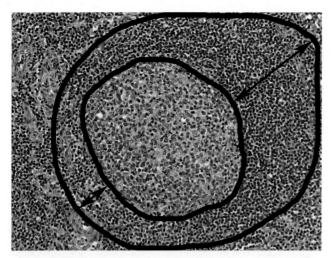

Figure 1.19. The mantle zone is outlined. Arrows indicate the variable thickness of the polarized mantle zone.

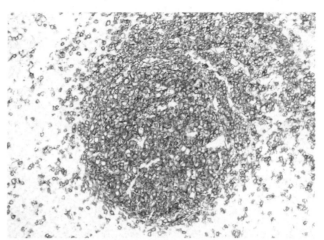

Figure 1.20. CD20 marks B-cells. The germinal center B-cells are slightly larger with slightly brighter expression of CD20 as compared with the mantle zone B-cells.

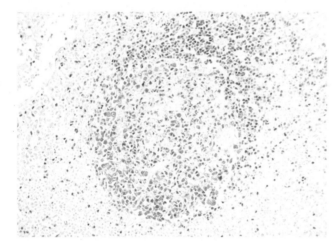

Figure 1.21. Pax-5 also marks B-cells. The germinal center cell nuclei are larger with slightly dimmer Pax-5 expression than the nuclei of mantle zone B-cells.

Figure 1.22. CD10 marks germinal center B-cells. A few small follicular helper T-cells show bright expression of CD10.

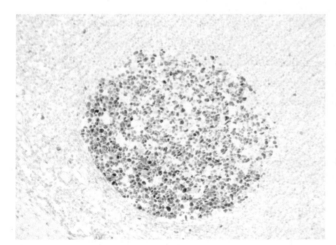

Figure 1.23. The germinal center B-cells are also positive for Bcl-6.

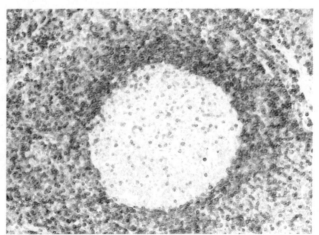

Figure 1.24. Bcl-2 expression is downregulated in germinal centers, but Bcl-2 is brightly expressed in the mantle zone B-cells. Both follicular helper T-cells and the surrounding T-cells are also Bcl-2-positive.

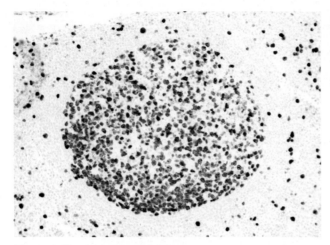

Figure 1.25. The proliferation index is high in the germinal center and is slightly higher in the dark zone.

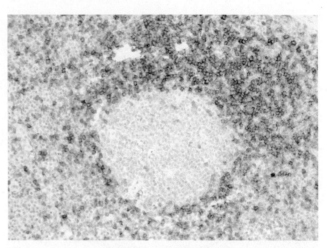

Figure 1.26. The polarized mantle zone B-cells are highlighted by IgD.

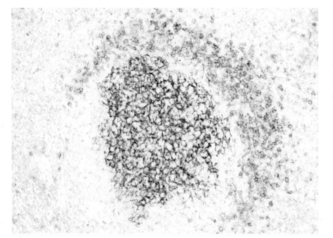

Figure 1.27. CD23 marks the mantle zone B-cells, as well as follicular dendritic cell meshworks that underlie the follicles.

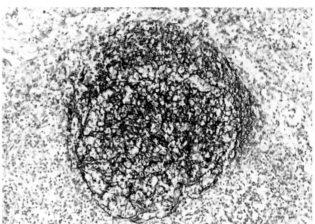

Figure 1.28. CD21 is positive in the follicular dendritic cell meshworks.

KEY FEATURES of an Abnormal Lymph Node
- Monotonous follicles (similar size and shape) present throughout the lymph node
- Germinal centers lack polarization or lack tingible-body macrophages
- Absent or unpolarized mantle zones surrounding the germinal centers
- Abnormal immunophenotype of germinal center cells (ie, Bcl-2+, low Ki-67)
- Follicles are disrupted, peripheralized, or absent due to a paracortical expansion

PARACORTEX

The **paracortex** comprises the area between follicles and the medullary cords near the hilum and is composed of a mixture of lymphocytes, small vessels, and scattered activated lymphocytes known as **immunoblasts** (Figure 1.30). The paracortex also contains antigen-presenting cells, including Langerhan cells, interdigitating dendritic cells, and histiocytes.[9,10]

The majority of the cells in the paracortex are CD3-positive T-cells (Figure 1.7) which express CD43, CD2, CD4 or CD8, CD5, and CD7. Of note, reactive T-cells can occasionally

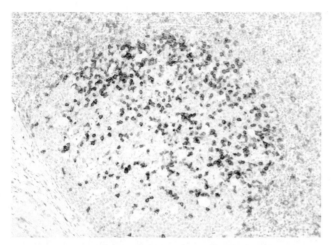

Figure 1.29. The follicular helper T-cells are highlighted by PD1.

show partial loss of CD7. T-cells in the paracortex are also typically positive for Bcl-2, but with a slightly dimmer intensity than the Bcl-2 expressed on the mantle zone B-cells (Figure 1.31). Lack of expression of Bcl-2 on the T-cells is unusual and, assuming that the Bcl-2 control tissue stains appropriately, should prompt further workup for involvement by a T-cell lymphoma.

Within the lymph node, the T-cells are a mixture of CD4 and CD8-positive cells. The ratio of CD4-positive cells to CD8-positive cells can be affected by several factors. In normal lymph nodes, the **CD4:CD8 ratio** usually ranges between 1:1 and 5:1. It should be noted that if there are numerous histiocytes within the paracortex, then enumeration of CD4-positive T-cells via immunohistochemical stains may not be straightforward since histiocytes are also positive for CD4. If needed, a CD68 immunohistochemical stain can be performed to help visualize histiocytes in the paracortex.

Unusually low CD4:CD8 ratios (<1:1) can be seen in HIV and other viral infections, or rarely in lymphomas such as CD8-positive peripheral T-cell lymphoma or T-cell–/histiocyte-rich large B-cell lymphoma. Unusually high CD4:CD8 ratios (>5:1) can be seen in benign reactive conditions, such as dermatopathic lymphadenopathy (Figures 1.32 and 1.33), but are also characteristic of some lymphomas including nodular lymphocyte predominant Hodgkin lymphoma and Epstein-Barr virus (EBV)–negative classical Hodgkin lymphoma (CHL). Additionally, abnormal CD4:CD8 ratios can be seen in the setting of nodal involvement by nonhematolymphoid neoplasms, as tumor-reactive lymphocytes may skew toward either CD4 or CD8.

Often, the paracortex contains singly scattered activated T- or B immunoblasts, which are large cells with prominent nucleoli that may very rarely be binucleate (Figure 1.34). These T- and B immunoblasts express variably intense CD3 or CD20, respectively. These immunoblasts also exhibit variable expression of CD30 (Figure 1.35) and MUM-1.

MEDULLA

The **medullary sinuses** are near the center of the lymph node and are surrounded by an area rich in lymphocytes, plasmacytoid lymphocytes, and plasma cells. This area, known as the **medullary cords**, is the site where plasma cells proliferate and produce antibodies (Figures 1.36-1.38). The plasma cells in the medullary cords are a mixture of kappa and lambda light chain-positive cells ("polytypic"). Kappa light chain–positive plasma cells often slightly outnumber lambda-positive cells, and the **kappa:lambda ratio** of plasma cells in normal lymph nodes ranges from 1:1 to 4:1.

Figure 1.30. Paracortical region of a normal lymph node with small vessels, histiocytes, and small lymphocytes.

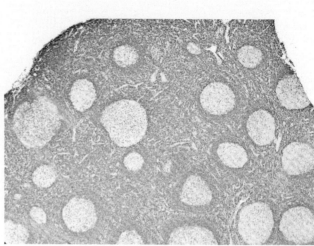

Figure 1.31. The T-cells in the paracortex are Bcl-2-positive, as are B-cells in primary follicles and mantle zones. (same lymph node as Figures 1.5-1.7)

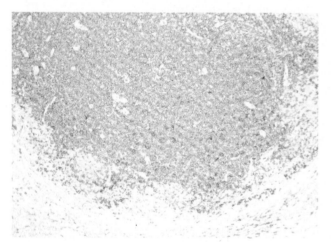

Figure 1.32. The vast majority of T-cells in the paracortex of this lymph node with dermatopathic lymphadenopathy are CD4-positive.

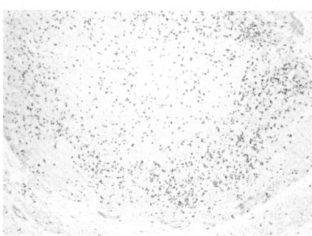

Figure 1.33. The same lymph node contains very few CD8+ T-cells in the paracortex.

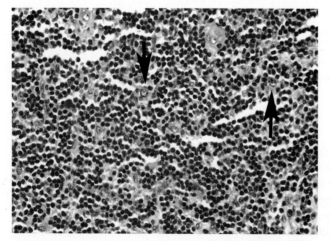

Figure 1.34. Paracortex composed of small lymphocytes, small vessels, and occasional histiocytes with scattered immunoblasts. Two of the most readily identified immunoblasts are marked with arrows.

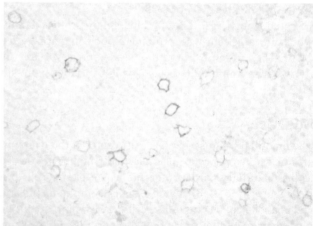

Figure 1.35. Variable CD30 expression is seen on singly scattered immunoblasts.

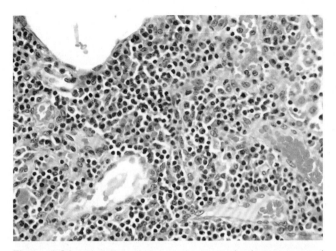

Figure 1.36. Medullary cords in a reactive node abut sinuses and are composed of a mixture of plasma cells, plasmacytoid cells, and small lymphocytes.

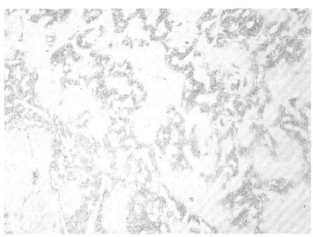

Figure 1.37. MUM-1 marks the plasma cells in this lymph node. The staining pattern shows the serpiginous arrangement of the expanded medullary cords.

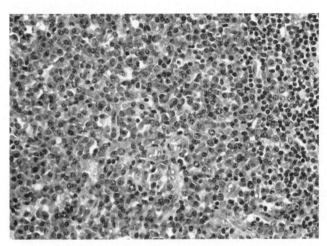

Figure 1.38. A lymph node involved by dermatopathic lymphadenopathy shows medullary plasmacytosis, which is characteristic of this entity.

Normal Lymph Node Architecture Checklist

☐ An intact, thin **capsule**

☐ **Sinuses** are patent and not distended with abnormal cells

☐ The **cortex** contains scattered primary or secondary follicles of various sizes and shapes

☐ Secondary follicles have polarized germinal centers with tingible-body macrophages and polarized mantle zones

☐ The **paracortex** is not expanded and contains small T-cells, histiocytes, and scattered immunoblasts

SPECIMEN PREPARATION

FIXATION

In order to fully appreciate the architectural features of a lymph node, appropriate sample preparation is essential. Adequate preparation requires thin sectioning of the lymph node specimen and immersion in fixative solution for a sufficient period of time. Poor fixation of lymph node specimens makes morphologic evaluation difficult or even impossible. While grossing large specimens, it is sometimes tempting to fill the cassettes with as much tissue as possible; however, thick sections are often not well-fixed due to the slow penetration of tissues by the fixative. The resulting tissue is difficult to section and does not stain well. This "fixation artifact" makes assessment of cytomorphology very difficult and can even hinder the evaluation of the overall nodal architecture (Figures 1.39 and 1.40). Ideally, relatively thin tissue sections (ie, the thickness of a nickel) are submitted to allow for adequate fixation. If the tissue is poorly fixed, then asking the histology lab to cut thin (4 μm) sections can be somewhat helpful.

Neutral buffered formalin is the preferred fixative in most histology labs and has the advantage of allowing polymerase chain reaction (PCR)–based molecular studies to be performed on fixed tissue; however, lymph nodes are sometimes fixed in metal-based fixatives, including B5 neutral Zenker solution and zinc sulfate formalin. These alternative fixatives allow for a shorter fixation time (2-6 hours) and are known for producing excellent nuclear morphologic features. A downside of using acidic fixatives is that molecular testing cannot be performed on the tissue because these fixatives impair the binding of PCR primers to DNA.[2]

> **PEARLS & PITFALLS**
>
> Clinical teams often want a diagnosis as quickly as possible and may request that a lymph node specimen be "rushed." Unfortunately, this request often backfires: poorly fixed tissue hinders morphologic assessment, necessitating the use of numerous ancillary studies to compensate for poor cytomorphology and extending the time needed to establish a final diagnosis. The clinical team should be forewarned that rushing lymph node specimens is not advisable.

FROZEN SECTIONS

Morphologic evaluation of lymph nodes can also be challenging on **frozen sections** (Figures 1.41 and 1.42). As with other tissues, when lymph node tissue is frozen, the cells become distorted, making it difficult to assess both the overall architecture of the node and the cytomorphology of the lymphocytes. Morphology is only marginally improved when the frozen sections are subsequently fixed in formalin and processed (Figures 1.43 and 1.44). Subclassification of lymphomas relies on evaluation of the lymph node architecture, cellular morphology, and cell size; therefore, freezing artifact can result in significant diagnostic challenges.

One of the best ways to avoid freezing artifact is to discourage frozen section analysis when there is a high clinical suspicion for lymphoma. However, if a frozen section is requested on a suspected lymphoma, then it is advisable to only freeze part of the specimen, create a touch preparation or smear, and reserve the remainder of the specimen for normal processing. In general, it is preferable to defer diagnosis until the pathologist examines the permanent sections.

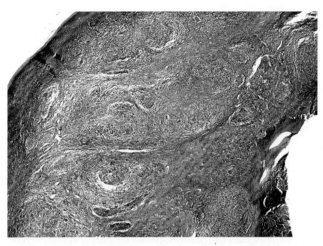

Figure 1.39. Poor fixation limits evaluation of the architectural features in lymph nodes. Ultimately, this lymph node was found to be involved by classical Hodgkin lymphoma.

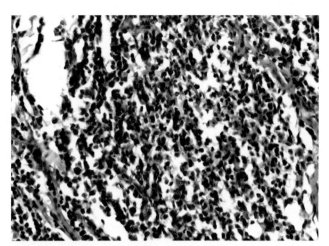

Figure 1.40. Poor fixation limits evaluation cytomorphology. Hodgkin/Reed-Sternberg cells are very difficult to appreciate on this specimen, and immunohistochemical stains were required for diagnosis.

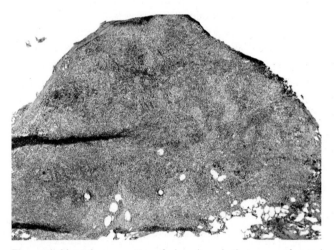

Figure 1.41. A frozen section of a lymph node that was performed to "rule out lymphoma."

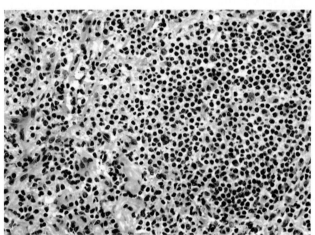

Figure 1.42. The same lymph node at high power (400×). The assessment of cytomorphology is affected by freezing artifact.

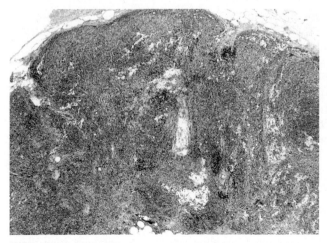

Figure 1.43. Even after fixation, it is difficult to evaluate the nodal architecture on previously frozen tissue in Figure 1.41.

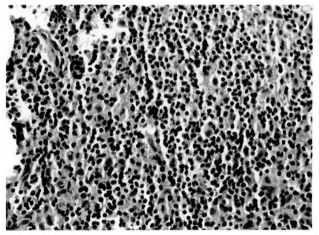

Figure 1.44. The same lymph node at high power (400×) after fixation. Cytomorphology remains distorted.

SAMPLE FROZEN SECTION SIGN OUT

Cervical biopsy:

• Lymphoid tissue present, defer to permanents sections. See note.

Note: A portion of the lymph node is submitted for flow cytometric analysis.

When lymphoma is suspected in a lymph node sent for frozen section analysis, immuno-histochemical and molecular analysis can be used to clarify structure, immunophenotype, and clonality. Unfortunately, however, the use of numerous ancillary techniques may extend the time that it takes to make a final diagnosis.

One way to encourage our surgical colleagues to forgo a frozen section or discourage the clinical team from "rushing" specimens is via clear communication. For instance, if flow cytometry is performed in-house, then a preliminary diagnosis on a lymph node biopsy may be available via flow cytometric analysis within a few hours, allowing for complete histologic evaluation of the adequately fixed specimen at a later time.

In all suspected lymphoma cases, a portion of the tissue should be submitted for flow cyto-metric evaluation if possible. Ideally, a portion of tissue approximately the size of a pencil eraser should be minced into 1 to 2 mm cubes and placed in cell culture media (ie, RPMI) or saline and submitted immediately to the flow cytometry lab. In practice, however, much less tissue is often submitted, particularly with needle core biopsies. An attempt at flow cytometric evaluation is, however, encouraged even in minute specimens, since the results can sometimes be informative, particularly in the case of low-grade B-cell lymphomas.

If clinical suspicion for lymphoma is low, then a small portion of the node can be stored in cell culture media (ie, RPMI) in the refrigerator. The tissue can then be submitted to the flow cytometry lab if review of the H&E sections raises the possibility of nodal involvement by lymphoma. This strategy reduces both costs and unnecessary work in the flow cytom-etry lab. However, it is important to remember that any delay in processing may result in cell loss, particularly in aggressive lymphomas. Short delays typically do not preclude the diagnosis of low-grade B-cell lymphomas via flow cytometry, since these cells remain viable for longer periods of time.

FAQ: Do I need to perform immunohistochemical stains on a lymph node that looks reactive?

Answer: The answer to this frequently asked question, like many answers in pathology, is—it depends. There are many factors that are in play, including the clinical history and morphologic findings on the H&E. For example, if the lymph node in question is 1 of the 12 reactive lymph nodes in a colon resection for inflam-matory bowel disease, then it's most likely safe to rely on the H&E. If, however, an enlarged lymph node with no known etiology is sampled, then it may be prudent to perform a short immunohistochemical panel or to consult an expert hemato-pathologist. The addition of flow cytometry is also helpful in the case of enlarged nodes and will help rule out partial involvement by non-Hodgkin lymphoma.

LIMITED SPECIMENS

Increasingly, core or needle biopsies of lymph nodes are submitted for histologic evaluation. This practice is easier for patients, but the evaluation of small biopsies poses diagnostic challenges to pathologists including limited sampling, variable fixation, and scant tissue that does not allow for a full immunohistochemical or molecular workup.[11-14] Crush artifact can also pose significant challenges in the interpretation of core biopsies and should be noted in the report (Figure 1.45).

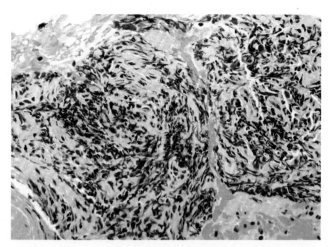

Figure 1.45. This core biopsy of a peripancreatic lymph node shows extensive crush artifact. Evaluation of an excisional biopsy demonstrated involvement by classical Hodgkin lymphoma.

Additionally, the workup of core biopsies often takes longer than the workup of larger specimens because stains must be ordered sequentially in order to preserve the scant remaining tissue. If possible, a portion of the specimen should also be sent for flow cytometric analysis. If flow cytometric evaluation was not performed or was unrevealing, and if there is morphologic or clinical concern for involvement by lymphoma, then a short immunohistochemical stain panel is useful.

Example of a Short Immunohistochemical Panel for a Lymph Node Needle Core Biopsy
• CD20, CD3, CD30, Ki-67

Core biopsies from lymph nodes should reveal normal nodal architecture (Figures 1.46-1.48), with clearly defined follicles that predominantly contain B-cells (Figure 1.49) and a paracortex rich in T-cells (Figure 1.50). Germinal centers can often be seen on the CD20 stain because the germinal center B-cells are larger with slightly brighter expression of CD20 than mantle B-cells. The germinal centers will also be highlighted by Ki-67, as the proliferation index in normal germinal centers is high (Figure 1.51). Depending on the tissue orientation, Ki-67 may also highlight the polarity of the germinal center.

PEARLS & PITFALLS

A low Ki-67 proliferation index in an apparent germinal center is abnormal and should trigger further workup for a low-grade B-cell lymphoma, such as follicular lymphoma or follicular colonization by a nodal marginal zone lymphoma (NMZL) (see Near Misses at the end of the chapter).

The CD30 immunohistochemical stain will highlight scattered immunoblasts that are present in normal reactive lymph nodes and confirm the absence of Hodgkin/Reed-Sternberg cells (HRS cells) (Figure 1.52). If the morphologic and immunophenotypic findings cannot definitively distinguish immunoblasts from HRS cells on a core biopsy, then an excisional biopsy is recommended. Clinical correlation is also important; if biopsies were performed to evaluate involvement by metastatic disease, then the appropriate immunohistochemical stains (ie, cytokeratins) should be performed.

Overall, reactive lymphoid tissue can usually be confirmed in core biopsies. However, small biopsies are notoriously difficult to evaluate and lesional tissue may have been missed; thus, it is prudent to make a note of the limitations in the pathology report.

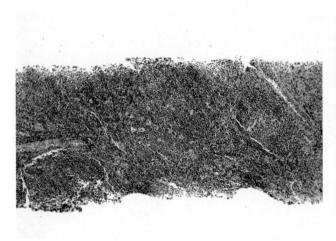

Figure 1.46. Core biopsy of a 2 cm cervical node in a 23-year-old man. Several reactive follicles are seen.

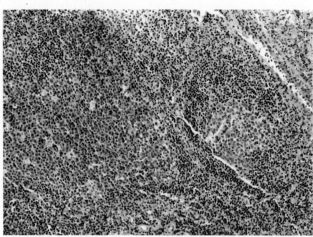

Figure 1.47. The reactive follicles have polarized mantle zones, though the polarity of the germinal center is difficult to appreciate.

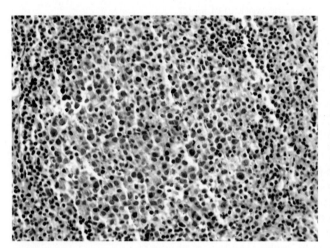

Figure 1.48. The germinal centers contain scattered tingible-body macrophages.

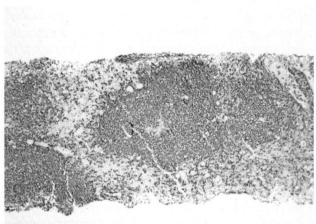

Figure 1.49. A CD20 immunohistochemical stain highlights B-cells, which are concentrated in follicles.

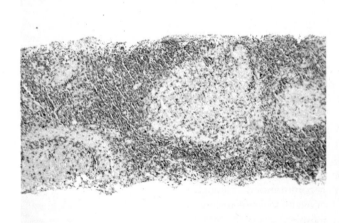

Figure 1.50. CD3-positive T-cells predominate in the interfollicular areas.

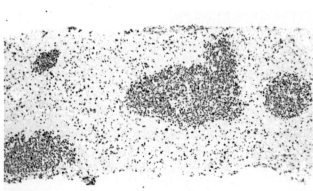

Figure 1.51. The Ki-67 proliferation index is appropriately high in the germinal centers, but it is relatively low in the interfollicular areas.

SAMPLE SIGN OUT

Right axilla, needle core biopsy:

• Reactive lymphoid tissue. See note.

Note: The findings in this scant specimen do not suggest involvement by lymphoma or metastatic carcinoma; however, if clinical suspicion for involvement by a neoplastic process is high, then evaluation of a more generous specimen is recommended.

CLINICAL CONTEXT

ANATOMIC SITE

Pathologists occasionally receive cases that lack pertinent clinical information. A laconic clinical history of "lymph node" or "lymphadenopathy" may be the only information given, with the location of the lymph node omitted. Conversely, the location of the biopsy may be provided, but the type of tissue that was biopsied is not supplied.

Fortunately, even limited information, such as the location of the lymph node, can be of value. For instance, supraclavicular lymph nodes deserve special attention, as enlarged nodes at this site often represent a pathologic process. Additionally, the anatomic site provides some context for interpreting the lymph node size. In general, lymph nodes >1 cm are considered enlarged; however, normal inguinal and pelvic lymph nodes may be significantly larger than 1 cm. Pelvic lymph nodes in older patients often show fibrosis and may even exhibit calcifications in the fibrotic areas (Figure 1.53).

Lymph nodes can also show benign epithelial inclusions, including thyroid and salivary gland tissue in cervical nodes, and endosalpingiosis involving pelvic lymph nodes (Figures 1.54 and 1.55). Lymph nodes that drain the skin may contain inclusions of benign nevus cells, which are often associated with the capsule and are referred to as "capsular nevi" (Figure 1.56).

PATIENT DEMOGRAPHICS

Patient demographics, including the patient age and sex, are important information for pathologists when examining lymph nodes. Younger patients, particularly children and adolescents, can exhibit very vigorous lymphoid hypertrophy, with reactive lymph nodes reaching several centimeters in size. Older patients are less likely to develop exuberant reactive lymphoid hypertrophy, and lymph nodes that are larger than 1 cm in size should be regarded with more suspicion in older adults. Older patients also frequently show lipomatous replacement of lymph nodes (Figure 1.57). While this is a normal finding, pathologic changes may still be present in the remainder of the lymph node, and careful morphologic evaluation of the remaining rim of lymphoid tissue is still essential.

CLINICAL INFORMATION

Electronic medical records (EMR) certainly have drawbacks, but they can be especially helpful for pathologists when evaluating a lymph node specimen. As previously noted, the clinical information provided on specimen requisitions is often sparse; therefore, review of the EMR for pertinent patient history is critical. A prior history of lymphoma, autoimmunity, inflammation, or infection can be of value. For instance, while mesenteric lymph nodes are typically rather small, they can show marked reactive changes and become greatly enlarged in the setting of inflammation, such as diverticulitis or inflammatory bowel disease.

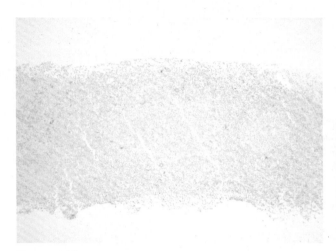

Figure 1.52. CD30 stains only rare immunoblasts in this core biopsy.

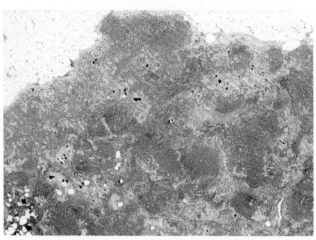

Figure 1.53. Pelvic lymph nodes from older patients often show normal degenerative changes, including significant fibrosis and focal calcifications. This is a pelvic lymph node that was sampled at the time of a radical prostatectomy in a 67-year-old man.

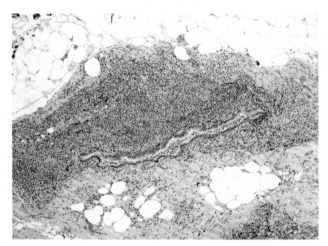

Figure 1.54. Lymph node with focal endosalpingiosis in a 55-year-old woman with a history of high-grade serous carcinoma.

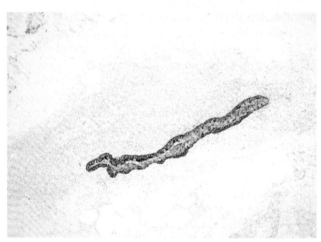

Figure 1.55. A keratin (AE1/AE3) immunohistochemical stain of pelvic lymph node, highlighting the endosalpingiosis.

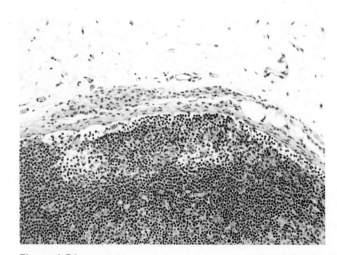

Figure 1.56. A subtle capsular nevus.

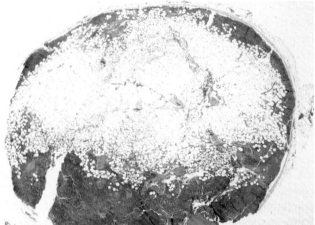

Figure 1.57. Fatty replacement of the hilum is a normal degenerative change that is frequently seen in the lymph nodes of older patients. This lymph node was part of an axillary node dissection in a 65-year-old woman with untreated invasive ductal carcinoma of the breast.

IMPORTANT PATIENT HISTORY TO OBTAIN

- Prior history of a hematolymphoid neoplasm
- History of infection or inflammatory condition
- Immunodeficiency, autoimmunity, or treatment with immunosuppressant medications
- B-symptoms (weight loss, fevers, night sweats)

Radiology reports are also informative to pathologists, indicating the location or extent of the patient's lymphadenopathy. Review of radiology reports may reveal that the most accessible lymph node (rather than the largest or obviously abnormal lymph node) was sampled. If the radiology report indicates the presence of markedly enlarged lymph node(s), but the sampled lymph node is small and shows nonspecific histologic findings, then it may be prudent to recommend biopsy of a specific enlarged node in the note of the pathology report. This will alert the clinical team that a lymph node with a low probability of involvement by disease was sampled.

SAMPLE SIGN OUT

Cervical lymph node, biopsy:
- Lymph node with reactive lymphoid hyperplasia. See note.

Note: While the sampled lymph node shows only reactive changes, the presence of a contralateral 3 cm cervical node is noted. Sampling of this lymph node may be of value, if clinically indicated.

Positron-emission tomography (PET) scans are usually performed after a diagnosis of malignancy is established; however, PET scan results are occasionally available at the time of histopathologic evaluation of the lymph node. If available, the presence of lymph nodes with a maximum standardized uptake value (SUV max) of greater than 9 or 10 should raise the possibility of an aggressive lymphoma. Additionally, the SUV max of the sampled lymph node should be confirmed and correlated with the histologic findings, if possible. If there are any nodes with an unusually high SUV max that were not sampled, this can also be indicated in a note.

Finally, laboratory values may be helpful. For instance, review of the CBC and differential may reveal that a patient has a long-standing lymphocytosis, which could raise suspicion for a low-grade B-cell lymphoma such as chronic lymphocytic leukemia/small lymphocytic lymphoma (CLL/SLL). Anemia and/or other cytopenias may indicate bone marrow involvement or peripheral destruction. An elevated lactate dehydrogenase (LDH) is often seen in aggressive lymphomas. Ferritin is characteristically markedly elevated (>20,000 ng/mL) in hemophagocytic lymphohistiocytosis. Low-level monoclonal gammopathies identified on serum protein electrophoresis (SPEP) and serum immunofixation electrophoresis (SIFE) studies can be present in patients with low-grade B-cell lymphomas. For instance, low-level IgM paraproteins can be seen in CLL/SLL. On the other hand, a high IgM spike should alert the pathologist to the possibility of lymphoplasmacytic lymphoma, and high immunoglobulin levels suggest a plasma cell neoplasm.

Microbiology and serology studies can also assist in the interpretation of lymph node specimen, including rapid plasma reagin (RPR) for syphilis, as well as serology for EBV, cytomegalovirus (CMV), or *Bartonella henselae* (cat scratch lymphadenitis). EBV viral levels may also be increased in patients with EBV-positive lymphomas.

PERTINENT LAB FINDINGS

- CBC (WBC, HGB, PLTS, and WBC differential)
- LDH
- Ferritin
- Erythrocyte sedimentation rate
- Total protein/SPEP/SIFE

ANCILLARY STUDIES

FLOW CYTOMETRY

In a perfect world, all lymph node specimens suspicious for lymphoma would be submitted for flow cytometric evaluation. While Hodgkin lymphomas cannot be detected by routine flow cytometry assays, this ancillary test is very useful in the evaluation of reactive lymph nodes and non-Hodgkin lymphomas.[15-19]

When evaluating flow cytometry plots from a lymph node specimen, the first step should be to note the cellular composition of the sample. A specimen from a normal lymph node will be predominantly composed of CD45-bright lymphocytes (Figure 1.58). The lymphocytes will be a mixture of T-cells and B-cells with only rare NK cells. Often T-cells predominate, but there may be more B-cells than T-cells in lymph nodes with follicular hyperplasia or in a specimen where a follicle-rich area was submitted for flow cytometric analysis.

If there are numerous neutrophils with some monocytes, it may indicate peripheral blood contamination, which can occur during the biopsy procedure (Figure 1.59). If there is significant peripheral blood contamination, then the findings may not accurately reflect the composition of the lymph node. Alternatively, numerous neutrophils can also be seen in the setting of acute lymphadenitis, so morphologic correlation is needed.

The B-cells in a reactive node will express a mixture of kappa and lambda light chains, with a kappa:lambda ratio of 1:1 to 4:1 (Figure 1.60). If a significant number of B-cells lack expression of light chains in an otherwise normal node, this could reflect insufficient washing of the specimen rather than an unusual B-cell population. Germinal center B-cells tend to be underrepresented on flow cytometry plots. They are slightly larger than background CD19-positive B-cells and show a distinct phenotype with expression of CD10, slightly brighter CD20, and slightly brighter CD38. They are usually polytypic with expression of both kappa and lambda light chains (Figure 1.61), but will rarely lack light chain expression.

Flow cytometry is also an excellent way to characterize T-cells.[20] The CD4:CD8 ratio can be ascertained, and the possibility of antigen loss can be assessed (Figure 1.62). Of note, a normal population of T-cells will show some variability in the expression of CD7, but T-cells with loss of CD7 should be a minority of the cells. Doublets, which represent flow cytometric analysis of two cells that are stuck together, can rarely cause some confusion in the interpretation of T-cells because when CD4+ T-cells are bound to CD8+ T-cells, these doublets can cause an apparent increase in CD4+CD8+ T-cells. Doublets can usually be excluded using light scatter characteristics (FSC-A vs FSC-H). Thus, if double-positive T-cells are increased but do not show any specific phenotypic abnormalities, review of the gating strategy may be warranted. Alternatively, a true increase in phenotypically unremarkable double-positive T-cells can be seen in nodular lymphocyte predominant lymphoma and the benign entity progressive transformation of germinal centers, emphasizing the need for correlation of flow cytometry findings with morphology.[21,22]

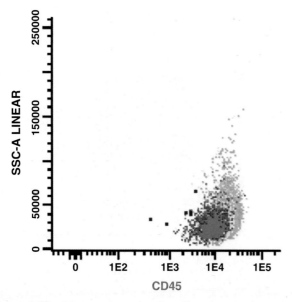

Figure 1.58. Flow cytometry dot plot of lymphocytes from a normal lymph node (CD45 vs SSC). Lymphocytes have bright CD45 expression and low side scattered (red, dark green, and orange).

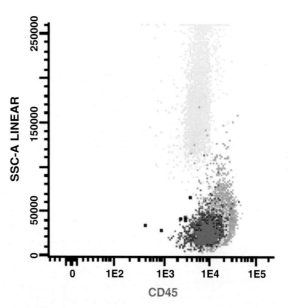

Figure 1.59. Flow cytometry dot plot from the same lymph node in Figure 1.58. This plot includes granulocytes from peripheral blood contamination. The myeloid cells (yellow) have slightly dimmer CD45 expression and higher side scatter than lymphocytes.

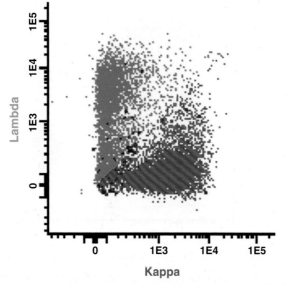

Figure 1.60. Flow cytometry dot plots of a lymph node with a mixture of kappa-positive (red) and lambda-positive (green) B-cells. Kappa-positive cells outnumber lambda-positive cells, with a ratio of 2:1 (kappa vs lambda; gated on B-cells).

Flow Cytometry Checklist for a Normal Lymph Node

☐ Predominantly lymphoid cells (exclude peripheral blood contamination)

☐ Mixture of T-cells and B-cells (T-cells > B-cells, except in follicular hyperplasia)

☐ T-cells are a mixture of CD4- and CD8-positive cells (CD4:CD8 ratio 1:1-5:1)

☐ B-cells are a mixture of kappa- and lambda-positive cells (K:L ratio 1:1-4:1)

☐ No abnormal monoclonal B-cell population or phenotypically abnormal T-cell population

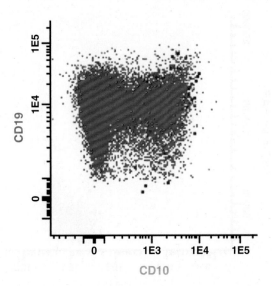

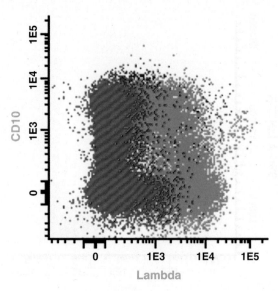

Figure 1.61. Flow cytometry dot plots of a lymph node with a CD10-positive B-cell population comprised of a mixture of red kappa-positive and green lambda-positive cells (CD10 vs CD19; gated on B-cells).

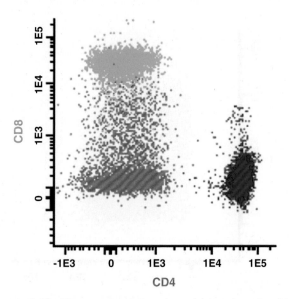

Figure 1.62. Flow cytometry dot plots of a lymph node with a mixture of CD4-positive and CD8-positive T-cells. CD4-positive cells, which are a mixture of CD7-positive (red) and CD7-negative (blue) cells outnumber the green CD8-positive cells, with a ratio of 3:1. NK cells (pink) are also present (CD4 vs CD8; gated on T & NK cells).

FAQ: Can Hodgkin lymphoma be detected by flow cytometry?

Answer: Flow cytometry is not a sensitive method for the detection of classical Hodgkin lymphoma (CHL) or nodular lymphocyte predominant Hodgkin lymphoma (NLPHL) using standard techniques; however, several flow cytometric findings may suggest a higher likelihood of CHL or NLPHL. For instance, NLPHL can show a high CD4:CD8 ratio with a distinct increase in CD4+/CD8+ ("double-positive") T-cells. Likewise, EBV-negative CHL is also often associated with a high CD4:CD8 ratio.

CYTOGENETIC/FISH STUDIES

In certain diagnostic settings, cytogenetic and FISH studies are recommended, as some specific lymphoma subtypes are categorized based on cytogenetic findings.[23] For instance, most follicular lymphomas exhibit a translocation t(14;18), which results in the fusion of *BCL2* and *IGH* genes. Burkitt lymphoma is associated with t(8;14), or less commonly t(8;22) or t(8;2), resulting in an *MYC* gene rearrangement. High-grade B-cell lymphomas may have translocations involving *MYC* and *BCL2* and/or *BCL6* (colloquially known as "double/triple-hit lymphomas")[24,25]; FISH studies are recommended to assess for these rearrangements in all new diagnoses of large B-cell lymphomas, as the presence of these cytogenetic abnormalities alters the patient prognosis and may influence the choice of chemotherapeutic regimens. Specific lymphomas with associated cytogenetic abnormalities will be discussed at length in later chapters.

Fresh lymph node samples may be submitted upfront for cytogenetic studies in RPMI. More often, however, FISH studies are ordered after morphologic and immunohistochemical evaluation generates a differential diagnosis. In these instances, formalin-fixed, paraffin-embedded unstained slides are acceptable for most routine lymphoma FISH studies.

MOLECULAR STUDIES

Molecular studies are performed with increasing frequency in the evaluation of lymph nodes in order to assess for B-cell or T-cell clonality. These findings are very helpful in making a diagnosis of lymphoma, but the results must be interpreted with caution and with the appropriate morphologic correlation, as clonal patterns can be seen in reactive lymph nodes, and polyclonal patterns may be seen in lymph nodes involved by lymphoma.

Normal B-cells rearrange two or three immunoglobulin genes, including the heavy chain gene (*IGH*) and the kappa (*IGK*) or lambda (*IGL*) light chain genes. The heavy chain (*IGH*) gene is most frequently assayed because this gene rearranges before the light chain genes.

The heavy chain is comprised of variable (V), diverse (D), joining (J), and constant (C) regions. Most PCR assays use primers that bind to the V and J regions to amplify a certain region of the gene (CDR III). Normal lymph nodes show a full repertoire of the rearrangement products of this region, which vary in size, as represented on the molecular electropherogram. This is often described as a "polyclonal pattern" (Figure 1.63). However, if the B-cells are clonal, the assay will show one dominant peak, representing the gene rearrangement products of only one clone (Figure 1.64).[26,27]

Clonal patterns can rarely be seen in reactive specimens. This frequently occurs in limited samples that contain very few B-cells, leading to very few peaks in the IGH assay. This mimics a clonal pattern, but is not truly clonal, and is referred to as a "pseudoclone."

It should be noted that polyclonal patterns can also be seen in some B-cell lymphomas, especially follicular lymphoma and some diffuse large B-cell lymphomas, because the PCR primers can no longer hybridize in the neoplastic cells due to ongoing somatic hypermutation. Thus, the presence of a polyclonal pattern should not be taken, by itself, as proof that a node lacks involvement by B-cell lymphoma, and morphologic correlation remains critical.

The addition of an assay for IGK clonality improves the sensitivity of molecular assays for B-cell clonality, but this test is not routinely performed or available in all labs.

T-cell receptor gene rearrangement (TCR) studies are performed similarly. T-cell gamma (TCRG) gene rearrangements are more commonly performed than T-cell beta (TCRB) assays.[28,29] Reactive lymph nodes most commonly show a polyclonal pattern (Figure 1.65); however, clonal patterns can occasionally be seen in reactive lymph nodes. Thus, clonal TCR studies must be interpreted along with clinical, morphologic, and immunophenotypic findings and are best reserved for confirming a morphologic diagnosis of T-cell lymphoma.

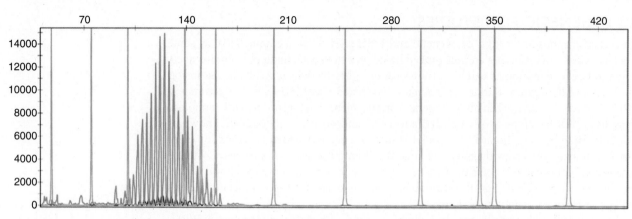

Figure 1.63. IGH electropherogram demonstrating a polytypic B-cell population in a normal Gaussian distribution.

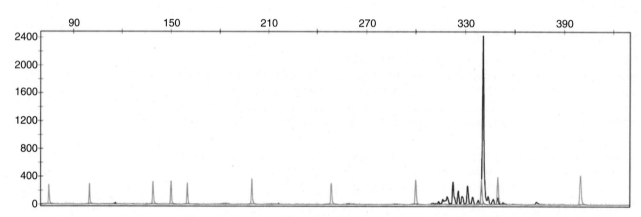

Figure 1.64. IGH electropherogram demonstrating a clonal B-cell population (peak; approximately 341) with a slight background of polytypic B-cells.

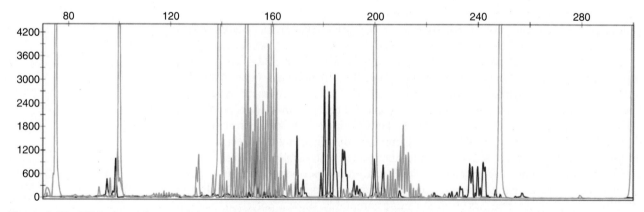

Figure 1.65. TCRG electropherogram demonstrating a polytypic T-cell population showing a normal Gaussian distribution.

FAQ: If a T-cell clone is detected by molecular tests, can I diagnose a T-cell lymphoma?

Answer: Maybe. As noted above, morphologic and clinical correlation is necessary to diagnose a clonal T-cell population as a T-cell lymphoma. Reactive lymph nodes can show T-cell clones. Additionally, B-cell lymphomas can also exhibit clonal T-cell populations, which are likely tumor-reactive lymphocytes. Moreover, clonal T-cell populations are occasionally not detected by T-cell receptor gene rearrangement studies in morphologically apparent T-cell lymphomas. To further complicate matters, both clonal T- and B-cell populations are often seen in angio-immunoblastic T-cell lymphoma. Therefore, while molecular studies are highly useful in difficult cases and/or in cases with limited material when there is a high suspicion for malignancy, these ancillary tests need to be interpreted with caution and in the correct clinical and morphologic context.

PEARLS & PITFALLS

IgG4-positive cells can be increased in other conditions, including marginal zone lymphomas; therefore, a full diagnostic workup is recommended. When lymphoma has been ruled out, a diagnosis of "reactive lymphoid hyperplasia with increased IgG4-positive cells" is appropriate. A note suggesting clinical and microbiologic studies, as well as measurement of serum Ig4 levels, should be included.

NEAR MISSES

Reactive-appearing lymph nodes occasionally harbor subtle histologic findings that, when correctly identified, allow the pathologist to provide a more specific diagnosis or avoid a clinically important misdiagnosis. The following examples are just a few of the numerous entities that should be considered in the differential diagnosis of benign or reactive lymph nodes.

IGG4-REACTIVE LYMPHADENOPATHY

The diagnosis of IgG4-related lymphadenopathy (discussed in detail later) is complicated, as the morphologic findings are protean and often nonspecific.[30-33] Lymph nodes can show several different morphologic patterns, including follicular hyperplasia, interfollicular expansion, progressive transformation of germinal centers, a multicentric Castleman disease–like appearance, and an inflammatory pseudotumor-like pattern with fibrosis. Most cases have increased eosinophils, and all show increased IgG4-positive cells, with the current formal criteria including an IgG4:IgG ratio >40% and >100% IgG4 plasma cells/high power field.

Some cases of IgG4-reactive lymphadenopathy with the follicular hyperplasia–type pattern show prominent curved epithelioid granulomas that partially encircle reactive follicles (Figures 1.66-1.68). The IgG4-positive plasma cells can be increased in both the follicles (Figures 1.69 and 1.70) and the interfollicular areas (Figures 1.71 and 1.72). Some cases of IgG4-related lymphadenopathy are quite subtle, and immunostains for IgG and IgG4 may be of value in reactive-appearing lymph nodes with increased eosinophils and/or plasma cells.

NODAL MARGINAL ZONE B-CELL LYMPHOMA WITH COLONIZATION OF REACTIVE FOLLICLES

Colonization of reactive germinal centers by NMZL may be subtle. In these cases, the lymphoma partially involves reactive germinal centers, but the overall nodal architecture remains largely intact (Figure 1.73) and the sinuses may be patent. Clues to this diagnosis

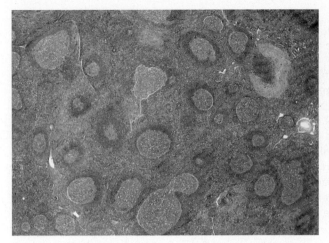

Figure 1.66. A lymph node at low power showing numerous reactive-appearing follicles. At the upper right corner, a large crescent-shaped granuloma partially surrounds a follicle.

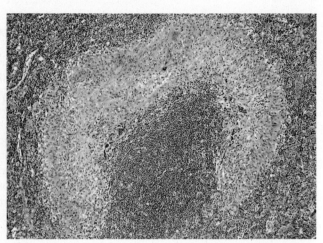

Figure 1.67. Crescent-shaped noncaseating granuloma composed of epithelioid histiocytes with a rare multinucleated giant cell surrounds a follicle.

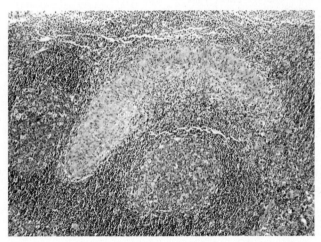

Figure 1.68. A reactive follicle with a germinal center, a mantle zone, and a surrounding epithelioid granuloma.

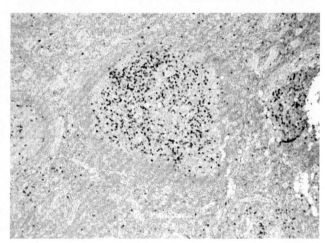

Figure 1.69. IgG-positive plasma cells in the reactive follicles.

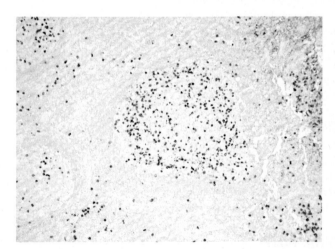

Figure 1.70. IgG4-positive plasma cells in the same follicle seen in Figure 1.70. The IgG4:IgG ratio is elevated.

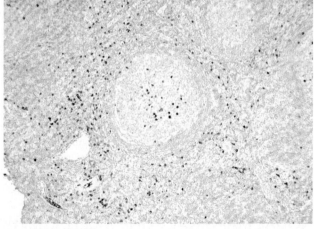

Figure 1.71. IgG-positive plasma cells in the interfollicular zones.

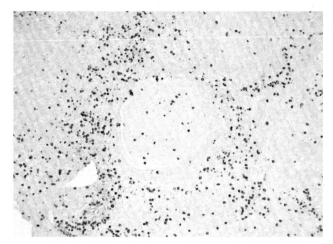

Figure 1.72. IgG4-positive plasma cells in the same interfollicular zone seen in Figure 1.71. The IgG4:IgG ratio is elevated.

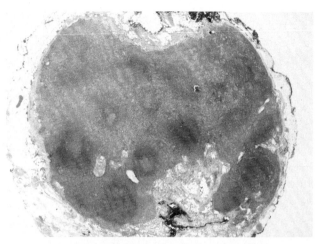

Figure 1.73. A lymph node at low power showing numerous follicles. The follicles are slightly disrupted and show blurring between the germinal centers and the mantle zones.

include germinal centers and mantle zones that are not crisply defined on the H&E, with blurring of the boundaries between the two zones (Figure 1.74). Immunohistochemical stains often show a predominance of B-cells (Figures 1.75 and 1.76), germinal centers with an unusually low Ki-67 proliferation index (Figure 1.77), and frequent Bcl-2-positive cells in germinal centers. Flow cytometry can be helpful in this situation and may identify a clonal population of CD5-negative, CD10-negative B-cells, typically in a background of polyclonal B-cells (Figures 1.78 and 1.79).[34]

However, when flow cytometry is not available or is unrevealing, this diagnosis can be challenging, particularly given the nonspecific immunophenotype of the neoplastic B-cells and the subtle morphologic findings in NMZL with follicular colonization. In cases with plasmacytic differentiation of the abnormal B-cells, immunohistochemical stains for kappa and lambda may be helpful for proving clonality (Figures 1.80 and 1.81). Sometimes, NMZL may show scattered epithelioid histiocytes, although well-formed granulomas are not typically seen (Figure 1.82).

INTRAFOLLICULAR NEOPLASIA

Occasionally, reactive-appearing lymph nodes contain Bcl-2-positive germinal center cells, with no other immunophenotypic or morphologic evidence of follicular lymphoma (Figures 1.83-1.91).[35,36] This phenomenon, previously called in situ follicular lymphoma and now referred to as in situ intrafollicular neoplasia, is a rare finding that is usually incidentally discovered when immunohistochemical stains are performed on an otherwise reactive-appearing lymph node.

While the diagnosis is likely often missed, approximately 60% of patients with interfollicular neoplasia reportedly have had no evidence of follicular lymphoma at other sites and never go on to develop follicular lymphoma. The other ~40% of patients were either diagnosed with follicular lymphoma at another site or later developed follicular lymphoma. Based on these findings, some experts believe that these "in situ" cells represent colonization of follicles by a follicular lymphoma clone from another site. Others believe that this simply represents non-malignant clonal B-cells with rearranged BCL-2, but none of the other cytogenetic abnormalities that typify frank follicular lymphoma.

The World Health Organization suggests using the term "intrafollicular neoplasia" to maintain consistency with other neoplastic diagnostic categories, and these cases should not be diagnosed as follicular lymphoma. However, it is prudent for the pathologist to suggest further clinical workup in a note.

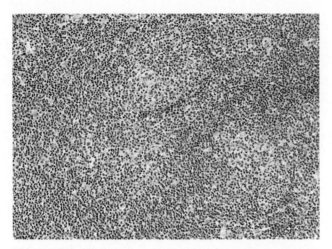

Figure 1.74. The center of one of the abnormal follicles. There is no crisp boundary between germinal center cells and mantle cells.

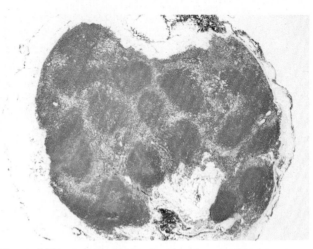

Figure 1.75. CD20 highlights the abundant B-cells in the abnormal follicles.

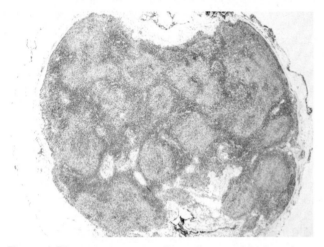

Figure 1.76. CD3 staining T-cells in the same lymph node as Figures 1.73-75. There are fewer T-cells than B-cells present.

Figure 1.77. Follicles show an abnormally low Ki-67 proliferation index, indicating a replacement of germinal center cells by neoplastic cells.

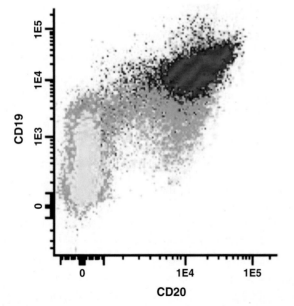

Figure 1.78. Flow cytometry dot plots of the lymph node in Figure 1.73 with an abnormal B-cell population (cyan) with very few background polytypic B-cells (red and green). The abnormal population expresses CD19 and CD20 (CD20 vs CD19; gated on all lymphocytes).

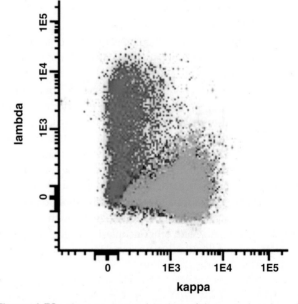

Figure 1.79. Flow cytometry dot plots of the same lymph node. The population is kappa-restricted (kappa vs lambda; gated on B-cells).

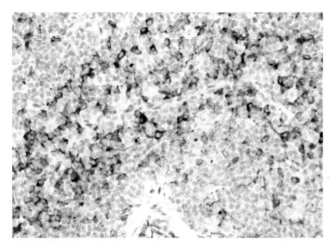

Figure 1.80. A kappa immunohistochemical stain highlights increased plasmacytoid B-cells and plasma cells.

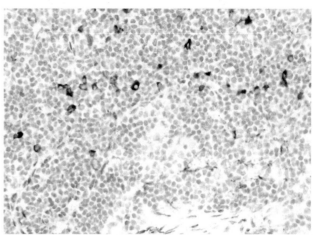

Figure 1.81. A lambda immunohistochemical stain highlights only scattered plasma cells.

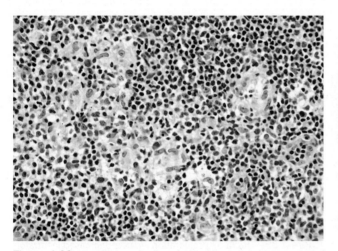

Figure 1.82. Small clusters of epithelioid histiocytes are scattered among small lymphoid cells in this case of nodal marginal zone lymphoma.

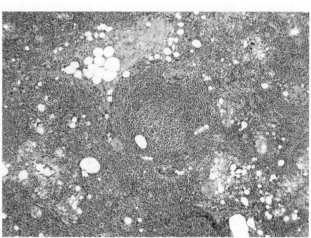

Figure 1.83. Low-power view of an apparently reactive follicle in a peripancreatic lymph node involved by lipid lymphadenopathy.

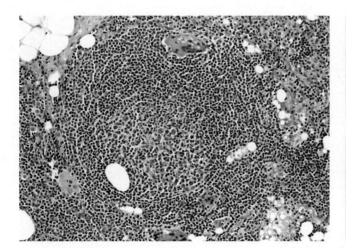

Figure 1.84. High-power view of the same follicle as Figure 1.83.

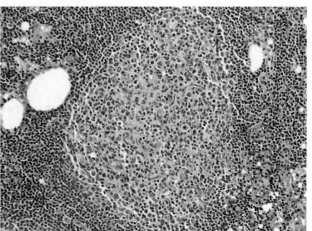

Figure 1.85. A normal follicle in the same lymph node.

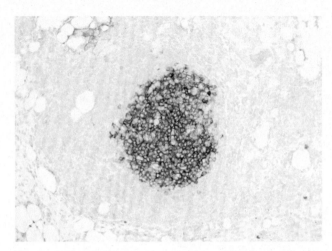

Figure 1.86. CD10 expression on an intrafollicular neoplasia in Figure 1.84. The cells are strongly positive for CD10.

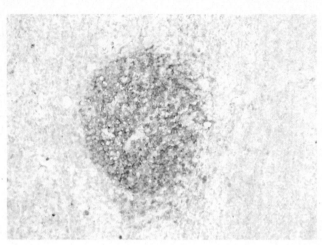

Figure 1.87. In comparison to Figure 1.86, the reactive germinal center in Figure 1.85 shows weaker staining for CD10.

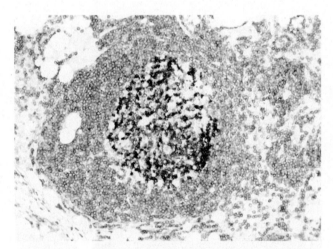

Figure 1.88. Bcl-2 is strongly positive on the abnormal follicle cells in intrafollicular neoplasia. Bcl-2 is also positive on the surrounding mantle zone B-cells.

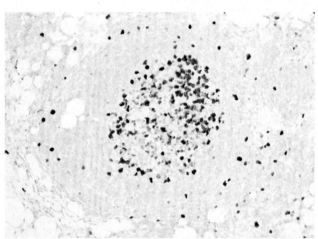

Figure 1.89. The Ki-67 proliferation index is decreased in intrafollicular neoplasia.

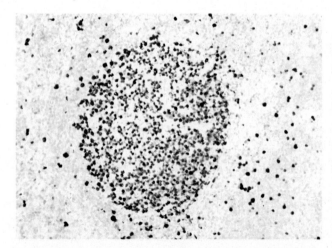

Figure 1.90. In comparison to Figure 1.89, the Ki-67 proliferation index in normal reactive germinal centers is high.

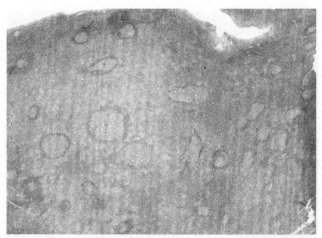

Figure 1.91. Low-power view of a lymph node with intact follicles and a mild interfollicular expansion.

SAMPLE SIGN OUT

Lymph node, excisional biopsy:

- Lymph node with in situ follicular neoplasia. See note.

Note: The overall lymph node architecture is intact with several reactive-appearing follicles. Germinal centers cells are focally positive for Bcl-2 (bright), in addition to CD10 (bright) and Bcl-6. The atypical cells are limited to the germinal centers, and the significance of this focal finding is uncertain. Clinical evaluation for evidence of overt follicular lymphoma at other anatomic sites is recommended.

INTERFOLLICULAR CLASSICAL HODGKIN LYMPHOMA

CHL is separated into four well-known subtypes based on lymph node architecture and cellular morphology: nodular sclerosis, mixed cellularity, lymphocyte-rich, and lymphocyte-depleted. While the other subtypes are usually easily identified on H&E-stained slides, lymphocyte-rich classical Hodgkin lymphoma (LRCHL) may be difficult to visualize initially, as the neoplastic cells can be scattered among a lymph node with relatively preserved architecture.

Two patterns of LRCHL are recognized based on the arrangement of the neoplastic HRS cells in relation to follicles. In the so-called "follicular" pattern, HRS cells are distributed in follicles, usually in the eccentric mantle zones of atretic follicles. In the "interfollicular" pattern, HRS cells are scattered in the interfollicular spaces in a background of T-cells.

Likewise, partial involvement of any type of CHL may resemble this interfollicular pattern (Figures 1.92-1.99),[37] especially in lymph nodes at the periphery of a lymph node conglomerate. There is some debate about whether LRCHL simply represents an early phase of nodular sclerosis or mixed cellularity or is in fact a distinct entity.

EARLY ANGIOIMMUNOBLASTIC T-CELL LYMPHOMA

Early lymph node involvement by angioimmunoblastic T-cell lymphoma (AITL) is easy to miss, as it shows morphologic features that are similar to reactive lymph nodes (Figure 1.100). In early AITL (so-called "Pattern 1"), the lymph node contains follicles with reactive germinal centers, and the neoplastic T-cells loosely surround the follicles. A morphologic clue to Pattern 1 AITL is thin, absent or disrupted mantle zones (Figure 1.101). Immunohistochemical stains are necessary for the diagnosis, highlighting the abnormal T-cell population surrounding the follicles; these T-cells exhibit a helper T phenotype (CD4-positive, CD10/BCL-6-positive, PD1-positive). EBER ISH may highlight scattered positive B immunoblasts (Figures 1.102-1.109) in AITL.

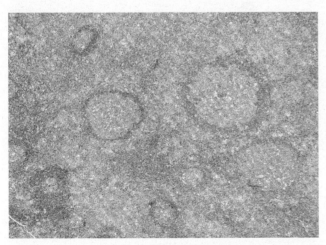

Figure 1.92. The follicles contain reactive germinal centers, but the surrounding mantle zones are disrupted and irregular. The interfollicular zones are expanded.

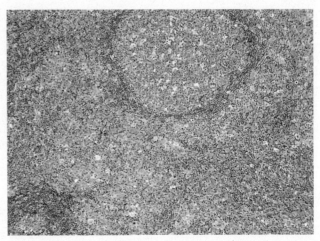

Figure 1.93. The interfollicular zones show a mixed inflammatory infiltrate.

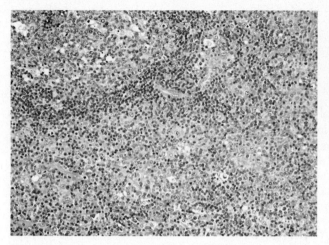

Figure 1.94. On closer inspection, the interfollicular zones show increased histiocytes and eosinophils in addition to large atypical cells.

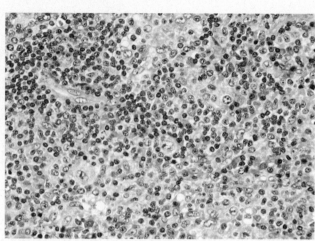

Figure 1.95. Scattered atypical cells have large irregular nuclei and vesicular chromatin with prominent nucleoli.

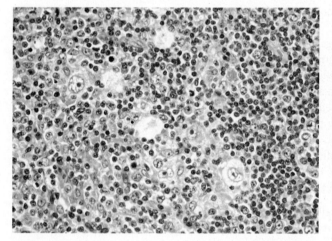

Figure 1.96. Typical large cells admixed with eosinophils, lymphocytes, and histiocytes.

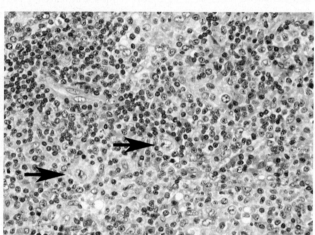

Figure 1.97. Some of the large cells show Hodgkin Reed-Sternberg (HRS) morphology, with monolobation and prominent eosinophilic macronucleoli.

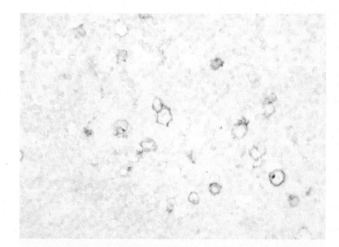

Figure 1.98. CD30 highlights the Hodgkin Reed-Sternberg cells in the interfollicular zones.

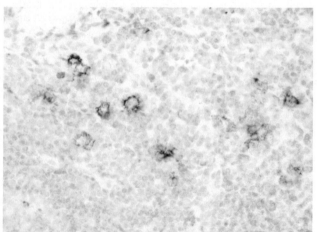

Figure 1.99. Hodgkin Reed-Sternberg cells in the interfollicular zones are also positive for CD15.

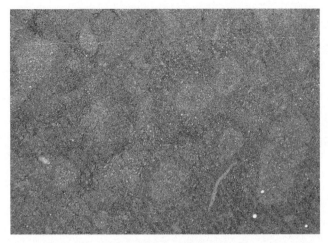

Figure 1.100. A 3.5 cm inguinal lymph node in a 72-year-old man. There are numerous reactive germinal centers.

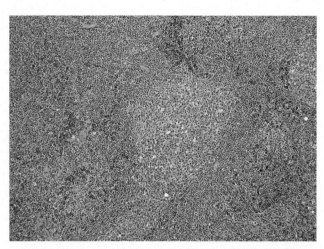

Figure 1.101. The germinal centers show somewhat attenuated and disrupted mantle zones that are not well-polarized.

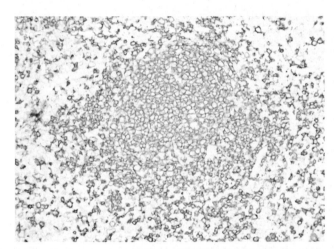

Figure 1.102. CD20 highlights the follicles, including the somewhat attenuated and disrupted mantle zones, as well as the germinal centers.

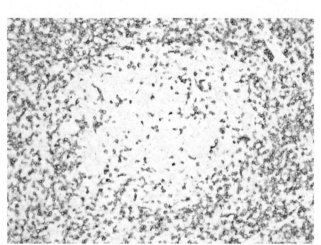

Figure 1.103. CD3-positive atypical T-cells predominate in the interfollicular area.

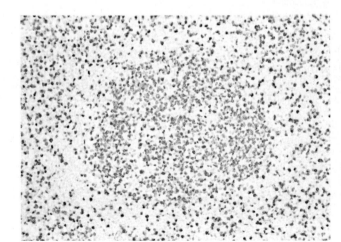

Figure 1.104. The Ki-67 proliferation index is appropriately high in the germinal center, low in the attenuated mantle zone, and moderately high in the interfollicular area.

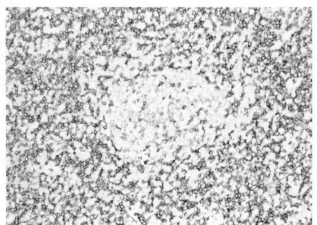

Figure 1.105. Most of the T-cells are CD4-positive.

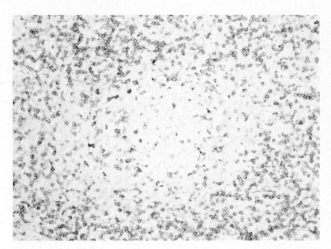

Figure 1.106. The T-cells show some loss of CD7.

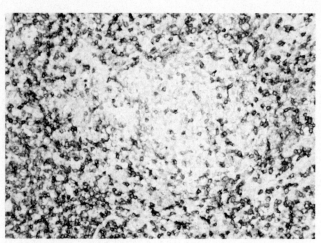

Figure 1.107. Many of the T-cells in the interfollicular area are PD1-positive. This pattern is abnormal (contrast with the normal reactive follicle in Figure 1.29).

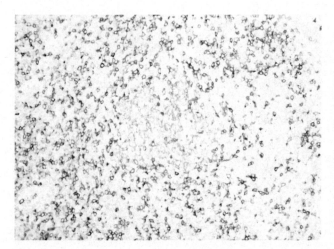

Figure 1.108. CD10 shows relatively dim staining in the germinal center and is brightly expressed on the neoplastic T-cells surrounding the germinal center (contrast with the pattern of CD10 staining in the normal reactive follicle in Figure 1.22).

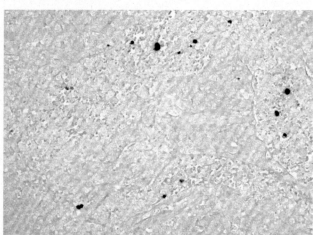

Figure 1.109. An *in situ* hybridization for Epstein-Barr virus (EBV) demonstrates that the interfollicular area contains scattered EBV-positive B-cells, including both small cells and larger immunoblasts. EBV-positive cells are frequently seen in angioimmunoblastic T-cell lymphoma.

An abnormal T-cell population may be detected on flow cytometry in these cases, consisting of CD4-positive T-cells with loss of CD7 and dim or absent surface CD3. A subset of these atypical T-cells usually show partial expression of CD10. These lymphomas are often associated with a certain molecular mutational profile, which will be discussed at length in later chapters.[38-40]

References

1. Willard-Mack CL. Normal structure, function, and histology of lymph nodes. *Toxicol Pathol.* 2006;34(5):409-424.

2. Medeiros LJ, O'Malley D, Caraway NP, Vega F, Elenitoba-Johnson KSJ, Lim MS. *AFIP Atlas of Tumor Pathology, Fourth Series; Tumors of the Lymph Nodes and Spleen.* Washington, DC: American Registry of Pathology; 2017.

3. Swerdlow SH, Campo E, Harris NL, et al. *World Health Organization Classification of Tumours of Haematopoietic and Lymphoid Tissues.* Lyon, France: International Agency for Research on Cancer; 2017.

4. Jaffe ES, Harris NL, Vardiman JW, Campo E, Arber DA. *Hematopathology.* St. Louis, MO: Saunders, Elsevier; 2011.

5. Ioachim HL, Medeiros LJ. *Lymph Node Pathology*. Philadelphia, PA: Lippincott Williams & Wilkins; 2009.

6. Gretz JE, Anderson AO, Shaw S. Cords, channels, corridors and conduits: critical architectural elements facilitating cell interactions in the lymph node cortex. *Immunol Rev*. 1997;156:11-24.

7. Camacho SA, Kosco-Vilbois MH, Berek C. The dynamic structure of the germinal center. *Immunol Today*. 1998;19(11):511-514.

8. Liu YJ, Grouard G, de Bouteiller O, Banchereau J. Follicular dendritic cells and germinal centers. *Int Rev Cytol*. 1996;166:139-179.

9. Kaldjian EP, Gretz JE, Anderson AO, Shi Y, Shaw S. Spatial and molecular organization of lymph node T cell cortex: a labyrinthine cavity bounded by an epithelium-like monolayer of fibroblastic reticular cells anchored to basement membrane-like extracellular matrix. *Int Immunol*. 2001;13(10):1243-1253.

10. Kelly RH. Functional anatomy of lymph nodes: I. The paracortical cords. *Int Arch Allergy Appl Immunol*. 1975;48(6):836-849.

11. Ben-Yehuda D, Polliack A, Okon E, et al. Image-guided core-needle biopsy in malignant lymphoma: experience with 100 patients that suggests the technique is reliable. *J Clin Oncol*. 1996;14(9):2431-2434.

12. Caraway NP. Strategies to diagnose lymphoproliferative disorders by fine-needle aspiration by using ancillary studies. *Cancer*. 2005;105(6):432-442.

13. de Larrinoa AF, del Cura J, Zabala R, Fuertes E, Bilbao F, Lopez JI. Value of ultrasound-guided core biopsy in the diagnosis of malignant lymphoma. *J Clin Ultrasound*. 2007;35(6):295-301.

14. Zeppa P, Marino G, Troncone G, et al. Fine-needle cytology and flow cytometry immunophenotyping and subclassification of non-Hodgkin lymphoma: a critical review of 307 cases with technical suggestions. *Cancer*. 2004;102(1):55-65.

15. Craig FE, Foon KA. Flow cytometric immunophenotyping for hematologic neoplasms. *Blood*. 2008;111(8):3941-3967.

16. Craig FE. Flow cytometric evaluation of B-cell lymphoid neoplasms. *Clin Lab Med*. 2007;27(3):487-512, vi.

17. Davis BH, Holden JT, Bene MC, et al. 2006 Bethesda international consensus recommendations on the flow cytometric immunophenotypic analysis of hematolymphoid neoplasia: medical indications. *Cytometry B Clin Cytom*. 2007;72(suppl 1):S5-S13.

18. Stetler-Stevenson M, Davis B, Wood B, Braylan R. 2006 Bethesda International Consensus Conference on flow cytometric immunophenotyping of hematolymphoid neoplasia. *Cytometry B Clin Cytom*. 2007;72(suppl 1):S3.

19. Demurtas A, Stacchini A, Aliberti S, Chiusa L, Chiarle R, Novero D. Tissue flow cytometry immunophenotyping in the diagnosis and classification of non-Hodgkin's lymphomas: a retrospective evaluation of 1,792 cases. *Cytometry B Clin Cytom*. 2013;84(2):82-95.

20. Craig JW, Dorfman DM. Flow cytometry of T cells and T-cell neoplasms. *Clin Lab Med*. 2017;37(4):725-751.

21. Rahemtullah A, Reichard KK, Preffer FI, Harris NL, Hasserjian RP. A double-positive CD4+CD8+ T-cell population is commonly found in nodular lymphocyte predominant Hodgkin lymphoma. *Am J Clin Pathol*. 2006;126(5):805-814.

22. Rahemtullah A, Harris NL, Dorn ME, Preffer FI, Hasserjian RP. Beyond the lymphocyte predominant cell: CD4+CD8+ T-cells in nodular lymphocyte predominant Hodgkin lymphoma. *Leuk Lymphoma*. 2008;49(10):1870-1878.

23. Medeiros LJ, Carr J. Overview of the role of molecular methods in the diagnosis of malignant lymphomas. *Arch Pathol Lab Med*. 1999;123(12):1189-1207.

24. Li S, Lin P, Fayad LE, et al. B-cell lymphomas with MYC/8q24 rearrangements and IGH@ BCL2/t(14;18)(q32;q21): an aggressive disease with heterogeneous histology, germinal center B-cell immunophenotype and poor outcome. *Mod Pathol*. 2012;25(1):145-156.

25. Li S, Desai P, Lin P, et al. MYC/BCL6 double-hit lymphoma (DHL): a tumour associated with an aggressive clinical course and poor prognosis. *Histopathology*. 2016;68(7):1090-1098.

26. Inghirami G, Szabolcs MJ, Yee HT, Corradini P, Cesarman E, Knowles DM. Detection of immunoglobulin gene rearrangement of B cell non-Hodgkin's lymphomas and leukemias in fresh, unfixed and formalin-fixed, paraffin-embedded tissue by polymerase chain reaction. *Lab Invest*. 1993;68(6):746-757.

27. Hughes J, Weston S, Bennetts B, et al. The application of a PCR technique for the detection of immunoglobulin heavy chain gene rearrangements in fresh or paraffin-embedded skin tissue. *Pathology*. 2001;33(2):222-225.

28. Vega F, Medeiros LJ, Jones D, et al. A novel four-color PCR assay to assess T-cell receptor gamma gene rearrangements in lymphoproliferative lesions. *Am J Clin Pathol*. 2001;116(1):17-24.

29. Khokhar FA, Payne WD, Talwalkar SS, et al. Angioimmunoblastic T-cell lymphoma in bone marrow: a morphologic and immunophenotypic study. *Hum Pathol*. 2010;41(1):79-87.

30. Bookhout CE, Rollins-Raval MA. Immunoglobulin G4-related lymphadenopathy. *Surg Pathol Clin*. 2016;9(1):117-129.

31. Cheuk W, Yuen HK, Chu SY, Chiu EK, Lam LK, Chan JK. Lymphadenopathy of IgG4-related sclerosing disease. *Am J Surg Pathol*. 2008;32(5):671-681.

32. Deshpande V, Zen Y, Chan JK, et al. Consensus statement on the pathology of IgG4-related disease. *Mod Pathol*. 2012;25(9):1181-1192.

33. Chen YR, Chen YJ, Wang MC, Medeiros LJ, Chang KC. A newly recognized histologic pattern of IgG4-related lymphadenopathy: expanding the morphologic spectrum. *Am J Surg Pathol*. 2018;42(7):977-982.

34. Naresh KN. Nodal marginal zone B-cell lymphoma with prominent follicular colonization – difficulties in diagnosis: a study of 15 cases. *Histopathology*. 2008;52(3):331-339.

35. Carbone A, Gloghini A. Emerging issues after the recognition of in situ follicular lymphoma. *Leuk Lymphoma*. 2014;55(3):482-490.

36. Carbone A, Gloghini A. Intrafollicular neoplasia/"in situ" lymphoma: a proposal for morphology and immunodiagnostic classification. *Am J Hematol*. 2011;86(8):633-639.

37. AbdullGaffar B, Seliem RM. Hodgkin lymphoma with an interfollicular growth pattern: a clinicopathologic study of 8 cases. *Ann Diagn Pathol*. 2018;33:30-34.

38. Lemonnier F, Couronne L, Parrens M, et al. Recurrent TET2 mutations in peripheral T-cell lymphomas correlate with TFH-like features and adverse clinical parameters. *Blood*. 2012;120(7):1466-1469.

39. Lemonnier F, Mak TW. Angioimmunoblastic T-cell lymphoma: more than a disease of T follicular helper cells. *J Pathol*. 2017;242(4):387-390.

40. Wang M, Zhang S, Chuang SS, et al. Angioimmunoblastic T cell lymphoma: novel molecular insights by mutation profiling. *Oncotarget*. 2017;8(11):17763-17770.

THE LYMPH NODE CAPSULE

CHAPTER OUTLINE

Although often overlooked, routine examination of the lymph node capsule, including confirming its presence and evaluating the overall appearance, is recommended in the workup of all lymph node specimens. Identifying abnormalities of the capsule provides key diagnostic information to the pathologist and can be useful in formulating a differential diagnosis.

NORMAL LYMPH NODE CAPSULE

A normal lymph node is surrounded by a thin rim of fibrous tissue which forms the capsule (see Chapter 1). The presence of a capsule helps define the structure of the lymph node, and its appearance can point to pathologic processes. A normal lymph node capsule is thin and intact.

ABSENT CAPSULE

LYMPH NODE VERSUS LYMPHOID TISSUE

Lymphoid tissue that lacks a capsule does not represent a true lymph node and should be designated as "lymphoid tissue" in the pathology report even if the submitting radiologist or surgeon describes the tissue as a "lymph node." This is an important distinction because unencapsulated lymphoid tissue typically represents either a tissue inflammatory response or normal resident lymphoid tissue, such as the mucosa-associated lymphoid tissue, rather than a true lymph node. Differentiating between lymphoid tissue and a true lymph node can have significant clinical ramifications (see "Near Misses").

PEARLS & PITFALLS

In order to definitively identify lymphoid tissue as lymph node based on histology alone, associated capsule must be identified.

CAPSULAR INCLUSIONS

Rarely, the lymph node capsule can contain benign epithelial inclusions,[1-3] which may raise concern for metastatic carcinoma. It is important for the pathologist to consider the anatomic location of the lymph node, as distinct locations are associated with specific types of inclusions; for instance, thyroid tissue may be incidentally identified in cervical lymph nodes, and capsular nevi can be seen in superficial lymph nodes (see "Near Misses"). Careful cytomorphologic examination of the inclusions is also critical in order to rule out malignancy.

In pelvic lymph nodes, one of the most common inclusions is endosalpingiosis (Figure 2.1). Foci of endosalpingiosis within the capsule may be subtle and only apparent when highlighted with a cytokeratin immunohistochemical stain (Figures 2.2 and 2.3). Occasionally, however, these benign structures can mimic carcinoma, which is especially worrisome in specimens from patients undergoing staging for gynecological malignancies. However, unlike carcinoma, capsular endosalpingiosis is cytologically bland, and cilia can often be identified on a subset of the cells (Figure 2.4).

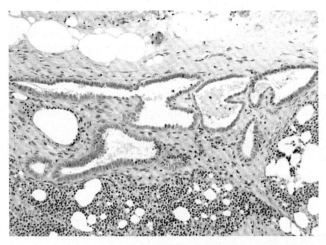

Figure 2.1. Capsular endosalpingiosis identified in a pelvic lymph node from a staging procedure for a 53-year-old woman with a malignant mesodermal mixed tumor of the uterus.

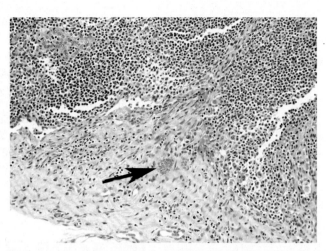

Figure 2.2. A benign lymph node with a minute focus of intra-capsular endosalpingiosis (arrow). The specimen was taken during a hysterectomy for endocervical adenocarcinoma.

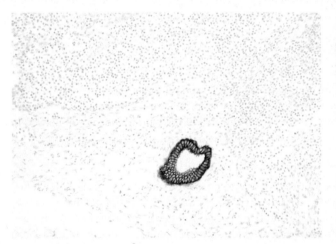

Figure 2.3. An immunostain for cytokeratin (AE1/AE3) highlights a focus of endosalpingiosis.

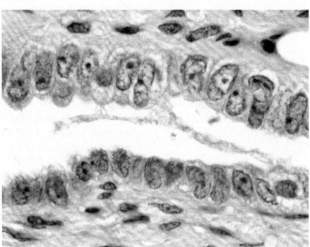

Figure 2.4. High-power view of the cells from the prior figure. There is no cytologic atypia, and cilia can be seen on some of the cells.

CHECKLIST: Benign Capsular Inclusions

☐ No cytomorphologic atypia
☐ Appropriate anatomic location
 o Cervical lymph nodes: Thyroid and salivary gland inclusions
 o Axillary lymph nodes: Breast tissue
 o Peritoneal lymph nodes: Benign glandular inclusions (endosalpingiosis) in women
 o Superficial lymph nodes draining skin: Nevus cells

DISRUPTED CAPSULE

A disrupted capsule is relatively uncommon in reactive lymph nodes and should raise suspicion for involvement by a neoplastic process. Any infiltrative process can disrupt the capsule, including metastatic tumors and lymphoma. Capsular disruption can be seen in both aggressive and low-grade lymphomas. Aggressive lymphomas tend to efface the lymph node architecture with diffuse infiltrates of abnormal, large, highly proliferative lymphoid cells that obliterate the capsule. Low-grade lymphomas, composed of small- or medium-sized atypical lymphoid cells with a low proliferative rate, may also obscure normal architecture, penetrate the capsule, and extend beyond the lymph node capsule. This is often seen in follicular lymphoma (Figures 2.5 and 2.6).

Rarely, the capsule is disrupted by a process that is not intrinsic to the lymph node. For instance, the lymph node capsule may be disrupted by the deposition of amyloid in systemic amyloidosis (Figures 2.7 and 2.8). While localized amyloid deposition can be seen within lymph nodes involved by low-grade B-cell lymphomas such as nodal marginal zone lymphoma, if the surrounding adipose tissue is also involved by amyloid deposition, then a systemic process should be considered (Figure 2.9).

THICKENED CAPSULE

A thickened capsule is a relatively frequent finding in lymph nodes that are submitted for pathologic evaluation. While it is a nonspecific finding that can be seen in both neoplastic and reactive processes, capsular thickening should prompt careful histologic evaluation of the node.

REACTIVE CONDITIONS
Chronic Inflammation

A thickened capsule in conjunction with reactive lymphoid hyperplasia likely indicates a chronic process, with long-standing antigenic stimulation (Figures 2.10 and 2.11). However, close examination of the other structural components of the lymph node is still needed to exclude a malignant process or suggest a possible etiology for the lymphadenopathy.

Syphilitic Lymphadenitis (Luetic Lymphadenitis)

Syphilitic lymphadenitis (luetic lymphadenitis) characteristically produces a thickened lymph node capsule. Patients with syphilis, which is caused by infection by the spirochete *Treponema pallidum*, can present with enlarged lymph nodes in all stages of the disease. Syphilitic lymphadenitis frequently involves the inguinal lymph nodes, although it can manifest in the cervical lymph nodes as well. The involved lymph nodes characteristically exhibit flagrant capsular thickening (Figure 2.12), which may "scallop" around germinal centers (Figures 2.13 and 2.14). Small vessels within the capsule are typically surrounded by a lymphoplasmacytic infiltrate (Figure 2.15). In addition to a marked follicular hyperplasia, plasma cells are often increased, and epithelioid granulomas or focal abscess formation may be seen.[4-7]

Special stains for microorganisms are recommended in lymph nodes with morphologic findings suggestive of syphilitic lymphadenitis, specifically a Warthin-Starry special stain, which highlights spirochetes (Figure 2.16). Although Warthin-Starry special stains may be difficult to interpret due to background staining, if organisms with the characteristic morphology of *T. pallidum* are identified, then a diagnosis of syphilitic lymphadenitis is likely. Use of a specific immunohistochemical stain directed against *T. pallidum* is also recommended, if available, to confirm the diagnosis. However, serologic studies are more sensitive than either a Warthin-Starry special stain or a syphilis immunostain.

It should be noted that, unless spirochetes are seen on an immunohistochemical or special stain, the morphologic findings of syphilitic lymphadenitis are nonspecific. Thus, it is advisable to sign these cases out as reactive lymph nodes, describing the thickened capsule and/or other unusual findings, with a note that syphilis may be included in the differential diagnosis.

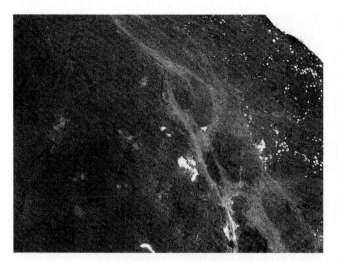

Figure 2.5. Follicular lymphoma, WHO grade 1-2 involving a 4 cm femoral lymph node in a 78-year-old man. The lymphoma disrupts the capsule and extends into the perinodal fat, maintaining its vaguely nodular architecture even beyond the capsule.

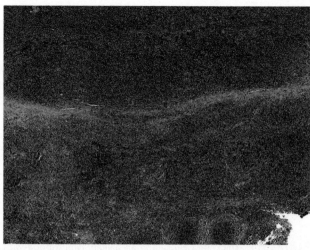

Figure 2.6. Higher power view of the disrupted capsule from the prior figure.

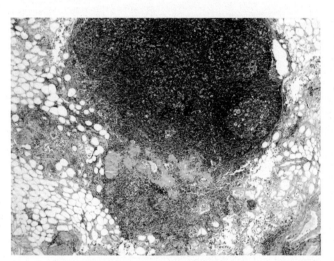

Figure 2.7. Amyloid deposition in the lymph node of a patient with systemic amyloidosis with focal disruption of the lymph node capsule. The sampled lymph node is reactive, and immunoglobulin heavy chain (IgH) gene rearrangements were polyclonal.

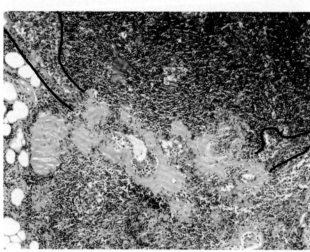

Figure 2.8. High-power view of the capsular disruption (black outline) by amyloid deposition.

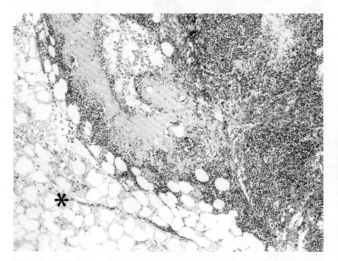

Figure 2.9. Perinodal adipose tissue that is also involved by amyloidosis (asterisk).

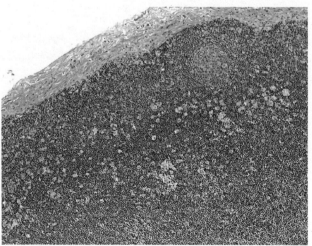

Figure 2.10. The capsule is thickened in a 2.6-cm inguinal lymph node from a 10-year-old boy. The patient had a history of seizure disorder treated with phenobarbital, which can be associated with lymphadenopathy.

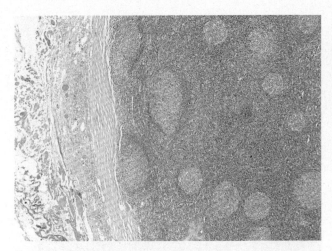

Figure 2.11. Thickened capsule in an axillary lymph node with reactive lymphoid hyperplasia. The 4.5-cm node was excised from the axilla of a 76-year-old woman.

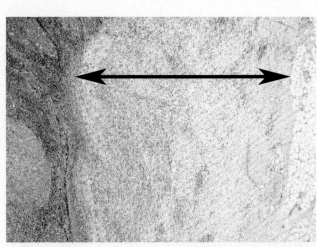

Figure 2.12. Markedly thickened capsule (double-headed arrow) of a 3.2-cm inguinal lymph node involved by syphilitic lymphadenitis.

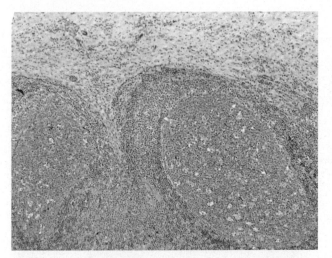

Figure 2.13. The thickened capsule of syphilitic lymphadenitis may "scallop" around prominent reactive germinal centers.

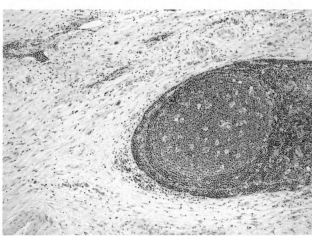

Figure 2.14. The secondary follicles in syphilitic lymphadenitis are prominent and well defined.

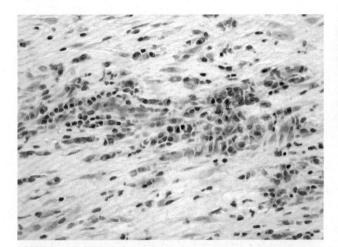

Figure 2.15. In syphilitic lymphadenitis, the capsule often shows significant chronic inflammation, including a lymphoplasmacytic infiltrate surrounding small vessels.

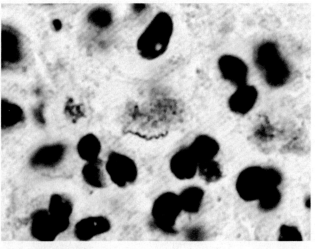

Figure 2.16. A Warthin-Starry silver stain highlights a spirochete in syphilitic lymphadenitis. The spirochetes are approximately 5 to 15 μM in length. The organisms can be difficult to identify on special stains, and immunostains directed against *Treponema pallidum* may be more sensitive.

SAMPLE NOTE

Inguinal lymph node (excisional biopsy):

- Reactive lymphoid hyperplasia with markedly thickened capsule and increased poly-typic plasma cells. See note.

Note: Some of the features of the node (ie, capsular fibrosis, perivascular lymphoplasma-cytic infiltrates, follicular hyperplasia, and increased plasma cells) raise the possibility of luetic lymphadenitis, but these findings are nonspecific. Serologic testing may be warranted if clinically indicated.

Sinus Histiocytosis With Massive Lymphadenopathy (Rosai-Dorfman Disease)

Sinus histiocytosis with massive lymphadenopathy (SHML) is best known for distinc-tively distended sinuses filled with abundant histiocytes displaying prominent emperip-olesis.[8] Lymph nodes in this disorder also typically display markedly thickened capsules (Figure 2.17). Bands of fibrosis often course through the lymph node and may extend into the perinodal fibroadipose tissue so that adjacent involved lymph nodes become matted together.

Fibrosis is not specific for SHML; however, and the diagnosis hinges on identifica-tion of dilated sinuses filled with S100-positive histiocytosis that exhibit emperipolesis. Emperipolesis refers to inflammatory cells passing through and "wandering around" the cytoplasm of the histiocytes (Figure 2.18). The inflammatory cells are most commonly lymphocytes, but can also include plasma cells, neutrophils, and red blood cells.

SHML can also involve nonnodal tissues, in which case it is typically referred to as Rosai-Dorfman disease. Emperipolesis tends to be relatively subtle in nonnodal disease, although fibrosis is seen in both nodal and nonnodal sites.

FAQ: How does Rosai-Dorfman Disease in lymph nodes differ from extranodal disease?

Rosai-Dorfman disease in extranodal locations typically shows scattered lymphoid follicles with intervening areas of fibrosis. The follicles are often scattered through-out the fibrotic background in a "checkerboard" pattern. The background fibro-sis typically contains scattered inflammatory cells, including small lymphocytes, plasma cells, and histiocytes. The histiocytes are S100+, but they can be difficult to see due to the fibrosis, and emperipolesis may relatively understated as com-pared to nodal disease.

IgG4-Related Lymphadenopathy

IgG4-related sclerosing disease is characterized by storiform fibrosis, obliterative phlebitis, and increased IgG4-positive plasma cells.[9-14] In general, the criteria for invoking IgG4-related sclerosing disease include a serum IgG4 level of >135 mg/dL and histopathologic evidence of lymphoplasmacytic infiltrates with >10 IgG4-positive plasma cells per high-power (X400) field. The IgG4:IgG ratio typically exceeds 0.4.

Almost any anatomic site may be involved, including lymph nodes. IgG4-related lymphadenopathy does not have a single characteristic morphologic appearance but can assume various morphologic appearances, resembling multicentric Castleman disease (CD), follicular hyperplasia, interfollicular lymphoplasmacytosis, progressive transfor-mation of germinal centers, and inflammatory pseudotumor (IPT)-like lesions (Figures 2.19-2.23). As expected with a sclerosing disease, capsular thickening may be seen in involved lymph nodes.

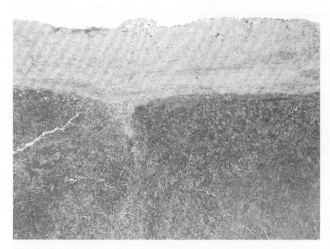

Figure 2.17. An otherwise asymptomatic 6-year-old girl presented with massive bilateral cervical lymphadenopathy. The thickened capsule and markedly dilated sinuses containing small lymphocytes and histiocytes that exhibit emperipolesis are characteristic of sinus histiocytosis with massive lymphadenopathy (Rosai-Dorfman disease).

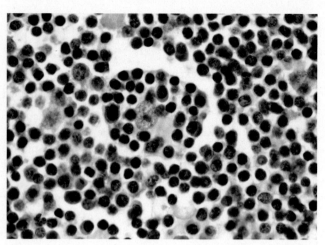

Figure 2.18. A histiocyte exhibiting emperipolesis.

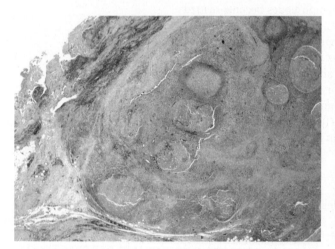

Figure 2.19. An enlarged cervical lymph node in a 60-year-old man. The capsule is thickened and the node contains bands of sclerosis.

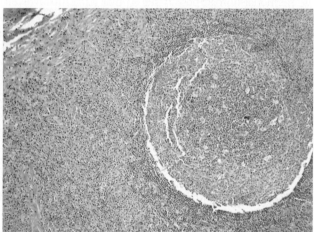

Figure 2.20. High-power view of the same lymph node in Figure 2.19 showing a thickened capsule.

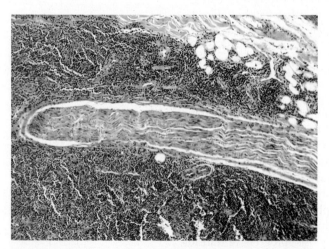

Figure 2.21. The infiltrate extends beyond the capsule into perinodal soft tissue and surrounds a nerve.

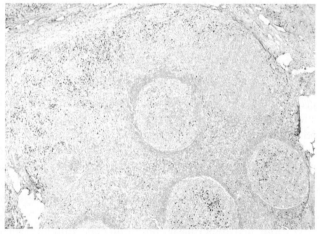

Figure 2.22. An immunostain for IgG highlights plasma cells in the lymph nodes.

SAMPLE NOTE

Cervical lymph node (excisional biopsy):

• Reactive lymph node with follicular and paracortical hyperplasia and increased IgG4+ plasma cells. See note.

Note: While IgG4+ cells are increased, this finding is not specific for IgG4-related disease. Clinical correlation is recommended, and measurement of serum IgG4 levels may be of value.

Kimura Lymphadenopathy

Kimura lymphadenopathy is a rare disorder. It most commonly affects patients of Asian descent but can be seen in other ethnicities as well.[8,15] The enlarged nodes are characteristically found in the cervical area or near the ears. The lymph node architecture is intact, displaying follicular hyperplasia and vascular proliferation. The capsule is typically thickened, and there may be bands of fibrosis (Figure 2.24), leading to aggregates of matted lymph nodes as the disease progresses (Figure 2.25).

The hallmark of Kimura lymphadenopathy is eosinophilia, involving both the peripheral blood and the lymph node. Eosinophils may be so abundant in the lymph node that they form eosinophilic microabscesses (Figure 2.26). The eosinophil-rich lymphoid infiltrate may also extend beyond the capsule of the node into the perinodal fibroadipose tissue (Figure 2.27). Multinucleated cells that resemble Warthin-Finkeldey cells can be seen in Kimura lymphadenopathy (Figure 2.28), but they are nonspecific as they can also be seen in viral lymphadenitis, including HIV and measles lymphadenitis. Warthin-Finkeldey-type cells in the setting of increased eosinophils strongly favor a diagnosis of Kimura lymphadenopathy.

While the morphologic findings in Kimura lymphadenopathy are relatively distinctive, it is difficult to make a definitive diagnosis without clinical correlation. In lymph nodes that exhibit features of Kimura lymphadenopathy, it is important to raise this possibility in the differential diagnosis.

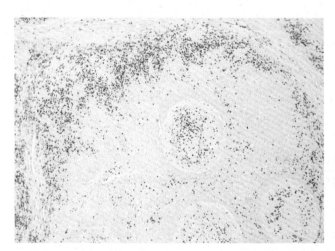

Figure 2.23. Virtually all of the IgG-positive plasma cells are IgG4-positive.

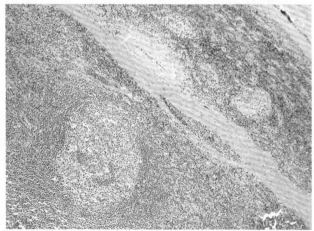

Figure 2.24. Lymph nodes involved by Kimura disease often have a thickened capsule. The lymph node architecture is intact with reactive germinal centers and a mildly expanded paracortex.

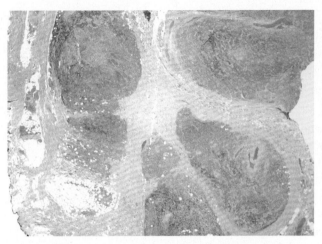

Figure 2.25. An infra-auricular mass in a 35-year-old man. The specimen contains matted lymph nodes. An eosinophil-rich lymphoid infiltrate extends beyond the capsule of the node into the perinodal fibroadipose tissue.

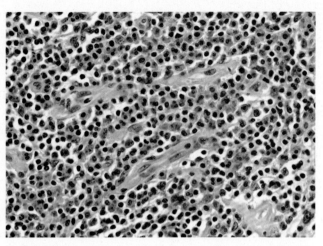

Figure 2.26. Increased eosinophils in a lymph node involved by Kimura lymphadenopathy.

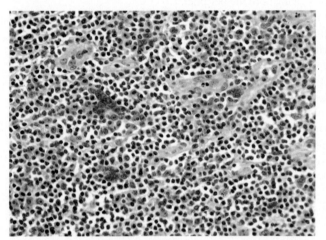

Figure 2.27. There are abundant eosinophils scattered throughout the lymph node, which form occasional eosinophilic microabscesses. Warthin-Finkeldey cells are readily identified.

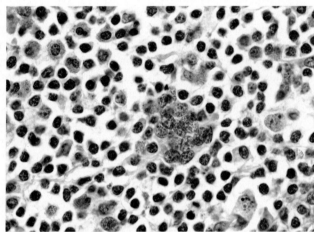

Figure 2.28. Warthin-Finkeldey-type cells are characteristically prominent in Kimura lymphadenopathy.

SAMPLE NOTE

Post auricular lymph node (excisional biopsy):

• Reactive lymphoid hyperplasia with increased eosinophils. See note.

Note: The findings in this case are strongly suggestive of Kimura disease, including the anatomic location, marked eosinophilia with eosinophilic microabscesses, moderate vascular proliferation, scattered Warthin-Finkeldey cells, and follicular hyperplasia. Kimura disease is associated with peripheral blood eosinophilia and elevated serum IgE. Laboratory correlation is recommended.

The differential diagnosis of Kimura lymphadenopathy includes angiolymphoid hyperplasia with eosinophilia (ALHE).[16,17] However, the inflammatory infiltrate of ALHE is concentrated in the dermis, whereas Kimura disease predominantly affects deep subcutaneous tissues and lymph nodes.

Castleman Disease

There are two main subtypes of CD: hyaline vascular Castleman disease (HV-CD) and the plasma cell variant (PC-CD).[8,18,19] There is also a "mixed variant" which shows some overlapping features of both subtypes. The hyaline vascular subtype (HV-CD) is more common and typically involves lymph nodes in a single location ("unicentric"), often within the mediastinum. In contrast, "multicentric" CD involves multiple sites and is usually the plasma cell variant.

The etiology of CD is unclear, although one known etiologic agent is human herpesvirus-8 (HHV-8), which is found in up to 50% of PC-CD, especially in patients with HIV. The presentation and clinical outcomes are variable. Many patients with unicentric CD are asymptomatic and present with isolated lymphadenopathy or an incidentally discovered mass. Patients with multicentric CD, on the other hand, typically present with systemic symptoms, including night sweats, fevers, and diffuse adenopathy, and may have splenomegaly and/or hepatomegaly.

The disease is histologically heterogeneous and shares many features with other reactive lymphadenopathies. In HV-CD, the capsule of an involved lymph node may be thickened. Alternatively, it may be totally disrupted, as in those cases of HV-CD that present as a large, destructive mass (Figure 2.29). The architecture of a lymph node involved by HV-CD often displays numerous follicles scattered through the cortex and paracortex with atretic germinal centers and concentrically layered mantle zones ("onion-skinning") (Figure 2.30). There may be two or more atretic germinal center present within one mantle zone ("twinning"). The interfollicular areas show increased high endothelial venules and variably increased polytypic plasma cells, and the medullary sinuses are often obliterated.

CHECKLIST: Differential Diagnosis of Lymph Nodes with Hyaline Vascular Castleman-like Changes

☐ Atretic follicles with concentrically layered mantle zones
  o Hyaline vascular CD
  o HHV-8+ CD
  o HIV lymphadenopathy
  o Interfollicular classical Hodgkin lymphoma
  o Mantle cell lymphoma ("mantle zone pattern" with neoplastic cells expanding mantle zones)
☐ Increased vascularity
  o Angioimmunoblastic T-cell lymphoma
  o Dermatopathic lymphadenopathy
  o Metastatic tumor

Inflammatory Pseudotumor

IPTs are proliferations that are composed of a mixture of fibroblasts and inflammatory cells, and while they form masses, they are not malignant neoplasms.[20]

Unfortunately, "IPT" and "inflammatory myofibroblastic tumor" are sometimes used interchangeably; however, it should be noted that they are different entities. IPT is reactive, whereas inflammatory myofibroblastic tumor is neoplastic.

IPT only rarely involves lymph nodes. The lymph nodes exhibit a thickened capsule with increased fibrosis and abundant inflammatory cells (Figures 2.31-2.35). Whorls of fibroblasts and collagen fibrosis can be seen (Figure 2.36). The uninvolved lymph node may show reactive changes.

The differential diagnosis of IPT includes spindled melanoma, metastatic carcinoma, Kaposi sarcoma (KS), inflammatory myofibroblastic tumor, follicular dendritic cell sarcoma, and the IPT pattern of IgG4 sclerosing disease. A panel of immunohistochemical stains is recommended to rule out these other entities before rendering a diagnosis of likely IPT.

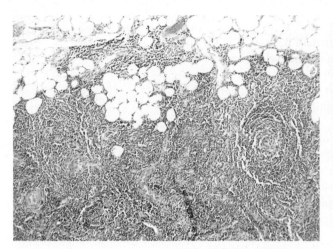

Figure 2.29. A 54-year-old woman was incidentally found to have mediastinal adenopathy during a chest X-ray for a positive tuberculosis screen. Histologic sections show largely unencapsulated lymphoid tissue that contains numerous and uniformly distributed follicles with atretic germinal centers.

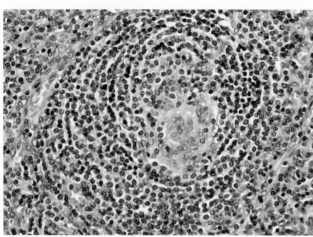

Figure 2.30. The mantle zones have a concentrically laminated appearance, and the interfollicular areas show a proliferation of high endothelial venules.

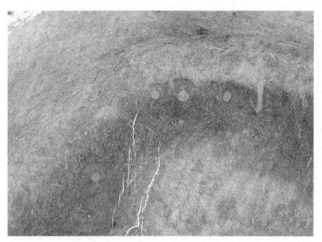

Figure 2.31. Enlarged cervical lymph node involved by inflammatory pseudotumor in a 27-year-old woman who presented with a history of a febrile episode and subsequent lymphadenopathy.

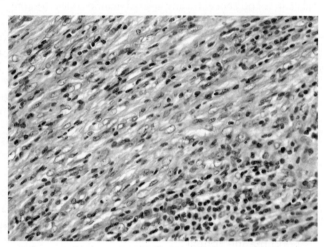

Figure 2.32. Higher power view of the markedly thickened capsule in prior figure.

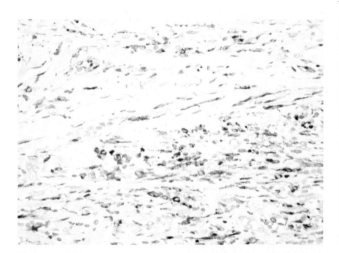

Figure 2.33. CD68 immunostain showing frequent histiocytes in prior figure.

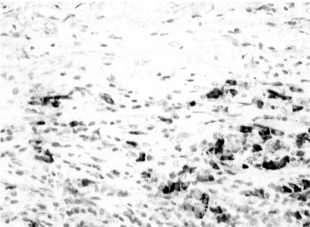

Figure 2.34. An immunohistochemical stain for IgG marks frequent plasma cells in the thickened capsule of an inflammatory pseudotumor.

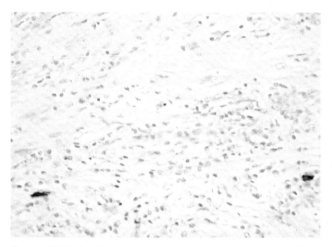

Figure 2.35. IgG4 lymphadenopathy can demonstrate an inflammatory pseudotumor (IPT)-like pattern; however, IgG4-positive plasma cells are rare in IPT.

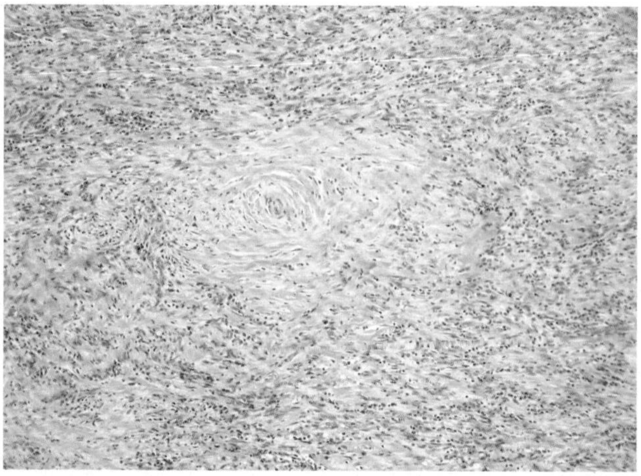

Figure 2.36. Higher power view of IPT. The spindled cells are negative for S100, HHV-8, ALK-1, CD21, actin, and CD34 (not shown).

KEY FEATURES: Immunophenotype of Spindled Cells in Lymph Nodes

Metastatic melanoma	Metastatic carcinoma	Kaposi sarcoma	Inflammatory myofibro-blastic tumor	Follicular dendritic cell sarcoma	IgG4 sclerosing disease
S100+	Keratin+	HHV-8+	ALK1+, Actin+	CD21+, CD35+	IgG4+

NEOPLASTIC CONDITIONS

Classical Hodgkin Lymphoma, Nodular Sclerosis Subtype

The nodular sclerosis variant of classical Hodgkin lymphoma (CHL) is the entity that is perhaps most closely associated with capsular fibrosis. The other three variants of CHL (mixed cellularity, lymphocyte-rich, and lymphocyte-depleted) do not typically show marked capsular fibrosis. The capsular fibrosis of the nodular sclerosis variant of CHL (NS-CHL) is often pronounced (Figure 2.37), and thick bands of sclerosis form the nodules that give this neoplasm its name and characteristic appearance (Figure 2.38). Early disease may not show capsular thickening (Figure 2.39), but over time, the involved lymph node capsule thickens and adjacent involved lymph nodes may become matted together (Figure 2.40).

The cellular areas of NS-CHL are composed of a mixed inflammatory infiltrate, including small lymphocytes, histiocytes, plasma cells, eosinophils, and/or neutrophils. The composition of the inflammatory infiltrate varies, and some tumors exhibit a preponderance of either histiocytes, eosinophils, or neutrophils. CHL is characterized by scattered atypical cells, some of which are mononuclear ("Hodgkin cells") and some of which are multinucleate ("Reed-Sternberg cells") (Figure 2.41). Hodgkin/Reed-Sternberg (HRS) cells, a term which encompasses both variant cell types, have a moderate-to-abundant amount of cytoplasm, which is often eosinophilic, and prominent nucleoli. HRS cells in the nodular sclerosing variant of CHL may have more subtle nucleoli than those seen in the mixed cellularity variant of CHL. While HRS cells are often singly scattered, they may form sheets with foci of necrosis. This architectural pattern is called the "syncytial variant" and is seen in NS-CHL.

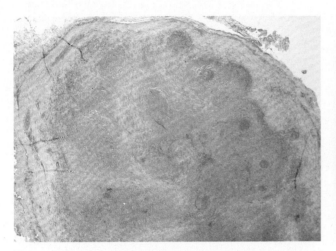

Figure 2.37. This supraclavicular lymph node from a 19-year-old woman shows the thickened capsule that is characteristic of the nodular sclerosis variant of classic Hodgkin lymphoma. Bands of sclerosis can also be seen extending throughout the node.

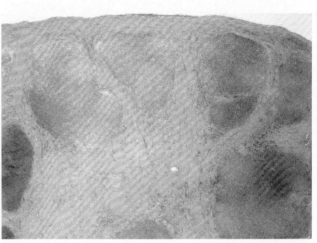

Figure 2.38. A supraclavicular lymph node from a 14-year-old boy with the nodular sclerosis variant of classic Hodgkin lymphoma shows a thickened capsule as well as well-developed bands of sclerosis that divide the node into nodules.

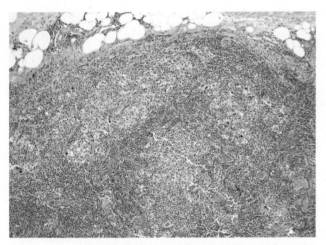

Figure 2.39. Mediastinal lymph node involved by recurrent nodular sclerosis classic Hodgkin lymphoma. While the nodular sclerosis variant of classic Hodgkin lymphoma characteristically has a thickened capsule, the capsule in early disease may be relatively thin.

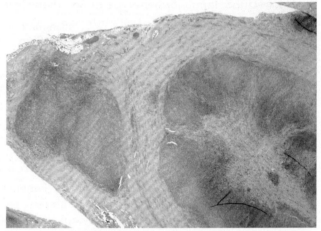

Figure 2.40. In long-standing nodular sclerosis classic Hodgkin lymphoma, adjacent nodes can become matted together.

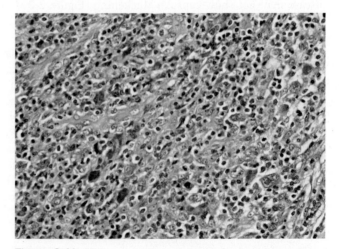

Figure 2.41. The nodules from the prior figure show a mixture of inflammatory cells as well as scattered large atypical cells. The Hodgkin Reed-Sternberg cells in the nodular sclerosis variant of classic Hodgkin lymphoma often have less prominent nucleoli than other subtypes of classic Hodgkin lymphoma. There are occasional mummified cells.

CHECKLIST: Differential Diagnosis of Lymph Nodes With Increased Eosinophils

☐ Classical Hodgkin lymphoma
☐ Mastocytosis
☐ T-cell lymphomas (peripheral T-cell lymphoma, NOS; angioimmunoblastic T-cell lymphoma)
☐ Myeloid sarcoma (often with inv(16) (p13.1q22))
☐ Myeloid and lymphoid neoplasms with *PDGFRA*, *PRGFRB*, or *FGFR1* rearrangement
☐ Langerhans cell histiocytosis
☐ Kimura disease
☐ IgG4 lymphadenopathy
☐ Drug reactions
☐ Dermatopathic lymphadenopathy

The immunophenotype of HRS cells in all CHL subtypes is characteristic: they are positive for CD30 (Figure 2.42) and MUM-1 and are often, but not necessarily, positive for CD15 (Figure 2.43). HRS cells also show dim expression of Pax-5 and exhibit variable expression of CD20, but are negative for CD45. If cells with otherwise classic HRS morphology and immunophenotype have strong, uniform expression of CD20, then a diagnosis of "B-cell lymphoma with features intermediate between diffuse large B-cell lymphoma and classical Hodgkin lymphoma" (so-called "gray zone lymphoma") may be entertained (see the chapter on diffuse nodal infiltrates for additional images and further details).

FAQ: Is it necessary to subtype classic Hodgkin lymphoma?

Answer: Subtyping classical Hodgkin lymphoma is recommended, but it may not be possible in small biopsy specimens. This is generally acceptable since all subtypes of classical Hodgkin lymphoma are currently treated with similar protocols. It is, however, absolutely critical to differentiate between classical Hodgkin lymphoma and nodular lymphocyte predominate Hodgkin lymphoma, as the treatments differ significantly.

Nodular Lymphocyte Predominant Hodgkin Lymphoma

Unlike NS-CHL, nodular lymphocyte predominant Hodgkin lymphoma (NLPHL) does not typically show marked capsular thickening. In long-standing cases of NLPHL, however, the capsule may thicken and bands of sclerosis may form (Figure 2.44), which raises the differential diagnosis of NS-CHL. NLPHL is characterized by expansive nodules of small lymphocytes with singly scattered large atypical lymphocyte predominant (LP) cells (Figure 2.45). The LP cells have abundant pale or clear cytoplasm and one or more large nuclei with irregular nuclear borders that can resemble "elephants' feet" or "popcorn cells." The nucleoli are conspicuous but are usually smaller than the nucleoli of CHL.

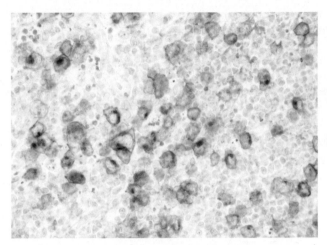

Figure 2.42. An immunostain for CD30 marks the Hodgkin/Reed-Sternberg cells from the lymph node in Figure 2.41.

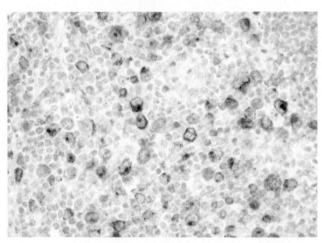

Figure 2.43. An immunostain for CD15 marks the Hodgkin/Reed-Sternberg cells as well as a few background inflammatory cells in the lymph node in Figure 2.41.

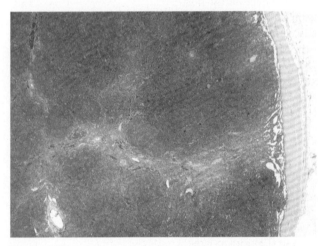

Figure 2.44. An enlarged (4.5 cm) node was reportedly present in the axilla of an 18-year-old woman for over 2 years. Long-standing nodular lymphocyte predominant lymphoma can show capsular thickening and even thin bands of fibrosis.

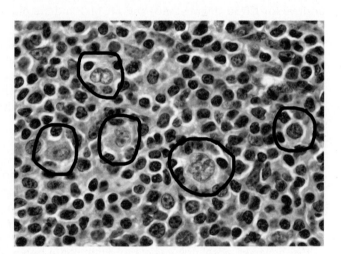

Figure 2.45. The large lymphocyte predominant (LP) cells are circled.

PEARLS & PITFALLS

Long-standing or recurrent NLPHL can show a thickened capsule and/or bands of sclerosis, similar to NS-CHL.

NLPHL can usually be differentiated from the nodular sclerosing and mixed cellularity variants of CHL based on morphologic findings, since the background cells in NLPHL are small lymphocytes (Figure 2.46), whereas CHL typically shows a distinctive mixed inflammatory background composed of small lymphocytes, histiocytes, eosinophils, plasma cells, and/or neutrophils.[21,22] However, since NLPHL can contain admixed histiocytes and epithelioid histiocytes, it is essentially impossible to differentiate NLPHL from the lymphocyte-rich variant of CHL based on morphologic findings alone, and an immunohistochemical panel is needed.

Unlike the HRS cells of CHL, the LP cells of NLPHL are characteristically positive for CD45 and bright CD20 (Figure 2.47) but are negative for both CD30 and CD15 and show only partial dim expression of MUM-1. Both PD-1-positive and CD57-positive small T-cells are increased in NLPHL. The LP cells are surrounded by distinctive rosettes of PD-1+ cells, and CD57+ T-cells may also occasionally rosette around the LP cells. See the chapter on nodular nodal infiltrates for further details.

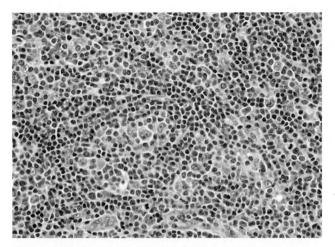

Figure 2.46. Nodular lymphocyte predominant lymphoma contains singly scattered large lymphocyte predominant (LP) cells in a background of small lymphocytes.

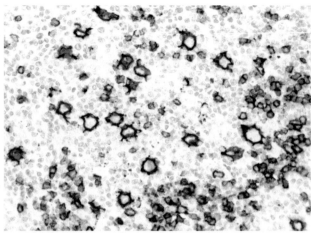

Figure 2.47. The lymphocyte predominant (LP) cells express bright CD20, and scattered small CD20-positive B-cells are present in the background.

KEY FEATURES: Immunophenotype of Hodgkin/Reed-Sternberg Cells in Classical Hodgkin Lymphoma (CHL) Versus Lymphocyte Predominant Cells in Nodular Lymphocyte Predominant (NLP) Hodgkin Lymphoma

	CD20	CD30	CD15	CD45	PAX-5	MUM-1	OCT2
CHL	–	+	+	–	+ Weak	+ Strong	–
NLPHL	+	–	–	+	+ Strong	–/+(Weak)	+ Strong

Non-Hodgkin Lymphoma

Thickened capsules are not limited to Hodgkin lymphomas and may also be seen in non-Hodgkin lymphomas, including diffuse large B-cell lymphoma (Figures 2.48-2.50). Careful morphologic assessment is necessary to reach a final diagnosis.

Metastatic Neoplasms

Lymph nodes that are involved by metastatic disease can also show thickening of the capsule (Figure 2.51) and may become matted together. If atypical cells in a lymph node are not hematolymphoid, then additional immunohistochemical workup is recommended, including cytokeratin (AE1/AE3, Cam5.2) and melanoma markers. It should be noted that normal lymph nodes contain scattered S100 histiocytes, and the use of additional markers (Sox10, Melan A, MART-1, HMB-45) is often helpful or even necessary in the identification of small foci of metastatic melanoma (Figures 2.52-2.54).

FAQ: What immunostain panel can be used to determine whether or not a cell is of hematolymphoid origin?

Answer: Nearly all hematolymphoid cells are positive for one or more of the following markers: CD45, CD43, MUM-1, and/or CD30. Further subclassification and characterization of the hematolymphoid cells will, however, likely require additional immunostains.

PEARLS & PITFALLS

Lymph nodes that contain metastatic tumor can show prominent reactive changes, including follicular and/or paracortical hyperplasia, as well as sinus histiocytosis and vascular proliferation. Additionally, the CD4:CD8 ratio in the paracortex may be unusually high (>5:1) or unusually low (<1:1).

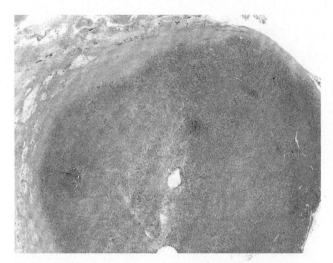

Figure 2.48. A 3-cm cervical lymph node in a 73-year-old man with a history of Crohn disease treated with methotrexate. The node has a markedly thickened capsule and is involved by Epstein-Barr virus (EBV)–negative diffuse large B-cell lymphoma, germinal center B-cell subtype.

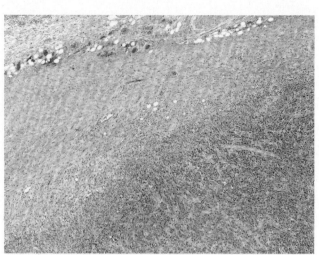

Figure 2.49. Higher power view of the prior figure. The subcapsular sinus is obliterated by the tumor cells.

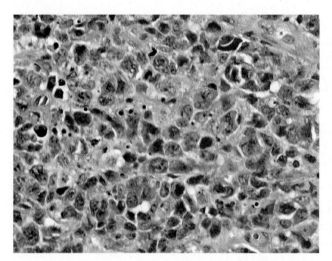

Figure 2.50. The atypical lymphocytes in the prior figure are large with a scant-to-moderate amount of eosinophilic cytoplasm, vesicular chromatin, and one or more variably prominent nucleoli.

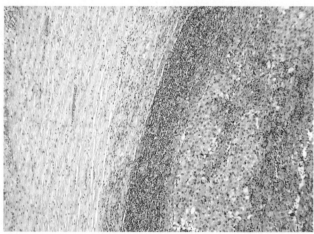

Figure 2.51. An enlarged node that is involved by metastatic melanoma from the axilla of an 85-year-old man. The capsule is thickened, with some of the nodes matted together.

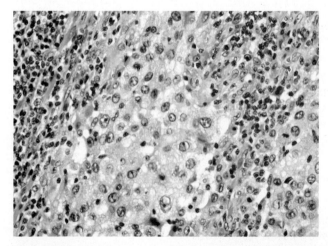

Figure 2.52. High-power view of the prior figure. The neoplastic cells are large with abundant pale cytoplasm, irregular nuclear border, and variably prominent nucleoli.

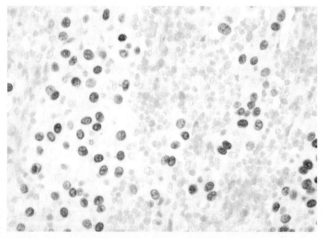

Figure 2.53. A Sox10 immunostain highlights the focus of metastatic melanoma in the prior figure.

NEAR MISSES

ANGIOIMMUNOBLASTIC T-CELL LYMPHOMA

Occasionally, focal extracapsular extension of lymphoid tissue can be seen in reactive lymph nodes, in which case the subcapsular sinus remains patent (Figure 2.55). As previously mentioned, lymphoma frequently effaces the nodal architecture, fills the sinuses, and extends beyond the lymph node capsule to involve the perinodal fibroadipose tissue. However, in some cases, an abnormal nodal infiltrate will "skip" the subcapsular sinus, leaving it largely patent, and continue on into the perinodal soft tissue.

These "skip lesions" with lymphomatous extension into the perinodal fat are particularly characteristic of angioimmunoblastic T-cell lymphoma (AITL) (Figures 2.56 and 2.57). AITL, as the name suggests, is a T-cell lymphoma that exhibits a characteristic vascular proliferation with scattered immunoblasts.

The neoplastic cells are medium-sized atypical lymphoid cells with clear cytoplasm. There are invariably admixed immunoblasts, B-cells, and plasma cells. A few eosinophils are also usually seen. The abnormal T-cells are CD4-positive with partial expression of follicular helper T-cell markers, including PD-1, CD10, and/or Bcl-6, and the T-cells usually show preservation of CD5 expression with significant loss of CD7. Additionally, the nodes show expansion of CD21 and/or CD23-positive follicular dendritic cell meshworks, and many cases also have scattered Epstein-Barr virus (EBV)–positive cells. Molecular studies for T-cell receptor gene rearrangements are particularly helpful in making a diagnosis of AITL, as they typically show a clonal pattern.

AITL can show various patterns of nodal involvement. This includes a relatively subtle paracortical expansion in the early stages of disease (see Chapter 1, "Near Misses"), which can be easy to overlook. Care is necessary when examining a lymph node with a paracortical expansion, and evaluation of the capsule may be helpful to assess for skip lesions. AITL can progress to completely efface the lymph node (see later chapter for details).[23-25]

KEY FEATURES: Angioimmunoblastic T-cell Lymphoma

- Partial or totally effaced lymph node architecture
- Extension of the infiltrate into the perinodal adipose tissue with sparing of the sinuses ("skip lesions")
- Prominent arborizing high endothelial venules
- Atypical small- to medium-sized lymphocytes with clear cytoplasm and mildly irregular nuclear borders
  - CD3+ (often slightly dim) and CD4+
  - Atypical T-cells often show preserved expression of CD5 with loss of CD7
  - Expression of PD-1, CD10, Bcl-6, ICOS, and/or CXCL13
- Admixed eosinophils, immunoblasts, and plasma cells
- Expanded CD21+ follicular dendritic cell meshworks that extend outside of the follicles
- Scattered EBV+ cells (many but not all cases)

KAPOSI SARCOMA

KS is a vascular neoplasm involving endothelial cells, which is associated with HHV-8 infection.[8,22,26,27] KS most frequently affects immunocompromised patients, specifically those with HIV/AIDS, but it is also found in patients from the Mediterranean region where HHV-8 infection is endemic.

Early KS lesions involve the lymph node capsule. A proliferation of endothelial cells in the capsule results in poorly formed slit-like vascular spaces (Figures 2.58 and 2.59), with extravasated red blood cells and hemosiderin-laden macrophages frequently identified. The endothelial cells do not show nuclear atypia, but do contain intracellular hyaline globules, though these may be difficult to identify on H&E. The remainder of the lymph node typically shows reactive changes, including follicular hyperplasia and a polytypic plasmacytosis.

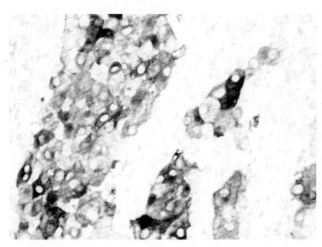

Figure 2.54. A Melan A immunostain highlights a focus of metastatic melanoma in Figure 2.53.

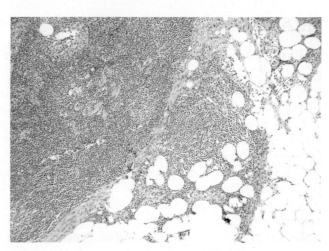

Figure 2.55. Focal extension beyond the capsule can be seen in reactive lymph nodes; however, the subcapsular sinus remains patent and the lymphocytes do not exhibit cellular atypia.

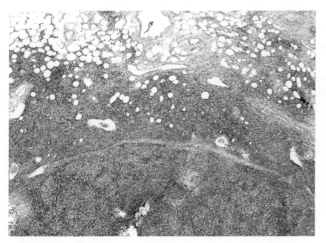

Figure 2.56. Angioimmunoblastic T-cell lymphoma with extension beyond the capsule and concomitant preservation of the sinuses.

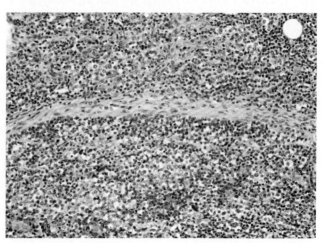

Figure 2.57. High-power view of the prior figure, showing preservation of the subcapsular sinus.

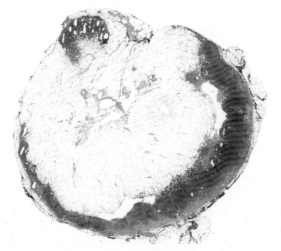

Figure 2.58. Kaposi sarcoma involving an axillary lymph node from a 44-year-old HIV-positive man. There is extensive fatty replacement of the hilum. The cortex contains scattered primary follicles, and the paracortex is mildly expanded with admixed plasma cells and immunoblasts. The medulla shows marked plasmacytosis. The subcapsular sinus is obliterated in areas by a vascular proliferation that extends down the lymph node trabeculae in a wedge-shaped pattern.

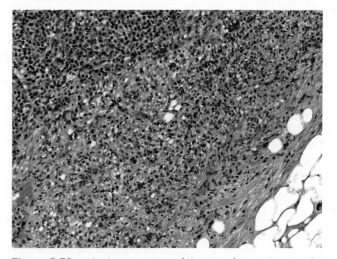

Figure 2.59. A high-power view of the prior figure, showing the atypical endothelial cells that form vascular clefts with extravasated red blood cells. The adjacent lymph node is notable for increased plasma cells.

Immunohistochemical stains may be required to confirm early involvement by KS. The neoplastic cells are invariably highlighted by an HHV-8 immunohistochemical stain and also express vascular markers including ERG, CD34, and CD31 (Figures 2.60-2.62). CD31 may be difficult to interpret in lymph nodes as there can be high background staining.

As KS advances, the endothelial proliferation extends into the lymph node in a wedge-shaped progression down fibrous septae (Figures 2.63 and 2.64). Ultimately, the neoplastic cells form dense whorls with associated fibrosis and may replace large portions of the lymph node (Figures 2.65-2.68).

TUMOR-INFILTRATING LYMPHOCYTES VERSUS METASTATIC DISEASE

It is important to note the presence or absence of a capsule when assessing both lymphoid and nonlymphoid malignancies. A variety of epithelial tumors may incite a vigorous inflammatory response, including breast cancer, colon cancer, melanoma, and soft tissue tumors (Figures 2.69-2.72).

In small core biopsy specimens, it is critically important to differentiate between a primary tumor with abundant infiltrating lymphocytes and nodal involvement by metastatic disease, as this distinction affects staging and treatment strategies. Thus, careful evaluation of the tissue for the presence of a capsule is paramount. In scant core biopsy specimens, clinical and/or radiographic correlation may be needed to determine if the findings represent primary tumor with a brisk inflammatory response or true metastatic disease.

CAPSULAR NEVI VERSUS METASTATIC MELANOMA

Superficial lymph nodes draining the skin occasionally have small, subtle collections of benign melanocytes on the surface of the capsule, within the capsule, or in the subcapsular area, known as capsular nevi (Figure 2.73). The cells should show no overt cytomorphologic atypia (Figure 2.74); however, occasionally, it may be difficult to distinguish capsular nevi from metastatic melanoma. In these settings, immunohistochemical stains can be helpful, as capsular nevi typically express S100 and Melan A (MART-1) but are negative for HMB-45 and have a low Ki-67 proliferation index. In contrast, metastatic melanoma is more likely to be positive for S100, Melan A/MART-1, and HMB-45, and has a high Ki-67 proliferation index.

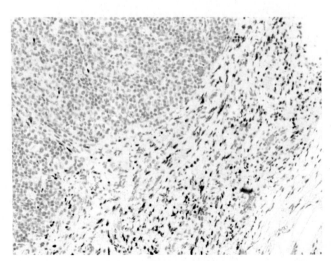

Figure 2.60. Human herpesvirus-8 (HHV-8) immunostain of the prior figure. HHV-8 highlights the nuclei of the neoplastic endothelial cells.

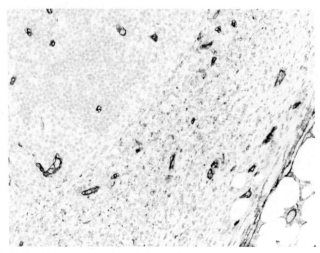

Figure 2.61. CD34 immunostain of the prior figure. The neoplastic endothelial cells may show unusual immunophenotypic features, as with this case in which CD34 is largely negative on the tumor cells.

KEY FEATURES: Immunophenotype of Capsular Nevi Versus Metastatic Melanoma

	S100	Melan A	HMB-45	Ki67
Capsular nevi	+	+	−	Low
Metastatic melanoma	+	+	+	High

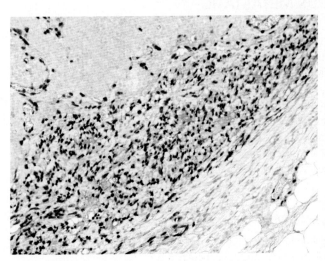

Figure 2.62. ERG immunostain of the prior figure. The endothelial marker ERG highlights the neoplastic endothelial cells.

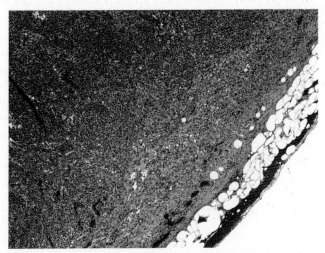

Figure 2.63. The subcapsular sinus of the prior figure is obliterated by a vascular proliferation that involves the capsule and extends down the lymph node trabeculae in a wedge-shaped pattern.

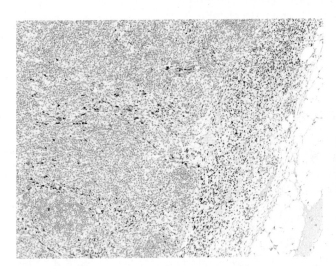

Figure 2.64. An HHV-8 stain highlights the wedge-shaped infiltrate as seen in the prior figure.

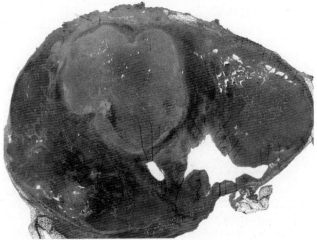

Figure 2.65. A 1.1-cm cervical lymph node from an HIV-negative 38-year-old man who was born in Cyprus. The node is largely replaced by tumor nodules. This represents sporadic Kaposi sarcoma in a patient of Mediterranean origin.

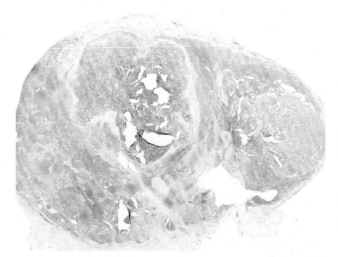

Figure 2.66. The neoplastic cells are HHV-8 positive.

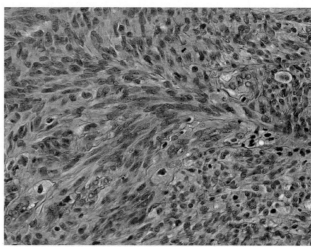

Figure 2.67. A high-power view of the prior figure, which shows the dense whorls of neoplastic endothelial cells.

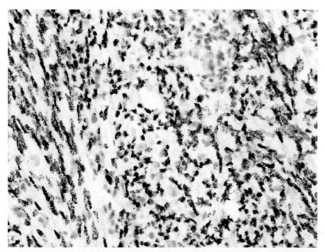

Figure 2.68. An HHV-8 stain highlights the neoplastic cells in the prior figure.

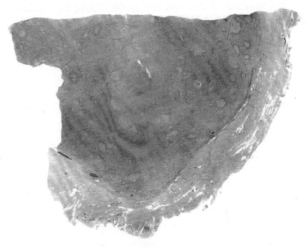

Figure 2.69. Thigh mass in a 78-year-old man. The excision consisted of a 4-cm mass of well-defined lymphoid tissue with reactive follicles and was ultimately diagnosed as a lymphocyte-rich well-differentiated liposarcoma.

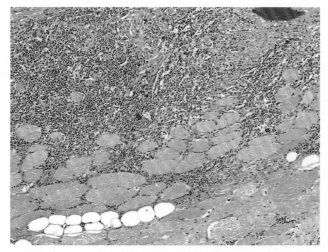

Figure 2.70. The lymphoid infiltrate involves the surrounding soft tissue and skeletal muscle. It lacks a capsule, and the inflammatory cells are a mixture of B-cells and T-cells with scattered secondary follicles.

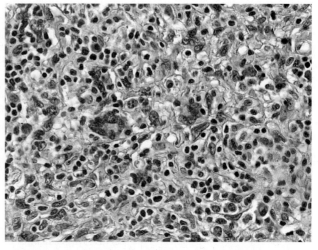

Figure 2.71. The lymphoid tissue in the liposarcoma contains markedly atypical cells that are MDM2-positive lipoblasts.

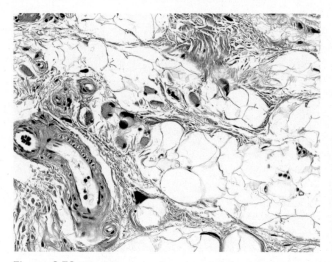

Figure 2.72. Lipoblasts are also scattered throughout the surrounding adipose tissue, many of which are highlighted by MDM2.

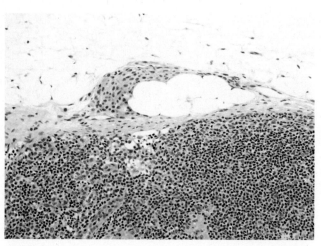

Figure 2.73. A capsular nevus in a sentinel node biopsy from a 65-year-old woman with microinvasive mammary carcinoma. The nevus cells may be associated with the outer surface of the capsule, within the capsule itself, or may have a subcapsular location.

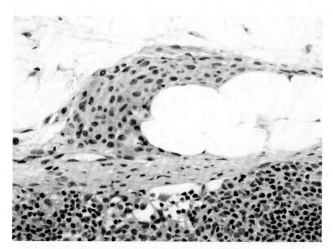

Figure 2.74. The cells in this capsular nevus do not show cytomorphologic atypia. Capsular nevi are typically S100- and MART-1-positive. In contrast to melanoma, they usually lack expression of HMB-45 and have a low Ki-67 proliferation index.

References

1. Fisher CJ, Hill S, Millis RR. Benign lymph node inclusions mimicking metastatic carcinoma. *J Clin Pathol*. 1994;47(3):245-247.

2. Norton LE, Komenaka IK, Emerson RE, Murphy C, Badve S. Benign glandular inclusions a rare cause of a false positive sentinel node. *J Surg Oncol*. 2007;95(7):593-596.

3. Corben AD, Nehhozina T, Garg K, Vallejo CE, Brogi E. Endosalpingiosis in axillary lymph nodes: a possible pitfall in the staging of patients with breast carcinoma. *Am J Surg Pathol*. 2010;34(8):1211-1216.

4. Wessels A, Bamford C, Lewis D, Martini M, Wainwright H. Syphilitic lymphadenitis clinically and histologically mimicking lymphogranuloma venereum. *S Afr Med J*. 2016;106(5):49-51.

5. Duffield AS, Borowitz MJ. Syphilitic lymphadenitis with abscess formation involving cervical lymph nodes. *Blood*. 2018;131(6):707.

6. Yuan Y, Zhang X, Xu N, et al. Clinical and pathologic diagnosis and different diagnosis of syphilis cervical lymphadenitis. *Int J Clin Exp Pathol*. 2015;8(10):13635-13638.

7. Liu Z, Zhang C, Kakudo K, et al. Diagnostic pitfalls in pathological diagnosis of infectious disease: patients with syphilitic lymphadenitis often present with inconspicuous history of infection. *Pathol Int.* 2016;66(3):142-147.

8. Ioachim HL. *Lymph Node Pathology*. Philadelphia, PA: Lippincott Williams & Wilkins; 2009.

9. Bledsoe JR, Della-Torre E, Rovati L, Deshpande V. IgG4-related disease: review of the histopathologic features, differential diagnosis, and therapeutic approach. *APMIS.* 2018;126(6):459-476.

10. Bookhout CE, Rollins-Raval MA. Immunoglobulin G4-related lymphadenopathy. *Surg Pathol Clin.* 2016;9(1):117-129.

11. Chen YR, Chen YJ, Wang MC, Medeiros LJ, Chang KC. A newly recognized histologic pattern of IgG4-related lymphadenopathy: expanding the morphologic spectrum. *Am J Surg Pathol.* 2018;42(7):977-982.

12. Cheuk W, Yuen HK, Chu SY, Chiu EK, Lam LK, Chan JK. Lymphadenopathy of IgG4-related sclerosing disease. *Am J Surg Pathol.* 2008;32(5):671-681.

13. Deshpande V, Zen Y, Chan JK, et al. Consensus statement on the pathology of IgG4-related disease. *Mod Pathol.* 2012;25(9):1181-1192.

14. Detlefsen S. [IgG4-related disease: microscopic diagnosis and differential diagnosis]. *Der Pathologe.* 2019;40(6):619-626.

15. Maehara T, Munemura R, Shimizu M, et al. Tissue-infiltrating immune cells contribute to understanding the pathogenesis of Kimura disease: a case report. *Medicine.* 2019;98(50):e18300.

16. Li SL, Han JD. Solitary nodule of angiolymphoid hyperplasia with eosinophilia of the back masquerading as pyogenic granuloma. *Mol Clin Oncol.* 2017;7(5):874-876.

17. Marka A, Cowdrey MCE, Carter JB, Lansigan F, Yan S, LeBlanc RE. Angiolymphoid hyperplasia with eosinophilia and Kimura disease overlap, with evidence of diffuse visceral involvement. *J Cutan Pathol.* 2019;46(2):138-142.

18. Abramson JS. Diagnosis and management of Castleman disease. *J Natl Compr Cancer Netw.* 2019;17(11.5):1417-1419.

19. Glick L, Xu H, Han TM, HooKim K, Vogel A, Lallas CD. Castleman disease: an uncommon mass in the retroperitoneum. *Urology.* 2019;136:e12-e15.

20. Perrone T, De Wolf-Peeters C, Frizzera G. Inflammatory pseudotumor of lymph nodes. A distinctive pattern of nodal reaction. *Am J Surg Pathol.* 1988;12(5):351-361.

21. Swerdlow SH, Campo E, Harris NL, et al. *World Health Organization Classification of Tumours of Haematopoietic and Lymphoid Tissues.* Lyon, France: International Agency for Research on Cancer; 2017.

22. Medeiros LJ, O'Malley DP, Caraway NP, Vega F, Elenitoba-Johnson KSJ, Lim MS. *AFIP Atlas of Tumor Pathology, Fourth Series; Tumors of the Lymph Nodes and Spleen.* Washington DC: American Registry of Pathology; 2017.

23. Ree HJ, Kadin ME, Kikuchi M, et al. Angioimmunoblastic lymphoma (AILD-type T-cell lymphoma) with hyperplastic germinal centers. *Am J Surg Pathol.* 1998;22(6):643-655.

24. Attygalle AD, Kyriakou C, Dupuis J, et al. Histologic evolution of angioimmunoblastic T-cell lymphoma in consecutive biopsies: clinical correlation and insights into natural history and disease progression. *Am J Surg Pathol.* 2007;31(7):1077-1088.

25. Tan LH, Tan SY, Tang T, et al. Angioimmunoblastic T-cell lymphoma with hyperplastic germinal centres (pattern 1) shows superior survival to patterns 2 and 3: a meta-analysis of 56 cases. *Histopathology.* 2012;60(4):570-585.

26. Cesarman E, Damania B, Krown SE, Martin J, Bower M, Whitby D. Kaposi sarcoma. *Nat Rev Dis Primers.* 2019;5(1):9.

27. Oksenhendler E, Boutboul D, Galicier L. Kaposi sarcoma-associated herpesvirus/human herpesvirus 8-associated lymphoproliferative disorders. *Blood.* 2019;133(11):1186-1190.

CHAPTER OUTLINE

INTRODUCTION

A basic knowledge of the functional histo-anatomy of the lymph node sinus is essential to understand abnormal pathologic processes involving the lymph node sinuses. The lymphatic sinuses serve in the process of carrying lymph containing antigens to the afferent lymphatics which enter and drain into the subcapsular/marginal/peripheral cortical sinus which invests the entire circumference of the lymph node. The subcapsular sinus further drains into the cortical sinus, which in turn drains into the medullary sinuses. The latter in turn drains into the efferent lymphatic channels. The cellular component of the sinuses includes lymphocytes, macrophages/histiocytes, dendritic cells/Langerhans cells (so-called "veiled" cells), and antigen-antibody complexes.[1]

Lymph nodes draining sites of inflammation or cancer reflect some of these findings in the form of dilated expanded sinuses which frequently contain cells reflective of these sites such as metastatic cancer cells, neutrophilic abscesses, sinus histiocytes, etc. Therefore, adequate knowledge of the clinical history is necessary whenever lymph node biopsies are performed in patients with localized lymphadenopathy so as to explain seemingly reactive but enlarged lymph nodes. This chapter will focus on entities associated with prominent dilated sinuses and those with obliteration of sinuses with discussion of pertinent differential entities.

CONDITIONS WITH DILATED PROMINENT SINUSES

SINUS HISTIOCYTOSIS AND DERMATOPATHIC LYMPHADENOPATHY

Patients with reactive/inflammatory dermatoses or cutaneous lymphomas are frequently reactive to proliferation of cutaneous epidermal Langerhans cells which react in response to antigens and travel to the subcapsular sinus of the draining lymph nodes bearing these antigens (so-called "veiled" cells) (Figure 3.1). These dendritic cells react with the paracortical T-cells and associated histiocytes and frequently form nodular clusters of paracortical/perisinusoidal T-cells in the outer cortex which demonstrate a mottled appearance at low power almost reminiscent of primary lymphoid follicles (Figure 3.2). Frequently, melanin pigment may be seen within macrophages, consistent with a dermatopathic lymphadenopathy (Figures 3.3 and 3.4).

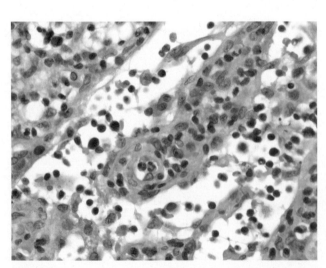

Figure 3.1. **Subcapsular sinus, H&E:** High-power view of the subcapsular/peripheral cortical sinus which is dilated and filled with lymph and incoming antigens as well as antigen/antibody complexes as well as tissue-resident dendritic ("veiled") cells with antigens.

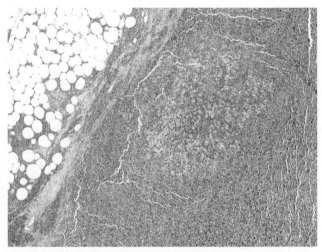

Figure 3.2. **Nodular paracortical hyperplasia, H&E:** Low-power view of focus of nodular paracortical hyperplasia with mottled areas comprising pale pink Langerhans cells/interdigitating dendritic cells and macrophages. Sometimes, these are confused for follicular structures. CD3 stain is helpful to confirm T-cell predominance within the nodules.

In other patients, there is prominent expansion of reactive sinus histiocytes without any obvious dermatopathic changes such as nodular paracortical hyperplasia and this is termed as sinus histiocytosis.[2] This latter phenomenon occurs frequently in response to recent surgery at the sites of draining lymph nodes and a nonspecific finding frequently seen in deep mesenteric lymph nodes (Figure 3.5). Likewise, prominent anthracosis may be observed in mediastinal and hilar nodes while axillary nodes can frequently harbor tattoo pigment–filled macrophages (Figure 3.6).

PEARLS & PITFALLS

Both S100 and CD1a immunostains will highlight interdigitating dendritic cells in the node that correspond the Langerhans cells homing to lymph nodes from tissues. These will be prominent in dermatopathic lymphadenitis and should not be called Langerhans cell histiocytosis (LCH).

SINUS HISTIOCYTOSIS WITH MASSIVE LYMPHADENOPATHY (SHML)

Prominently distended sinuses filled with histiocytes containing variable numbers of lymphocytes within the cytoplasm (emperipolesis) is a characteristic feature of Rosai-Dorfman disease (RDD)/sinus histiocytosis with massive lymphadenopathy.[3] These histiocytes are distinctively positive for S100 in addition to critical histiocytic markers including CD68 and CD163. There is often polytypic plasmacytosis in the background with numerous reactive small B-cells. A subset of these cases are now known to have increased IgG4+ plasma cells (Figures 3.7-3.11).[4]

LANGERHANS CELL HISTIOCYTOSIS (LCH)

Nodal involvement in LCH is generally part of multisystem involvement but rarely may occur as an isolated phenomenon. Early nodal involvement frequently takes the form of isolated sinus involvement by confluent clusters of neoplastic Langerhans cells and focal spillover into the paracortex in more advanced cases. The cellular cytomorphology is other characteristic with folded and grooved nuclei. Foci of necrosis with increased eosinophils are frequently seen. Immunostains including S100, CD1a, and Langerin (CD207) are all positive (Figures 3.12-3.16).

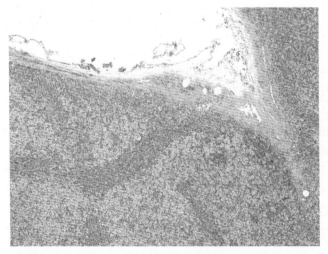

Figure 3.3. Nodular paracortical hyperplasia, dermatopathic changes, H&E, low power: Extensive nodular dermatopathic changes with melanin-laden macrophages in a patient with extensive cutaneous graft versus host disease after allogeneic bone marrow transplantation. Note that there is marked attenuation of follicular B-cell areas.

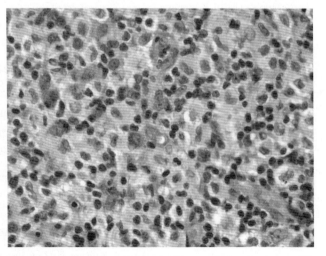

Figure 3.4. Nodular paracortical hyperplasia, dermatopathic changes, H&E, high power: High-power view of Figure 3.3 demonstrating deposits of melanin pigment of cutaneous origin. The pigment is phagocytosed by skin-resident Langerhans cells which travel to the T-cell areas of the draining lymph node which leads to these dermatopathic changes observed.

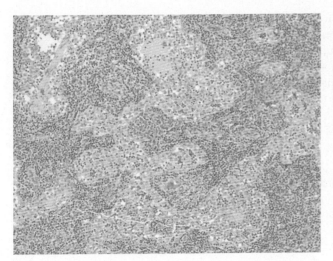

Figure 3.5. **Reactive sinus histiocytosis, H&E:** Typical pattern of sinus histiocytosis in a lymph node comprising pale bland reactive histiocytes in and around the sinuses.

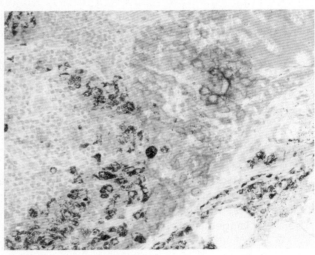

Figure 3.6. **Reactive paracortical hyperplasia, tattoo pigment, PD-L1 immunostain:** Tattoo pigment within the subcapsular macrophages and Langerhans cells extending into the paracortical areas. Note PD-L1-positive histiocytes on the right side of the field.

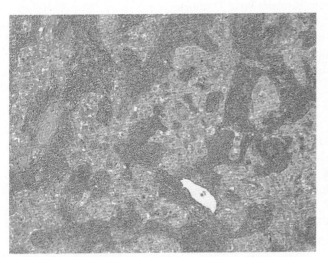

Figure 3.7. **Rosai-Dorfman disease, H&E, low power:** Striking sinus dilatation filled with numerous histiocytes containing abundant eosinophilic cytoplasm.

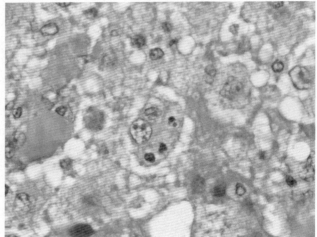

Figure 3.8. **Rosai-Dorfman disease, H&E, high power:** Rosai-Dorfman disease with distinctive histiocytes containing single small, central nucleoli and emperipolesis of lymphocytes within the abnormal sinus histiocytes.

KEY FEATURES of Histiocytic Lesions in Lymph Nodes

- CD68, S100, and CD1a are three important stains in this context
- Nuclear grooves apparent—order CD1a and S100 (possible Langerhans cells)
  - Round nuclei with small distinct nucleoli—S100+/CD1a– (Rosai-Dorfman disease)
- Unremarkable benign morphology (reactive sinus histiocytosis)
- Bizarre pleomorphic histiocytes—CD68+, S100–, CD1a– (histiocytic sarcoma, see Figure 3.17)

LYMPHOPLASMACYTIC LYMPHOMA

Among low-grade lymphomas, lymphoplasmacytic lymphoma characteristically exhibits dilated sinuses filled with histiocytes associated with clusters of lymphoplasmacytic cells located in the perisinusoidal areas (Figures 3.18-3.23). Sinusoidal involvement by lymphoma is usually absent (in contrast to follicular lymphoma which often involves the sinuses). Chronic lymphocytic leukemia and marginal zone lymphoma usually demonstrate

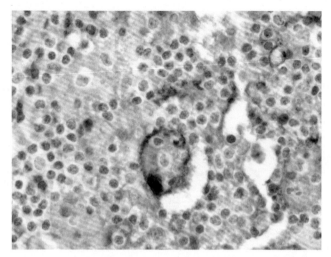

Figure 3.9. **Rosai-Dorfman disease, S100 immunostain, H&E, high power:** Rosai-Dorfman disease histiocytes express S100, an aberrant feature for macrophages/histiocytes. Only Langerhans cells and interdigitating dendritic cells in the node typically express S100 otherwise. This image highlights a histiocyte with several lymphocytes in the cytoplasm. This stain is especially useful for identifying emperipolesis.

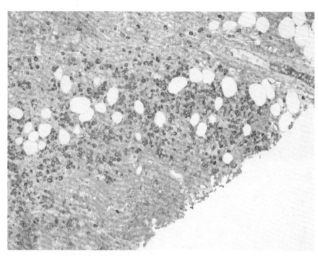

Figure 3.10. **Rosai-Dorfman disease, kappa immunostain:** Rosai-Dorfman disease with increased number of polytypic plasma cells expressing kappa light chain.

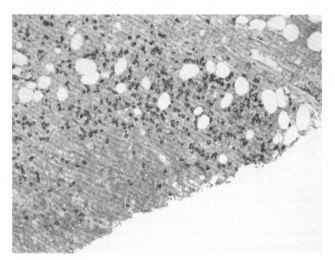

Figure 3.11. **Rosai-Dorfman disease, lambda immunostain (case in Figure 3.10):** There are scattered lambda-positive plasma cells with a normal kappa/lambda ratio. Often there is variable increase in IgG4+ plasma cells in RDD (not shown).

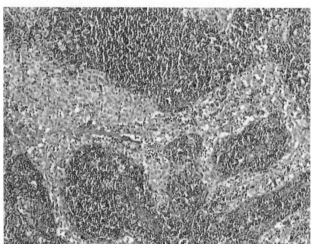

Figure 3.12. **Langerhans cell histiocytosis, H&E, low power:** Involving node with predominant sinus pattern. Areas with subtle involvement show a sprinkling of eosinophils seen at the top left of the image.

preserved sinuses without sinusoidal involvement by lymphoma cells in nodal locations although marrow sinusoidal involvement is frequently noted in marginal zone lymphoma, more so of splenic origin.[5]

NODE DRAINING SUPPURATIVE AREA

Lymph nodes draining an abscess frequently contain sinuses with abundant neutrophils and suppurative debris and usually these lymph nodes are not biopsied.

LIPID-ASSOCIATED LYMPHADENOPATHY (LYMPHANGIOGRAM, PROSTHESIS, OR STORAGE DISEASES)

Patients with breast implants (Figures 3.24 and 3.25) and lymphangiography (Figures 3.26-3.28) both result in foamy histiocytes in the sinuses containing large lipid vacuoles brought

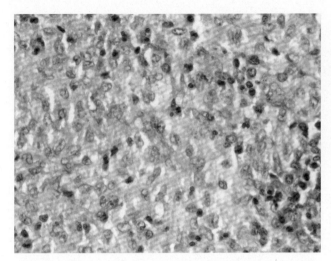

Figure 3.13. Langerhans cell histiocytosis (LCH), H&E, high power: LCH shows increased numbers of eosinophils associated the lesion.

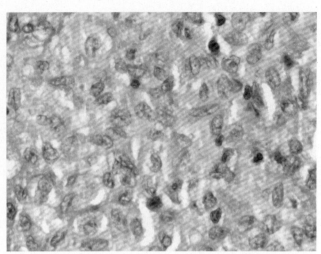

Figure 3.14. Langerhans cell histiocytosis (LCH), H&E, high power: High power of LCH histiocytes showing typically elongated nuclei with grooves abundant cytoplasm.

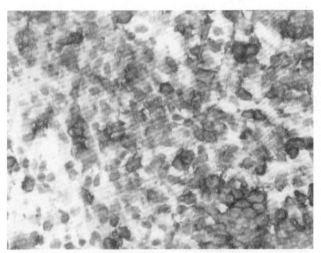

Figure 3.15. Langerhans cell histiocytosis (LCH), CD1a immunostain: CD1a-positive LCH histiocytes. S100 and CD1a are both positive in all LCH cells.

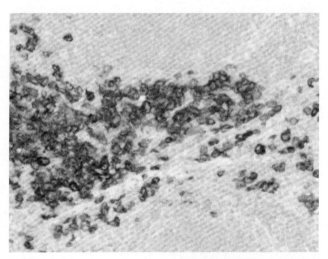

Figure 3.16. Langerhans cell histiocytosis (LCH), langerin (CD207) immunostain: Langerin (CD207), a C-type lectin receptor that induces Birbeck granules, is expressed by LCH cells in this case.

into these lymph nodes as a result of these procedures. Surrounding multinucleate giant cells may also be seen in the adjoining paracortex.

In addition, patients with Whipple disease demonstrate prominent lymph node sinus expansion with foamy histiocytes containing pale staining finely vacuolated diastase-resistant, periodic acid Schiff–positive structures within the cytoplasm (Figures 3.29-3.31). A high degree of clinical suspicion with clinical correlation for possible arthralgia, gastrointestinal involvement, and lymphangiectasia is necessary to make a diagnosis of Whipple disease.[2]

VASCULAR TRANSFORMATION OF SINUSES

Vascular transformation of sinuses (VTS) is frequently detected incidentally in lymph nodes resected as part of other procedures, and it is thought that this occurs as a result of vascular or lymphatic obstruction.[2] On histologic examination, the medullary, cortical, and, to a lesser extent, subcapsular sinuses are encased by thin-walled endothelium-lined vascular channels that frequently arborize and are filled with red blood cells (Figures 3.32-3.34).

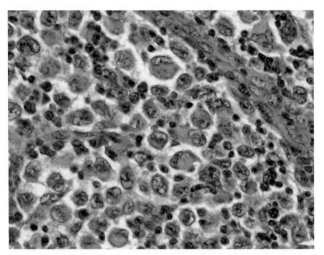

Figure 3.17. **Histiocytic sarcoma, H&E, high power:** Bizarre pleomorphic clusters of histiocytic cells effacing the node. Cases of histiocytic sarcoma sometimes borders on myeloid sarcoma and hence, additional examination of peripheral blood and marrow is necessary to make sure that it is not a myeloid sarcoma. NPM1 immunostain is useful in confirming the latter diagnosis since many such cases are often NPM1-mutated.

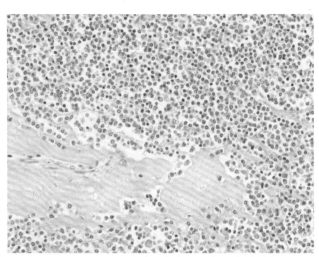

Figure 3.18. **Lymphoplasmacytic lymphoma, H&E, low power:** Patchy sclerosis with a surrounding monotonous lymphoid infiltrate of small lymphoid cells in lymphoplasmacytic lymphoma.

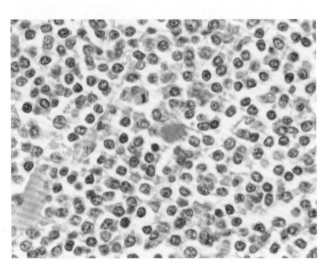

Figure 3.19. **Lymphoplasmacytic lymphoma, H&E, high power:** At higher power, a mix of lymphoid and plasmacytic cells is typical. A plasma cell filled with immunoglobulin is noted in the center of the field ("Mott cell").

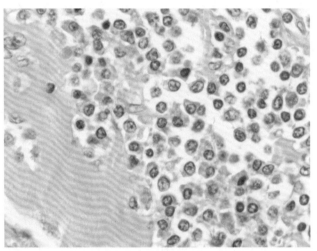

Figure 3.20. **Lymphoplasmacytic lymphoma, H&E, high power:** Sinus at the bottom right in lymphoplasmacytic lymphoma containing cells with plasmacytic differentiation.

NEAR MISS

SINUSOIDAL INVOLVEMENT BY KAPOSI SARCOMA MIMICKING VASCULAR TRANSFORMATION OF SINUSES

Sometimes, the distinction between VTS and Kaposi sarcoma becomes difficult morphologically. However, the lesions of Kaposi sarcoma are frequently centered in the subcapsular sinus and often extend into and beyond the confines of the lymph node capsule, in contrast to VTS which involves the subcapsular sinus less often and does not extend into the lymph node capsule. In difficult cases, staining for HHV8 confirms the diagnosis of Kaposi sarcoma (Figures 3.35-3.38).

SINUSOIDAL LYMPHOMATOUS INFILTRATES
Anaplastic Large Cell Lymphoma

Among T-cell lymphomas, anaplastic large cell lymphoma frequently involves the subcapsular sinus as well as cortical and medullary sinuses. Involvement may often be subtle

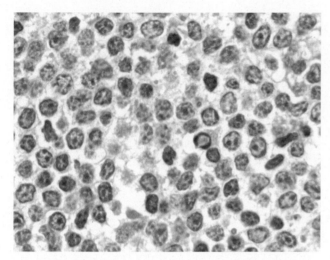

Figure 3.21. **Lymphoplasmacytic lymphoma, H&E, high power:** Intranuclear inclusion derived from cytoplasmic immunoglobulin (Dutcher body) is frequently seen in lymphoplasmacytic lymphoma besides mast cells.

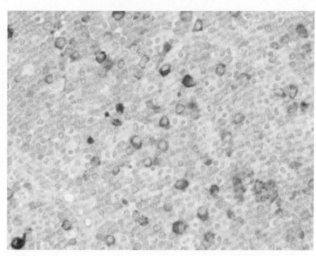

Figure 3.22. **Lymphoplasmacytic lymphoma, kappa immunostain:** The lymphoplasmacytic cells exhibit kappa light chain restriction by immunohistochemistry. See corresponding lambda in Figure 3.23.

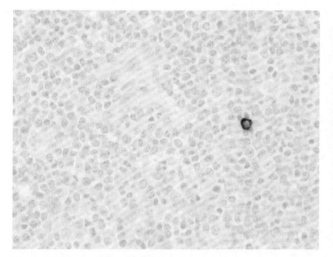

Figure 3.23. **Lymphoplasmacytic lymphoma, lambda immunostain:** Only rare lambda positive plasmacytic cells are present in this case.

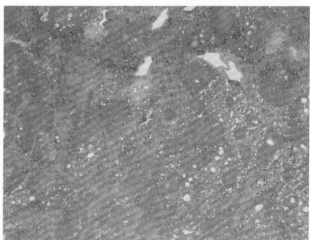

Figure 3.24. **Lipid-associated lymphadenopathy, H&E, low power:** Patient with recent lymphangiography with prominent dilated sinuses.

and difficult to recognize without immunostains since a subset of these lymphomas may be rather paucicellular as in histiocyte-rich anaplastic large cell lymphoma with near-exclusive sinusoidal involvement. Appropriate immunostaining with a comprehensive panel including CD30, cytotoxic markers, and other T-cell markers is helpful in arriving at the appropriate diagnosis.

NEAR MISS

ALCL MIMICKING METASTATIC CARCINOMA

This is a 45-year-old female with bilateral axillary lymph nodes, initially thought to be metastatic breast cancer. Frozen section slides were reviewed with clusters of cohesive sinusoidal large atypical cells, consistent with carcinoma. However, permanent sections revealed lymphoid cytomorphology with immunophenotype supporting the diagnosis of anaplastic large cell lymphoma. Frequently, sinusoidal involvement by anaplastic large cell lymphoma is mistaken for metastatic carcinoma (Figures 3.39-3.41).[6]

HHV8+/EBV+ Extracavitary Primary Effusion Lymphoma

Nodal involvement by solid extracavitary primary effusion lymphoma usually takes the form of solid confluent sheets, but rare cases are described with isolated sinusoidal involvement.[7] Confluent clusters of large pleomorphic, plasmablastic neoplastic lymphoid cells are seen within the subcapsular and cortical sinuses with focal spillover into the adjoining areas of the paracortex. By immunostaining, the neoplastic cells are negative for multiple B-cell markers including CD20 and PAX5.[8] However, a more extensive panel of stains including CD79a, kappa, lambda, IgG, IgA, and IgM, as well as confirmatory HHV8 and EBER are both useful in arriving at the appropriate diagnosis (Figures 3.42-3.47).

PEARLS & PITFALLS

HHV8+ extracavitary primary effusion lymphoma frequently expresses aberrant CD3 and may be confused with T-cell lymphoma if HHV-8 stain is not performed.

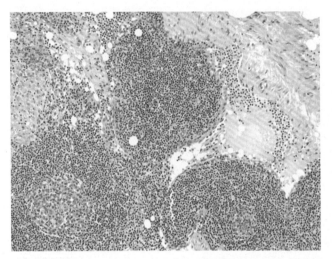

Figure 3.25. Lipid-associated lymphadenopathy, H&E, low power: Patient with recent lymphangiography with prominent dilated sinuses.

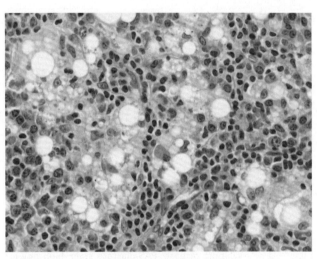

Figure 3.26. Lipid-associated lymphadenopathy, H&E, high power: Lipogranulomas with foamy macrophages are typically noted.

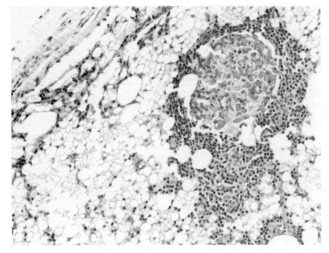

Figure 3.27. Silicone-related lymphadenopathy, H&E, low power: Extensive paracortical replacement by numerous macrophages filled with silicone. A single reactive follicle is seen.

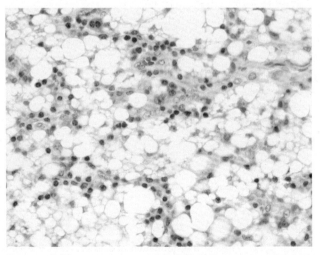

Figure 3.28. Silicone-related lymphadenopathy, H&E, high power: High-power view of Figure 3.27 showing macrophages.

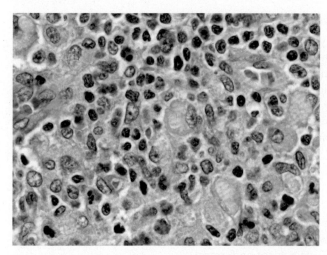

Figure 3.29. **Whipple disease, H&E, high power:** Lymph node paracortex demonstrating multiple histiocytes with granular amphophilic cytoplasmic structures.

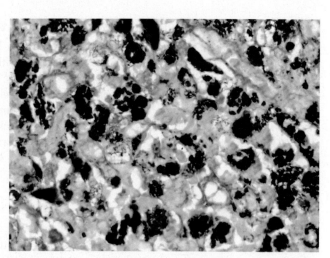

Figure 3.30. **Whipple disease, periodic acid Schiff (PAS) stain, high power:** All the cytoplasmic structures within the histiocytes are strongly positive for PAS.

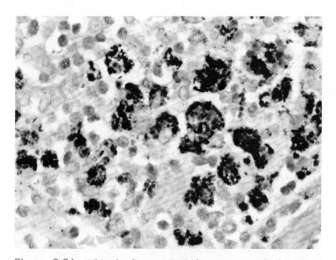

Figure 3.31. **Whipple disease, PAS-diastase stain, high power:** The cytoplasmic structures in the same case are diastase-resistant, typical of *Tropheryma whipplei* organism.

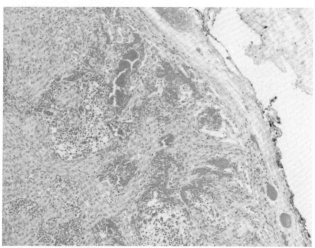

Figure 3.32. **Vascular transformation of sinuses (VTS), H&E, low power:** Lower power depicting extensive VTS extensively replacing the entire node. Note that the process does not extend beyond the capsular sinus.

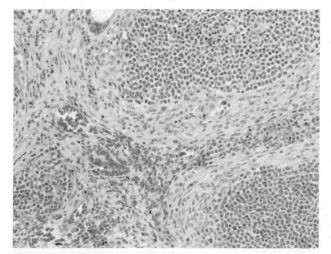

Figure 3.33. **Vascular transformation of sinuses, H&E, medium power:** At medium power, note endothelialized lining of the sinuses which are filled with red cells.

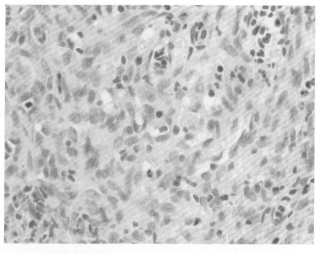

Figure 3.34. **Vascular transformation of sinuses, H&E, high power:** At high power, the lesion may resemble Kaposi sarcoma but hyaline globules are not seen.

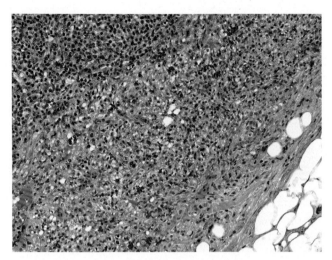

Figure 3.35. Kaposi sarcoma, H&E, low-power: A 35-year-old male with largely preserved lymphoid architecture demonstrating obliteration of the subcapsular sinus with increased numbers of blood vessels reminiscent of vascular transformation of sinuses. The stains depicted in the subsequent pictures confirmed involvement by Kaposi sarcoma.

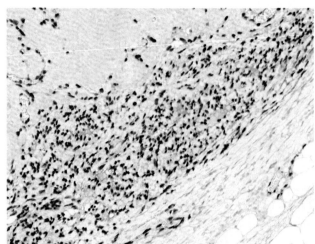

Figure 3.36. Kaposi sarcoma, ERG immunostain: ERG immunohistochemistry highlights numerous endothelial cell nuclei within this lesion confirming vascular origin.

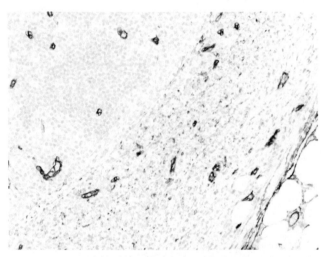

Figure 3.37. Kaposi sarcoma, CD34 immunostain: CD34 immunostain is mostly negative consistent with nascent blood vessels.

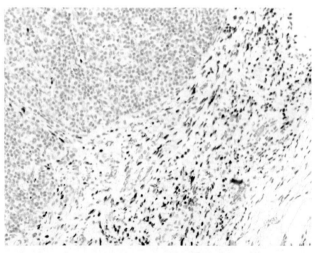

Figure 3.38. Kaposi sarcoma, HHV8 immunostain: HHV8 immunostain highlights infection by HHV8 in the spindle cell component, confirming the diagnosis of Kaposi sarcoma.

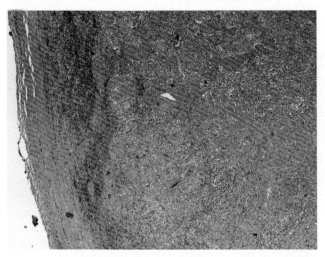

Figure 3.39. Anaplastic large cell lymphoma, H&E, low power: Anaplastic large cell lymphoma with capsular and cortical sclerosis.

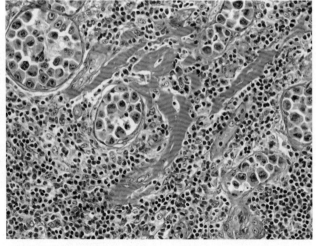

Figure 3.40. Anaplastic large cell lymphoma, H&E, high power: At higher power, there is a near-exclusive intrasinusoidal large lymphoid infiltrate reminiscent of plasmablasts.

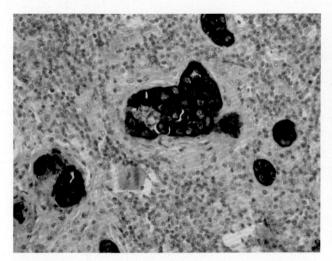

Figure 3.41. **Anaplastic large cell lymphoma (ALCL), CD30 immunostain:** ALCL strong CD30 expression in the intrasinusoidal/intravascular infiltrate. These cells were positive for CD2 but negative for CD3 as well as several other T-cell antigens.

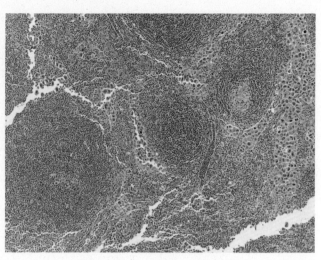

Figure 3.42. **Primary effusion lymphoma, H&E, low power:** At low power, there is preservation of the nodal architecture with scattered reactive lymphoid follicles.

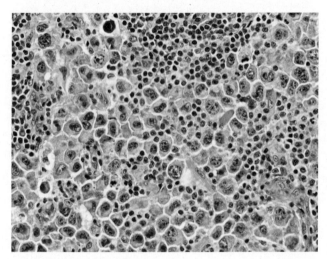

Figure 3.43. **Primary effusion lymphoma, H&E, high power:** At high power, however, there is a pleomorphic sinusoidal infiltrate.

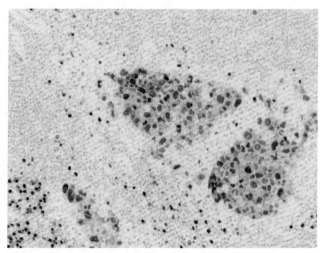

Figure 3.44. **Primary effusion lymphoma (PEL), MUM1 immunostain:** The large lymphoid cells are positive for MUM1. MUM1 confirms plasmacytic phenotype. CD138 is also sometimes positive.

Intravascular Large B-cell Lymphoma

Intravascular large B-cell lymphoma demonstrates similar near exclusive sinusoidal involvement by large B-cells that may not be conspicuous in many cases and can be easily missed.[8] High degree of clinical suspicion is necessary. CD20 immunostain is helpful in confirming the diagnosis (Figures 3.48 and 3.49).

METASTATIC CANCER

Among metastatic cancers, melanoma, breast carcinoma, renal cell carcinoma, and mesothelioma frequently involve the lymph node sinuses. Careful examination of the subcapsular sinus, which is often the first and only site of involvement, is necessary. Staining for epithelial, mesothelial, or melanoma-related markers including cytokeratin, calretinin, or SOX10, respectively, confirms the diagnosis of metastatic malignancy (Figures 3.50-3.53).

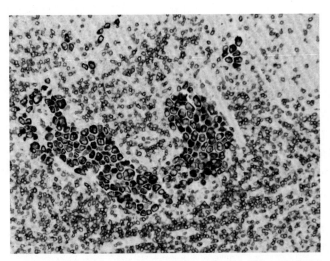

Figure 3.45. **Primary effusion lymphoma (PEL), CD3 immunostain:** The large lymphoid cells are positive for CD3. Background T-cells are positive in addition. Aberrant CD3 expression often leads to mistaken diagnosis of T-cell lymphoma or extranodal NK T-cell lymphoma when CD3 and EBER are both noted.

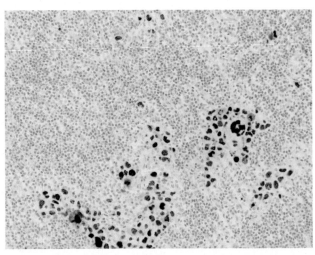

Figure 3.46. **Primary effusion lymphoma (PEL), HHV8 immunostain:** The large lymphoid cells are positive for HHV8 confirming the diagnosis of PEL. One must also look for spindly HHV8+ foci to carefully exclude concurrent Kaposi sarcoma in these cases.

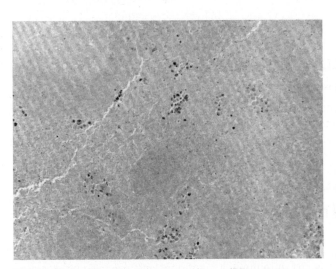

Figure 3.47. **Primary effusion lymphoma (PEL), EBER in situ hybridization, low power view:** The large lymphoid cells are positive for EBER confirming the diagnosis of PEL.

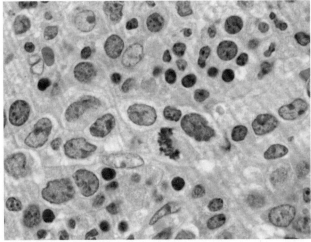

Figure 3.48. **Intravascular large B-cell lymphoma, H&E, high power:** Intravascular large B-cell lymphoma with large lymphoma cells within the sinuses.

NEAR MISS

BENIGN MESOTHELIAL CELLS

This is a 35-year-old female with breast cancer and axillary lymph nodes were excised. Scattered single cells of the subcapsular sinus were noted with concern for metastatic breast cancer. However, closer inspection and appropriate stains allow the exclusion of metastatic carcinoma and confirmation of benign mesothelial cells (Figures 3.54-3.56).

LEUKEMIC INFILTRATES

While most immature leukemic infiltrates such as lymphoblastic lymphoma mostly involve the paracortex and sinuses, exclusive sinusoidal involvement is not common. Nevertheless, patchy involvement in the lymph node with primary extramedullary presentation can be seen in lymphoblastic processes and must be kept in mind. Appropriate immunostaining with TdT and CD34 will highlight immature/blastic cellular populations for lymphoid malignancies but staining with MPO and CD117 and/or CD33 is helpful in cases of myeloid lineage (Figures 3.57-3.63).

Checklist of Immunostains for Large Atypical Sinusoidal Cellular Infiltrates

Panel to include CD45, CD20, CD3, CD30, keratin, and HHV8/LANA

☐ Intravascular large B-cell lymphoma (CD20+)
☐ Anaplastic large cell lymphoma (CD30+)
☐ Extracavitary primary effusion lymphoma (HHV8+)

Extended panel can include CD45, CD19, CD34, NPM1, and CD117 to cover myeloid sarcoma

☐ CD19+/CD34+ (B–lymphoblastic leukemia)
☐ CD34+/CD117+ (myeloid sarcoma)

PEARLS & PITFALLS

Myeloid sarcoma is often positive for abnormal cytoplasmic NPM1 localization since NPM1-mutated acute myeloid leukemias (AML) are overrepresented in myeloid sarcomas compared with cases of wild-type NPM1. CD34 is often negative in these cases and hence CD117 and NPM1 are more useful.[5]

OTHER PERISINUSOIDAL CELLULAR CLUSTERS

Monocytoid B-cells (Viral Infections)

Multifocal reactive perisinusoidal monocytoid B-lymphoid cells with moderate-abundant clear cytoplasm and convoluted nuclei are frequently observed in patients with autoimmune conditions and viral infections (Figures 3.64-3.66). Frequently, singly scattered neutrophils are often seen amidst such monocytoid B-cell clusters. Appropriate testing for cytomegalovirus, Epstein-Barr virus (with immunostains), and human immunodeficiency virus is recommended in these cases.

Reactive Plasmacytoid Dendritic Cell Clusters (Viral, Autoimmune, and Lymphomas)

The perisinusoidal areas may also contain clusters of plasmacytoid dendritic cells (PDCs) in patients with viral infections and autoimmune conditions and may also be increased in patients with certain lymphoma such as Hodgkin lymphoma. In lymph node sections, PDCs often appear somewhat blastoid in cytomorphology at low power and are often mistaken for reactive germinal centers of secondary lymphoid follicles. Frequently, apoptotic bodies are seen amidst touch clusters of PDCs. CD123 is strongly positive in these cells allowing confirmation of their phenotype (Figures 3.67-3.69).

Checklist of Reactive Cellular Infiltrates in the Sinusoidal/Perisinusoidal Areas

☐ Reactive sinus histiocytosis (localized to the sinuses and perisinusoidal areas)
☐ Dermatopathic changes (often nodular and mottled)
☐ Monocytoid B-cells (clear cells with scattered neutrophils)
☐ PDCs (blastoid cells resembling reactive germinal centers with scattered apoptosis)
☐ Florid immunoblastic reaction (often CD30-positive)

When it is hard to decide on H&E if the cellular clusters are monocytoid B-cells or PDCs, see the background. If there are apoptotic cells admixed, they are likely to be PDCs (Figures 3.70 and 3.71), whereas if they have scattered neutrophils amidst them, they are likely to be monocytoid B-cells (Figure 3.72).

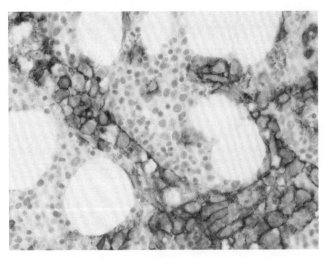

Figure 3.49. **Intravascular large B-cell lymphoma, CD20 immunostain:** High degree of suspicion is necessary and further CD20 immunostain confirms the diagnosis.

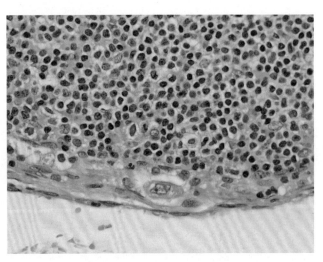

Figure 3.50. **Metastatic carcinoma, H&E, high power:** Micrometastases of single carcinoma cells within subcapsular and cortical sinuses.

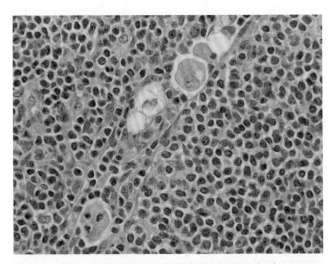

Figure 3.51. **Metastatic carcinoma, H&E, high power:** Micrometastases of single carcinoma cells within subcapsular and cortical sinuses.

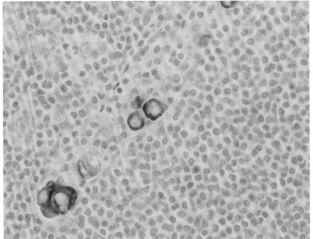

Figure 3.52. **Metastatic carcinoma, AE1/AE3 immunostain:** Cytokeratin stain highlights the carcinoma cells from Figure 3.51.

CONDITIONS WITH INCONSPICUOUS/OBLITERATED SINUSES

FOLLICULAR LYMPHOMA

Follicular lymphoma is a low-grade lymphoma that frequently involves not only follicular areas but also spills over extensively into the paracortical regions and extends into the lymph node sinuses obliterating them (Figures 3.73-3.75).[8]

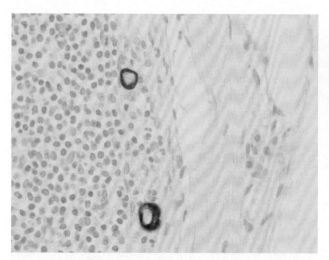

Figure 3.53. **Metastatic carcinoma, AE/AE3 immunostain:** Cytokeratin stain highlights the carcinoma cells from Figure 3.51.

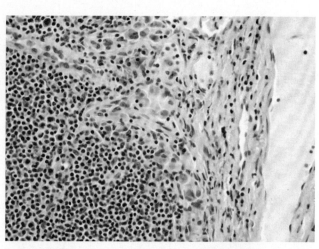

Figure 3.54. **Benign mesothelial cells, H&E, high power:** Mediastinal lymph node in the patient with breast cancer demonstrating singly scattered atypical epithelioid cells within the sinus with abundant cytoplasm.

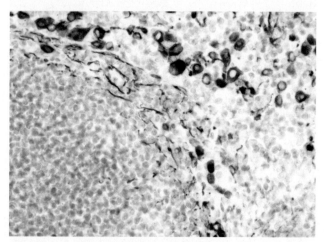

Figure 3.55. **Benign mesothelial cells, calretinin immunostain:** However, calretinin (mesothelial marker) is strongly positive in the cells confirming benign mesothelial origin.

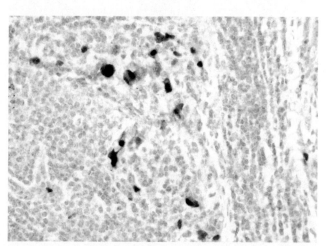

Figure 3.56. **Benign mesothelial cells, AE1/AE3 immunostain:** Immunostain for pankeratin (AE1/AE3) is positive in the cells suggesting metastatic carcinoma.

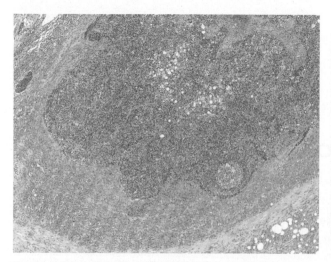

Figure 3.57. **Extramedullary myeloid tumor (myeloid sarcoma), H&E, low power:** Extramedullary myeloid tumor extensively involving subcapsular, cortical, and medullary sinuses.

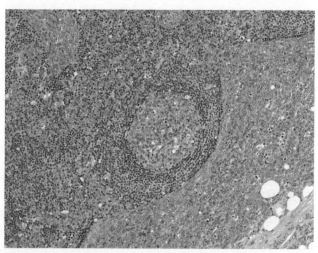

Figure 3.58. **Extramedullary myeloid tumor (myeloid sarcoma), H&E, medium power:** Extramedullary myeloid tumor extensively involving subcapsular, cortical, and medullary sinuses.

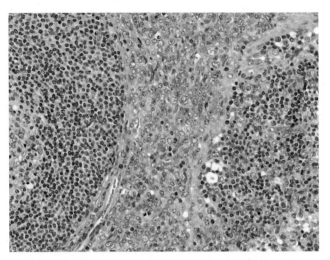

Figure 3.59. **Extramedullary myeloid tumor (myeloid sarcoma), H&E, high power:** Higher power Figure 3.47 shows typical blastic infiltrate in between the follicles.

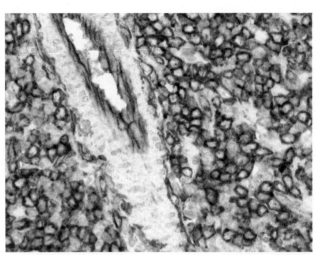

Figure 3.60. **Extramedullary myeloid tumor (myeloid sarcoma), CD34 immunostain:** Blasts in myeloid sarcoma are positive for CD34, Note endothelial staining for CD34 serving as internal control in the large blood vessel.

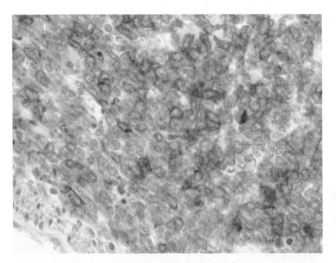

Figure 3.61. **Extramedullary myeloid tumor (myeloid sarcoma), CD117 immunostain:** Blasts in myeloid sarcoma are positive for CD117. Although not apparent here, scattered CD117-bright mast cells within the tumor serve as internal controls.

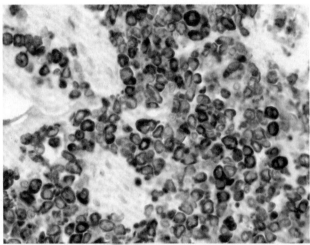

Figure 3.62. **Extramedullary myeloid tumor (myeloid sarcoma), myeloperoxidase immunostain:** Blasts in myeloid sarcoma are positive for myeloperoxidase.

CASTLEMAN DISEASE

Hyaline-vascular Castleman disease (HVCD) demonstrates typical morphology within follicles (described elsewhere). However, the interfollicular regions in advanced cases of HVCD are notable for prominent vascular proliferation lined by high endothelial venules with associated sclerosis while lymph node sinuses are conspicuously absent (Figures 3.76 and 3.77). This is in contrast to plasma cell variant of Castleman (including HHV8-negative and HHV8-positive cases) where sinuses are usually patent despite interfollicular vascular proliferation and lymphoid depletion.[2]

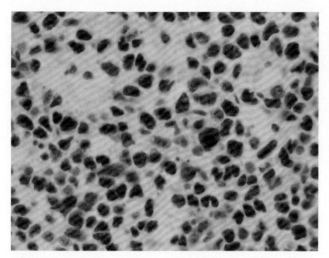

Figure 3.63. **Extramedullary myeloid tumor (myeloid sarcoma), NPM1 immunostain:** Blasts in myeloid sarcoma are positive for NPM1 stain (using clone 376 from DAKO) shows isolated nuclear staining indicating wild-type pattern. Mitotically active and apoptotic cells with open nuclear envelope show cytoplasmic staining as noted in the single apoptotic cell in the center.

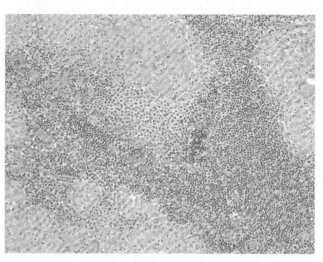

Figure 3.64. **Monocytoid B-cells, H&E, low power:** Patchy cluster of perisinusoidal monocytoid B-cells (in the center of the field) in a patient with toxoplasma with extensive granulomatous inflammation. The moderate amount of clear cytoplasm allows identification of monocytoid B-cells readily at low-power examination.

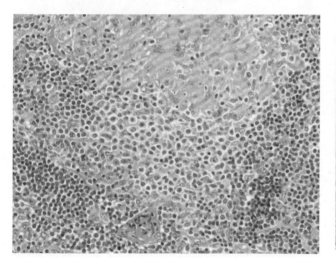

Figure 3.65. **Monocytoid B-cells, H&E, medium power:** Patchy cluster of perisinusoidal monocytoid B-cells in a patient with toxoplasma with extensive granulomatous inflammation.

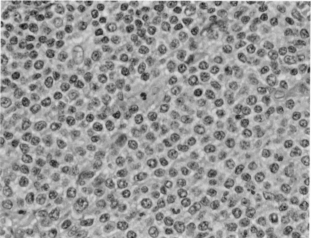

Figure 3.66. **Monocytoid B-cells, H&E, high power:** Patchy cluster of perisinusoidal monocytoid B-cells in a patient with toxoplasma with extensive granulomatous inflammation. Occasional neutrophils are often seen amidst such clusters.

ANGIOIMMUNOBLASTIC T-CELL LYMPHOMA

Frequently in angioimmunoblastic T-cell lymphoma (AITL), there is obliteration and/or retraction of the peripheral cortical sinus with linear subcapsular small B-cell aggregates. Paying attention to the subcapsular sinus is important in AITL (Figures 3.78 and 3.79).

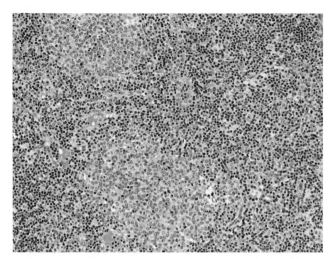

Figure 3.67. Plasmacytoid dendritic cells (PDCs), H&E, low power: Clusters of PDCs in patient with classical Hodgkin lymphoma. Reactive PDC proliferations accompany several reactive/autoimmune conditions as well as lymphomas. In lymph nodes, large clusters may be mistaken for germinal centers.

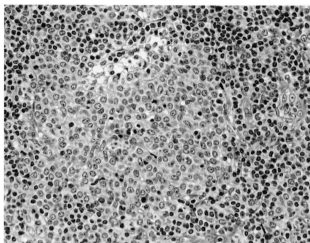

Figure 3.68. Plasmacytoid dendritic cells (PDCs), H&E, high power: Clusters of PDCs in patient with classical Hodgkin lymphoma. Reactive PDC proliferations accompany several reactive/autoimmune conditions as well as lymphomas. In lymph nodes, large clusters may be mistaken for germinal centers. However, the lack of any polarization or mantle cuffs coupled with distinctive blastoid, folded nuclei, and interspersed apoptotic bodies allows recognition of PDCs.

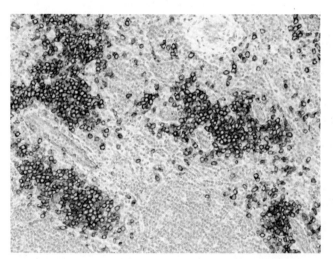

Figure 3.69. Plasmacytoid dendritic cells (PDCs), CD123 immunostain: CD123 (IL-3Ra) is strongly positive in the PDC clusters.

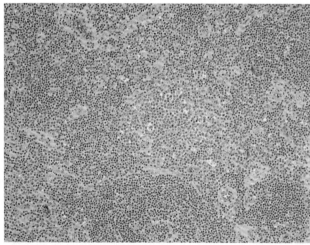

Figure 3.70. Plasmacytoid dendritic cells (PDCs), H&E, low power: Clusters of PDCs (seen in the center of the field) in a patient with hyaline-vascular Castleman disease.

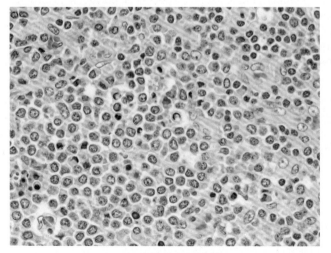

Figure 3.71. Plasmacytoid dendritic cells (PDCs), H&E, high power: Clusters of PDCs in a patient with hyaline-vascular Castleman disease. On high power, apoptotic cells are seen admixed with the PDCs.

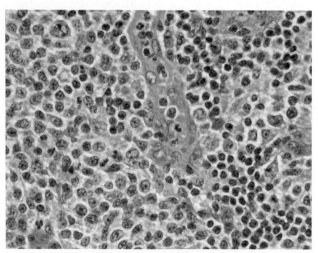

Figure 3.72. Monocytoid B-cells, H&E, high power: Monocytoid B-cells with neutrophils on the left side of field.

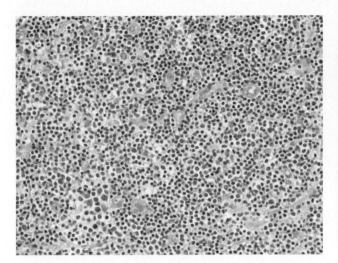

Figure 3.73. Follicular lymphoma, H&E, medium power: Follicular lymphoma with a diffuse pattern (inguinal location) showing obliteration of sinuses with infiltration by lymphoma cells.

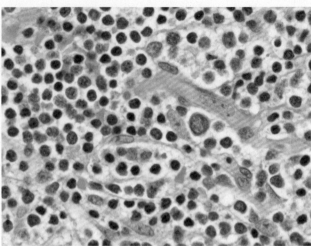

Figure 3.74. Follicular lymphoma, H&E, high power: Follicular lymphoma with a diffuse pattern (inguinal location) showing obliteration of sinuses with infiltration by lymphoma cells.

SAMPLE SIGN OUT LINES AND COMMENTS

Lymph node, axillary, excision:

- Reactive paracortical hyperplasia with prominent dermatopathic changes, see comment

    Comment: Please look for skin lesions in the site draining this lymph node since both benign and malignant skin conditions may be associated with dermatopathic changes including cutaneous T-cell lymphoma.

Lymph node, axillary, excision:

- Extramedullary myeloid tumor, so-called "myeloid sarcoma," see comment

    Comment: Abnormal cytoplasmic NPM1 localization is consistent with acute myeloid leukemia with underlying NPM1 mutation. Bone marrow biopsy and examination of peripheral blood is necessary prior to commencement of treatment as acute myeloid leukemia.

Lymph node, axillary, excision:

- Sinus histiocytosis with massive lymphadenopathy, so-called "Rosai-Dorfman disease", see comment

    Comment: There is prominent emperipolesis within distinct large polygonal histiocytes with round nuclei and small but distinct single nucleoli with an associated background of lymphocytes and plasma cells which are polytypic by immunohistochemistry. The Rosai-Dorfman histiocytes are positive for S100 and negative for CD1a.

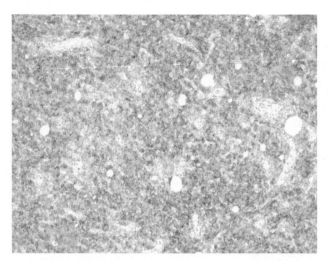

Figure 3.75. **Follicular lymphoma, CD10 immunostain:** CD10 is strongly positive in the follicular lymphoma cells.

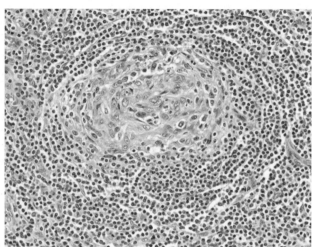

Figure 3.76. **Hyaline-vascular Castleman disease (HVCD), H&E, medium power:** HVCD with prominent regressed follicle and onion skinning by expanded mantle cuffs. There is sinus obliteration in this disease with prominence of paracortical postcapillary venules.

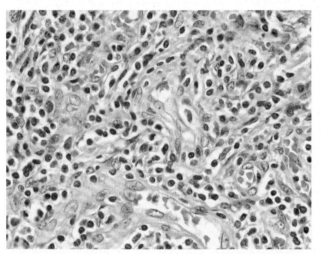

Figure 3.77. **Hyaline-vascular Castleman disease (HVCD), H&E, high power:** HVCD with prominent regressed follicle and onion skinning by expanded mantle cuffs. There is sinus obliteration in this disease with prominence of paracortical postcapillary venules.

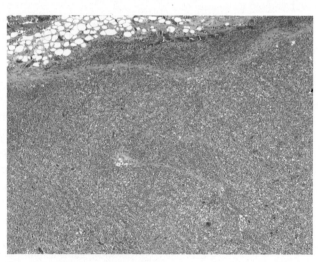

Figure 3.78. **Angioimmunoblastic T-cell lymphoma (AITL), H&E, low power:** In AITL, there is obliteration of the peripheral cortical sinus.

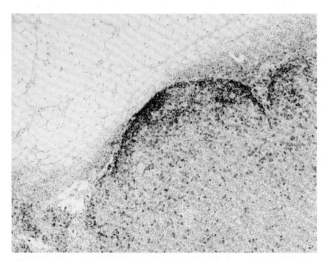

Figure 3.79. **Angioimmunoblastic T-cell lymphoma (AITL), CD20 immunostain:** The subcapsular sinus is seen to be lined by CD20+ aggregates of small B-cells in AITL.

FAQ:

1. What is the correct terminology to use (sinus vs sinusoid) in the lymph node, spleen and bone marrow?

   a. Answer: Sinus is primarily used in the lymph node to denote the subcapsular/peripheral cortical sinus as well as the trabecular sinus within the paracortex. Although the word "intrasinusoidal/perisinusoidal" may be used in the context of lymph nodes. Both spleen and bone marrow contain sinusoids. Sinusoids in the spleen are venous channels.

2. What is the best way to distinguish the lymph node from a spleniculi accessory spleen?

   a. Presence of a thick capsule and positivity for CD8 in the endothelium supports designation as splenic origin.

3. What is the best way to distinguish lymph node Langerhans cells from interdigitating dendritic cells?

   a. Dual expression of both S100 and CD1a is typical of Langerhans cells while the more mature dendritic cell, interdigitating dendritic cell in the lymph node paracortex, expresses only S100 without CD1a.

References

1. Delves PJ, Martin SJ, Burton DR, Roitt IM. *Roitt's Essential Immunology*. Chichester, West Sussex: John Wiley & Sons, Ltd; 2017.

2. Ioachim HL. *Lymph Node Biopsy*. Philadelphia, PA: Lippincott; 1982.

3. Foucar E, Rosai J, Dorfman R. Sinus histiocytosis with massive lymphadenopathy (Rosai-Dorfman disease): review of the entity. *Semin Diagn Pathol*. 1990;7:19-73.

4. Zhang X, Hyjek E, Vardiman J. A subset of Rosai-Dorfman disease exhibits features of IgG4-related disease. *Am J Clin Pathol*. 2013;139:622-632.

5. Swerdlow SH, Campo E, Harris NL, et al, eds. *WHO Classification of Tumours of Haematopoietic and Lymphoid Tissues*. Revised 4th ed. Lyons: IARC; 2017.

6. Vassallo J, Lamant L, Brugieres L, et al. ALK-positive anaplastic large cell lymphoma mimicking nodular sclerosis Hodgkin's lymphoma: report of 10 cases. *Am J Surg Pathol*. 2006;30:223-229.

7. Kim Y, Leventaki V, Bhaijee F, Jackson CC, Medeiros LJ, Vega F. Extracavitary/solid variant of primary effusion lymphoma. *Ann Diagn Pathol*. 2012;16:441-446.

8. Jaffe ES. *Hematopathology*. Philadelphia, PA: Saunders/Elsevier; 2011.

CHAPTER OUTLINE

INTRODUCTION

The cortex of the lymph node comprises mostly anatomically distinct nodular accumulations of unstimulated B-cells within primary follicles. The primary follicles are also notable for a rich meshwork of follicular dendritic cells. Subsequent to a T-cell-dependent antigenic challenge, the primary follicle is converted to a secondary follicle containing a germinal center and surrounding mantle zone. The germinal center is notable for two anatomic areas comprising a dark zone and a light zone. The dark zone comprises actively proliferating large B-cells called centroblasts which lack surface IgM and surface IgD characteristic of B-cells within the mantle zone/primary follicle. Centroblasts move to the basal light zone and form smaller resting cells called centrocytes which are non-cycling cells. A large fraction of centrocytes undergo apoptosis while the remaining that represent B-cells with the highest affinity for the antigen are destined to either become circulating/resting memory cells or convert to immunoblasts in the perifollicular location. These latter cells are then destined to become plasma cells that accumulate away from the follicles in the medullary cords that are present on either side of the medullary sinuses. It is notable that the plasma cells are anatomically separated away from the germinal centers. Disruption of this physical separation is a feature noted in autoimmune conditions detailed below.

Basic knowledge of the differences between primary and secondary lymphoid follicles is necessary to be able to recognize abnormal immunostaining patterns and lymphoma arising from follicular center cells. Normal primary follicles express B-cell markers including CD19, CD20, and PAX5 and, in addition, express IgM and IgD consistent with the phenotype expected for naïve unstimulated B-cells. These cells do not express CD10 and BCL6 (germinal center markers) but express BCL2 at levels similar to resting T-cells. The secondary lymphoid follicles on the other hand, express pan-B-cell antigens including CD19, CD20, and PAX5 but are negative for IgD and BCL2. They express weak-moderate levels of CD10.

CLINICAL CORRELATION

Several clinical aspects are important to know when examining lymph node biopsies representing follicular proliferations including the age, location, site of lymph nodes as well as presence or absence of systemic symptoms. In general, reactive lymphoid proliferations are localized and occur more commonly in younger populations (<40 years of age) and frequently are asymptomatic and detected on routine examination. Many of these are not biopsied typically, but persistent or progressive adenopathy may result in biopsies of these lymph nodes. Basic complete blood counts with differential count as well as some labs related to immune and/or viral studies are useful in assessing the etiology of reactive nodes with follicular-centered proliferations.

SITE-SPECIFIC VARIATIONS IN FOLLICLES

Lymph nodes in pelvic locations are notable for lack of distinct organization of nodal compartments as cortex and medulla and frequently show variable sclerosis and scattered primary follicles only without any secondary follicles (Figures 4.1-4.3). This can be confusing for the surgical pathologist when the expression of BCL2 further raises suspicion for FL and the needle core biopsies are taken from retroperitoneal locations. Neck nodes, on the other hand, contain more secondary follicles and are often easier to recognize as reactive.

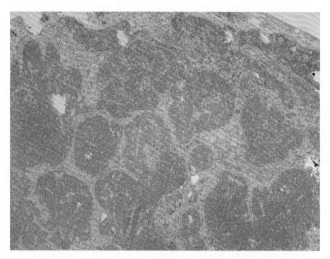

Figure 4.1. **Primary follicles, H&E:** Lymph node with multiple primary follicles at the periphery in an inguinal lymph node.

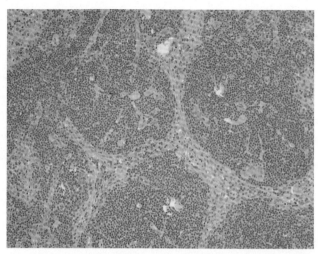

Figure 4.2. **Primary follicles, H&E:** Lymph node with multiple primary follicles at the periphery in an inguinal lymph node.

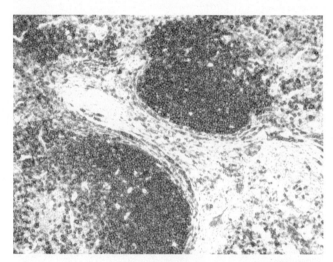

Figure 4.3. **Primary follicles, CD20 immunostain:** CD20 immunostaining highlights the follicles. Due to the somewhat monotonous morphology at low power, such back-to-back follicles may be confused with follicular lymphoma. However, basic immunostains will readily distinguish primary follicles from follicular lymphoma.

ABNORMAL FOLLICLES

REACTIVE FOLLICULAR HYPERPLASIA

The most important feature of reactive follicular hyperplasia is the presence of increased numbers of secondary follicles that extend geographically beyond the cortex encroaching into the medulla. These follicles are most often varying in size with occasional follicles exhibiting serpiginous patterns while still maintaining the sharp distinction of germinal center and mantle zones (Figures 4.4 and 4.5). Germinal centers exhibit typical polarization with dark and light zones containing centroblasts and centrocytes, respectively, with scattered reactive tingible body macrophages. Variable numbers of interspersed follicular dendritic cells may also be seen (Figure 4.6). Immunophenotypically, reactive follicles (germinal and mantle zones) express B-cell antigens including CD20, CD79a, and PAX5 with mantle zone expressing CD10–/IgD+/BCL2+ phenotype while germinal centers exhibit

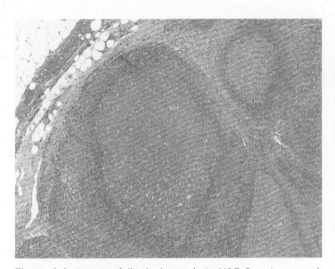

Figure 4.4. **Reactive follicular hyperplasia, H&E:** Reactive secondary lymphoid follicles which are varying in size. Note normal sized reactive second lymphoid follicle on the top right with large reactive secondary follicles at the bottom left.

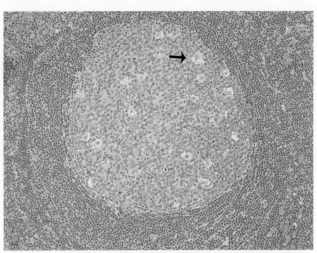

Figure 4.5. **Reactive follicular hyperplasia, H&E:** Higher power view of Figure 4.4 depicting reactive secondary lymphoid follicles with germinal centers polarized into light and dark zones (note the dark-zone on the right side of the field) with scattered tingible body macrophages (black arrow).

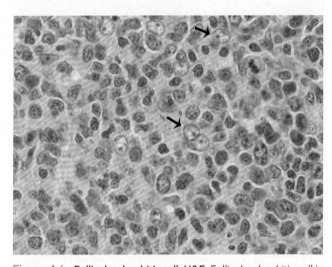

Figure 4.6. **Follicular dendritic cell, H&E:** Follicular dendritic cell in the center of the field within reactive germinal centers (black arrows). The follicular dendritic cell is readily recognized by the scattered bland-looking doublet nuclear structures with nuclear membranes and single small central nucleoli without any discernible cytoplasm. These cells are frequently confused for centroblasts and when present in excess, they may lead to upgrading of follicular lymphomas.

CD10+/IgD−/BCL2−phenotype. While most reactive follicular proliferations are confined to the nodes, the process may rarely spill over into the perinodal adipose tissue, especially in the salivary gland region, although in most other sites, clusters of B-cells in soft tissues is an abnormal finding.

GIANT FOLLICULAR HYPERPLASIA

Rarely, in children, there may be rather striking follicular hyperplasia beyond what is seen in reactive hyperplasia with numerous back-to-back geographic reactive follicles (Figure 4.7). These are often termed as "giant follicular hyperplasia" and such proliferations often resolve without therapy despite the worrisome morphology. A subset of cases like these often exhibit morphology compatible with grade 3b FL (with sheets of centroblasts, lacking germinal center light zone/dark zone distinction) with a BCL2-negative phenotype and are now thought to represent clonal follicular proliferations that fall within the so-called pediatric follicular lymphoma (Figures 4.8-4.11). These lymphomas harbor underlying mutations in *TNFRSF14* and *MAP2K1* mutations based on recent genomic studies.[1]

Rarely, lymph nodes in the pediatric age group in the tonsillar location may demonstrate follicular hyperplasia with clonal populations detected either by flow cytometry and/ or molecular studies. Such proliferations should not be considered as lymphoma as this represents abnormal skewed expansion of germinal center B-cells resulting in clonal B-cell populations.

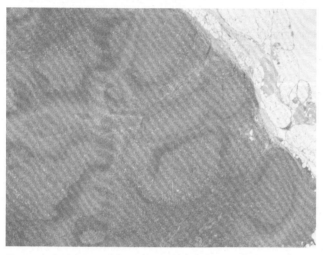

Figure 4.7. **Giant follicular hyperplasia, H&E:** Geographic reactive lymphoid follicles. Note the presence of multiple reactive secondary lymphoid follicles that are varying in size with serpiginous borders. Distinct mantle cuffs are present in all the follicles.

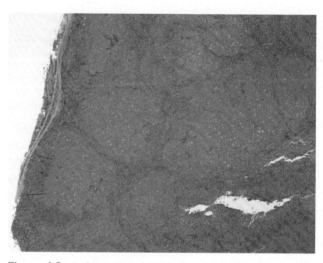

Figure 4.8. **Pediatric-type follicular lymphoma in an adult, H&E:** There are multiple expansile back-to-back monotonous follicular structures with indistinct mantle cuffs.

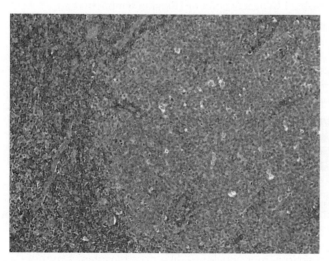

Figure 4.9. **Pediatric-type follicular lymphoma in an adult, H&E:** At higher power, there are sheets of large centroblastic cells within the follicular structures with high mitotic activity.

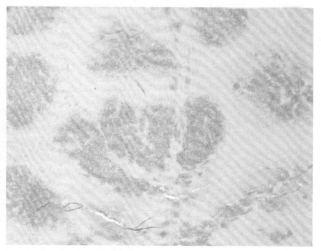

Figure 4.10. **Pediatric-type follicular lymphoma in an adult, CD10 immunostain:** Immunostain for CD10 is strongly positive within these follicular structures consistent with germinal center origin.

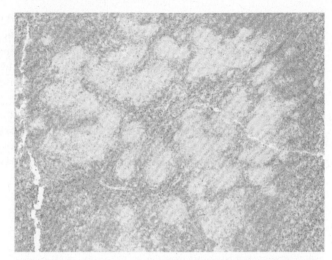

Figure 4.11. **Pediatric-type follicular lymphoma in an adult, BCL2 immunostain:** The follicular structures are negative for BCL2 which in turn, highlights the T-cell areas.

KEY FEATURES to Differentiate Primary and Secondary Lymphoid Follicles

- Primary follicles comprise a ball of mantle zone cells.
- Primary follicle immunophenotype reflects mantle zone phenotype with expression of BCL2 and IgD with negative CD10.
- Secondary lymphoid follicles contain germinal center and a peripheral corona of mantle zone cells.
- Germinal center of secondary lymphoid follicles lacked BCL2 and IgD but are positive for CD10.

KEY FEATURES for Choosing Immunostain Panels in Morphologically Reactive Lymph Nodes

- Basic panel*:
  - CD20, CD3, IgD/BCL2 (appreciation of immuno-architecture)
- Additional stains:
  - CD30 and EBER (for possible EBV reactivation or Hodgkin lymphoma)
  - IgG4 (IgG4-related adenopathy)

*Routine extensive immunostaining or flow cytometry of first time insignificant/localized adenopathy is not recommended.

NEAR MISS CASE 1: Infectious Mononucleosis–Like Posttransplant Lymphoproliferative Disorder Masquerading as Florid Follicular Hyperplasia

A 7-year-old boy with a history of a liver transplant 5 years ago developed bilateral tonsillar enlargement, which was biopsied. The sections demonstrated florid follicular hyperplasia without any other significant changes. Additional EBV in situ hybridization (EBER) demonstrated numerous paracortical EBV-positive cells of varying sizes along with increased numbers of CD20 positive immunoblasts, confirming the diagnosis of infectious mononucleosis–like posttransplant lymphoproliferative disorder with florid follicular hyperplasia (Figures 4.12-4.17). The case highlights the need to perform EBER in all posttransplant cases. Outside of the transplant setting, the morphologic findings are indistinguishable from infectious mononucleosis.

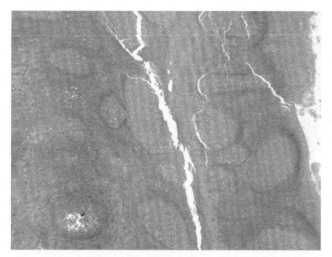

Figure 4.12. **IM-like PTLD, H&E:** Multiple scattered reactive lymphoid follicles are present on low power.

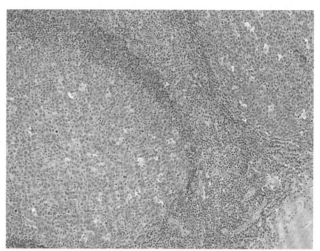

Figure 4.13. **IM-like PTLD, H&E:** High-power view demonstrates floridly reactive large secondary lymphoid follicles with tingible body macrophages.

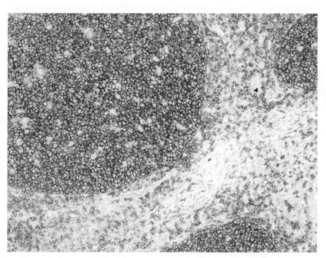

Figure 4.14. **IM-like PTLD, CD20 immunostain:** Follicles are positive for CD20 with some interfollicular B-cells.

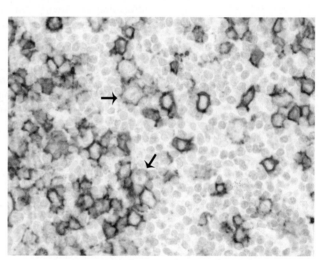

Figure 4.15. **IM-like PTLD, CD20 immunostain:** High-power view of the interfollicular areas demonstrates immunoblasts expressing weak CD20 (black arrows).

Figure 4.16. **IM-like PTLD, EBER in situ hybridization:** EBER, low-power view demonstrating numerous interfollicular EBV-positive small lymphoid cells.

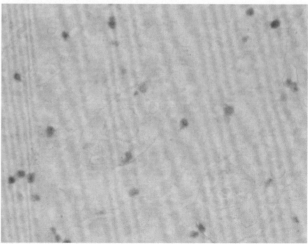

Figure 4.17. **IM-like PTLD, EBER in situ hybridization:** EBER, high-power view demonstrating EBER-positive cells that are varying sized.

REACTIVE FOLLICULAR HYPERPLASIA IN ALTERED IMMUNE STATES

Lymph node hyperplasia is a feature of several immune disorders including rheumatoid arthritis, early human immunodeficiency virus (HIV), and other autoimmune conditions (Figure 4.18). Notably, in the early stages of rheumatoid arthritis, follicular hyperplasia is a prominent feature, while in late stages, there is more interfollicular expansion with increased vascularity, numerous plasma cells, and distended subcapsular sinuses with neutrophils (Figure 4.19).

Likewise, in early HIV infection, there is prominent follicular hyperplasia, coinciding with primary generalized lymphadenopathy. With disease progression, there is regression of follicles due to collapse of the germinal centers with ingression of mantle zone cells. This latter stage is called follicular lysis, and beyond this stage, there is extensive interfollicular lymphoid depletion and vascular prominence noted typically in advanced HIV infection.

Many autoimmune conditions other than rheumatoid arthritis may also be associated with rather striking and florid follicular hyperplasia. These include systemic lupus erythematosus, in which there is variable follicular hyperplasia associated with interfollicular expansion and vascularity.

If careful attention is not patent to the clinical history, lymph nodes in patients with systemic lupus erythematosus may be misdiagnosed as angioimmunoblastic T-cell lymphoma, wherein follicular hyperplasia with interfollicular vascular proliferation are both features noted in this lymphoma.

FAQ: I have a lymph node that looks morphologically reactive but is noted to have clonal IGH rearrangement based on the report I have from the submitting institution. What is the next step?

Answer: False-positive clonal rearrangements may be observed in seemingly reactive lymph nodes, especially in patients with autoimmune conditions, and hence, unless there is absolute morphologic support for B-cell lymphoma, one must step back from calling such lymph nodes as lymphoma. Likewise, unnecessary polymerase chain reaction (PCR) studies must not be pursued unless there is a high degree of suspicion for lymphoma.

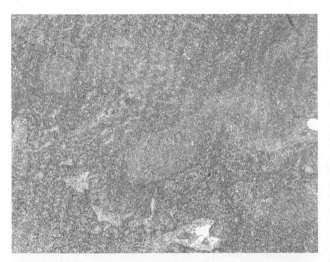

Figure 4.18. Lymph node morphology in advanced rheumatoid arthritis, H&E: Scattered small reactive secondary lymphoid follicles are noted with interfollicular expansion and prominent vascularity.

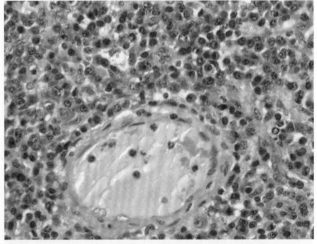

Figure 4.19. Lymph node morphology in advanced rheumatoid arthritis, H&E: At higher power, the paracortical regions are notable for sinusoidal dilation with scattered neutrophils associated with prominent plasmacytosis.

INTRAFOLLICULAR PLASMACYTOSIS-IGG4 DISEASE

More recently, another cause of recurrent generalized systemic lymphadenopathy includes the IgG4-related lymphadenopathy. Several patterns of involvement are noted in this disease. The common feature in all these patterns includes the presence of increased numbers of IgG4-positive plasma cells within the reactive lymphoid follicles as well as in the perifollicular and interfollicular regions of the lymph node (Figures 4.20-4.22). Frequently, circumferential with follicular granulomas with patchy areas of sclerosis and increased interfollicular vascularity and eosinophilic infiltrate are noted in these diseases. In some cases, this entity is often confused with hyaline vascular Castleman disease (hvCD) due to the prominent follicular regression noted in some follicles. Furthermore, significant interfollicular plasmacytosis may be mistaken for the plasma cell variant of Castleman disease.

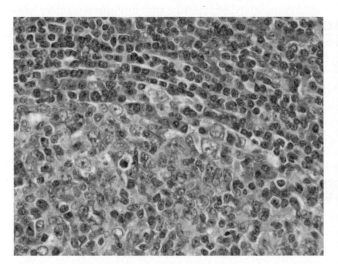

Figure 4.20. IgG4-related adenopathy, H&E: High-power view showing germinal center and mantle zones with prominent infiltrate of mature plasma cells.

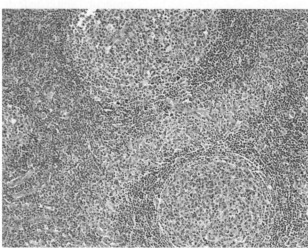

Figure 4.21. IgG4-related adenopathy, H&E: Low-power view showing linear perifollicular granulomas, morphologic feature commonly noted in IgG4-related adenopathy. These granulomas can often be circumferential.

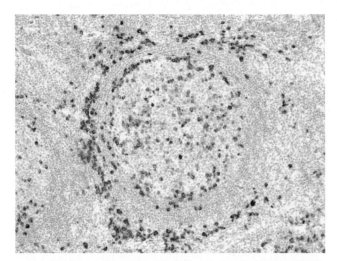

Figure 4.22. IgG4-related adenopathy, IgG4 immunostain: Immunostain for IgG4 highlights prominent intrafollicular and perifollicular IgG4+ polytypic plasmacytosis.

SAMPLE SIGN OUT FOR LYMPH NODES WITH INCREASED IGG4-POSITIVE PLASMA CELLS

Lymph node, right axillary, excision:

- Reactive follicular hyperplasia with increased IgG4-positive plasma cells, see comment.

Comment: There is moderate increase in IgG4-positive plasma cells (up to 40 per high-power field) in many areas including the interfollicular and occasionally interfollicular areas. Such increase may be seen in patients with autoimmune conditions and in patients with IgG4-related lymphadenopathy. Testing for serum IgG subclass and further autoimmune workup (such as ANA) may be performed to better assess this process.

Lymph node, right axillary, excision:

- Reactive lymphoid hyperplasia with markedly increased interfollicular IgG4-positive polytypic plasmacytosis, most consistent with IgG4-related lymphadenopathy, see comment.

Comment: Lymph node demonstrates preserved architecture with multiple secondary lymphoid follicles and focal follicles demonstrating perifollicular granulomas. At high-power, several follicles demonstrate increased numbers of mature plasma cells. Additional immunostains performed (CD20, CD3, kappa, lambda, and IgG4) highlight spatially appropriate staining for CD20 and CD3 within the lymphoid follicles and paracortex. There is polytypic plasmacytosis on kappa/lambda stains, and IgG4 immunostain highlights most of the intrafollicular plasma cells along with interfollicular areas with increased IgG4-positive plasma cells. The overall findings (specifically perifollicular granulomas and intrafollicular IgG4+ plasmacytosis) are in keeping with an IgG4-related lymphadenopathy.

NEAR MISS CASE 2: IgG4-Related Lymphadenopathy

A 75-year-old male with prominent cervical lymph node enlargement had a biopsy demonstrating prominent florid follicular hyperplasia with focal follicles demonstrating changes consistent with progressive transformation of germinal centers (Figures 4.23-4.26). Numerous intrafollicular plasma cells are the clue to perform IgG4 immunohistochemistry, and the presence of numerous intrafollicular IgG4-positive plasma cells coupled with perifollicular granulomas are both fairly specific features for IgG4-related lymphadenopathy. In patients with recurrent reactive follicular hyperplasia and subsequent biopsies, such testing must be performed to exclude the possibility of IgG4-related lymphadenopathy.

Figure 4.23. IgG4-related lymphadenopathy, H&E: Low-power view demonstrates single follicle in the center demonstrating indistinct germinal center-mantle zone interface with expanded mantle zones, consistent with progressive transformation of germinal centers. Note normal reactive secondary lymphoid follicle to the top right.

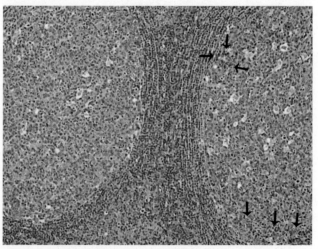

Figure 4.24. IgG4-related lymphadenopathy, H&E: High-power image demonstrating floridly reactive secondary lymphoid follicles. However, focal small clusters of plasma cells (black arrows) are seen throughout the germinal center.

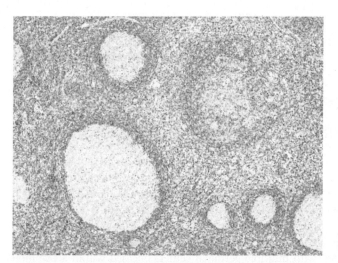

Figure 4.25. IgG4-related lymphadenopathy, BCL2 immunostain: BCL2 immunostain demonstrates multiple reactive secondary lymphoid follicles, negative for BCL2 with staining restricted to the mantle zones and the T-cell areas. Single follicle to the top right demonstrates progressive transformation of germinal center changes with evidence of BCL2-positive mantle zone cells within the germinal centers.

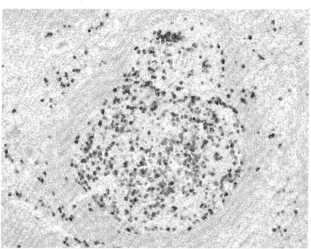

Figure 4.26. IgG4-related lymphadenopathy, IgG4 immunostain: IgG4 immunostain demonstrates numerous plasma cells positive for IgG4 within the follicles and at the periphery of the follicles in the paracortex.

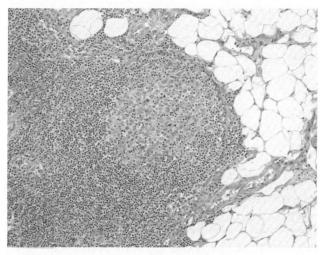

Figure 4.27. In situ follicular neoplasia (ISFN) in reactive-appearing lymph node adjoining another lymph node involved by diffuse large B-cell lymphoma, H&E: Morphologically reactive secondary lymphoid follicle with irregular borders between germinal center and mantle zones.

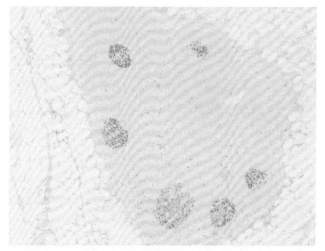

Figure 4.28. In situ follicular neoplasia (ISFN), CD10 immunostain: Low-power view demonstrating bright CD10 expression in small reactive-appearing follicles.

OTHER CLONAL CONDITIONS WITH REACTIVE HYPERPLASIA

Reactive Follicular Hyperplasia With Light Chain–Restricted Germinal Centers

Certain patients with immune conditions have been demonstrated to show morphologically reactive lymph nodes with follicular hyperplasia and light chain–restricted plasma cells or lymphoid cells within the germinal centers with molecular evidence of clonally rearranged immunoglobulin genes.[2] These light chain–restricted intrafollicular cells are usually BCL2 positive, but reported cases do not demonstrate evidence of any underlying IgH/BCL2 translocation allowing exclusion of in situ follicular neoplasia (ISFN).[3] These cases lack coinfection by EBV or HHV8 allowing exclusion of germinotropic lymphoproliferative disorder.

Insitu Follicular Neoplasia

Along these lines, cases of in situ follicular neoplasia exhibit reactive follicular hyperplasia with evidence of CD10bright/BCL2bright lymphoid cells within patchy germinal centers (Figures 4.27-4.29).[4] However, routinely testing all cases of reactive follicular hyperplasia with kappa/lambda and/or CD10, BCL2 is not warranted. It is possible that some of these cases would fall within the spectrum of IgG4-related lymphadenopathy recognized more recently.[5]

ABNORMAL EXPANDED MANTLE ZONES

CASTLEMAN-LIKE PROLIFERATIONS

1. **Hyaline-vascular Castleman disease, unicentric variant, HHV8-negative:** Clinically, this variant of Castleman disease presents as a solitary mass in superficial or deep sites including the neck, mediastinum, or abdominal regions. Histologically, there is marked distortion of the lymph node architecture by variably regressed lymphoid follicles which are notable for markedly expanded mantle zones with concentric rings of cells ("onion skinning") with small germinal centers that are frequently vascularized and lack polarization. In addition, there is frequent "twinning" with multiple germinal centers encased within a common mantle cuff beside "lollipop" lesions which comprise a single perpendicular blood vessel coursing through the germinal center with frequent hyalinization within the germinal center (Figures 4.30 and 4.31). Occasionally, follicular dendritic cell proliferations may be seen in the subcapsular areas coexisting, and hence, attention must be paid to these areas.

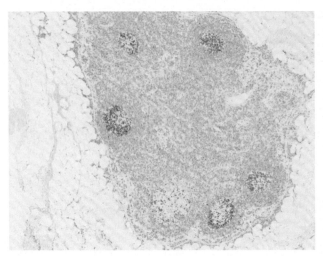

Figure 4.29. **In situ follicular neoplasia (ISFN), BCL2 immunostain:** There is coexpression of bright BCL2 within these follicles. BCL2 additionally stains mantle zone lymphocytes and T-cell areas with moderate intensity.

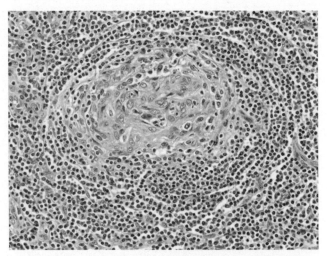

Figure 4.30. **Hyaline vascular Castleman disease, H&E:** Hyaline vascular Castleman disease demonstrating regressed and vascularized lymphoid follicles. There is prominent onion skinning of the mantle zone lymphocytes.

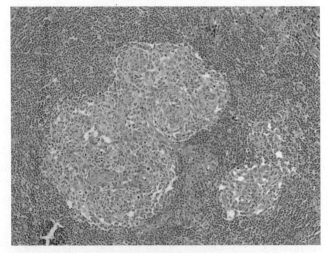

Figure 4.31. **Hyaline vascular Castleman disease, H&E:** HVCD with prominent twinning phenomenon comprising two germinal centers invested by a common mantle zone.

2. **Plasma cell variant of Castleman disease, unicentric, HHV8-negative:** Variable hvCD-like follicular changes may be observed in this variant of Castleman disease rich in interfollicular plasma cells. Occasionally, hybrid morphologic features with follicular regression and interfollicular plasmacytosis may be seen (Figures 4.32 and 4.33). Testing for KSHV/HH8 is important in these cases in order to exclude the multicentric variant of Castleman disease and to exclude focal involvement by Kaposi sarcoma, both of which are seen in the setting of HIV.

3. **Multicentric Castleman disease, plasma cell variant, HHV8+, HIV-related:** Although this entity is a clonal malignant neoplasm involving infection of plasmablasts by HHV8 virus, morphologically affected lymph nodes look reactive with relatively well-preserved architecture. Attention to clinical context is important in these cases so as to avoid the diagnosis. Patients with this entity typically have advanced HIV infection lymphadenopathy, splenomegaly, and cytopenias. Morphologically involved lymph nodes look reactive with variably regressed follicles and a variable amount of interfollicular plasmacytosis and lymphoid depletion associated with vascular prominence (Figures 4.34-4.38).

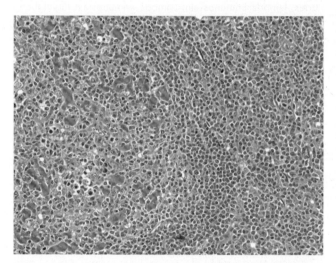

Figure 4.32. Plasma cell variant of Castleman disease, H&E: Plasma cell variant of Castleman disease demonstrating scattered hyalinized germinal centers on the left with interfollicular plasmacytosis on the right side.

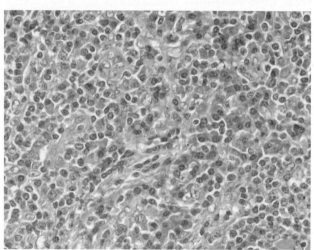

Figure 4.33. Plasma cell variant of Castleman disease, H&E: Higher power view of the interfollicular region with plasmacytosis.

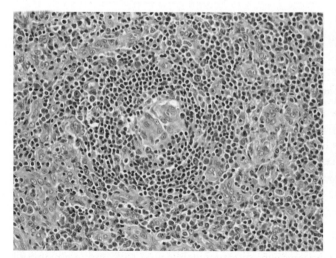

Figure 4.34. Multicentric Castleman disease involving lymph nodes, H&E: Scattered regressed lymphoid follicles with concentric rings of mantle zone cells reminiscent of hyaline vascular Castleman disease are noted.

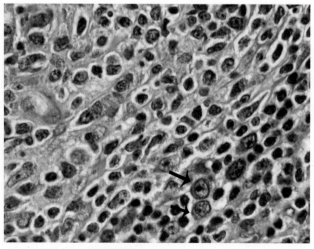

Figure 4.35. Multicentric Castleman disease involving lymph nodes, H&E: Higher power view of mantle zone showing singly scattered large plasmablastic cells (black arrows).

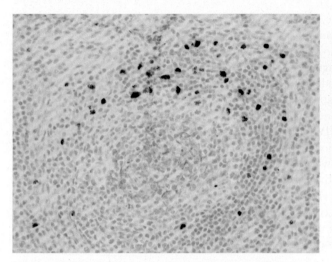

Figure 4.36. **Multicentric Castleman disease involving lymph nodes, HHV8 immunostain:** Immunostain for Kaposi sarcoma herpesvirus (KSHV) highlights infected mantle zone plasmablastic cells.

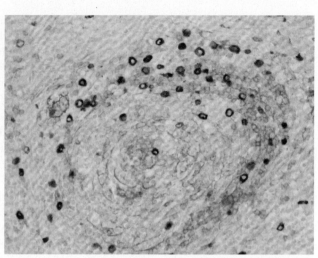

Figure 4.37. **Multicentric Castleman disease involving lymph nodes, lambda immunostain:** Lambda immunostain highlighting lambda-restricted phenotype in the neoplastic plasmablastic cells.

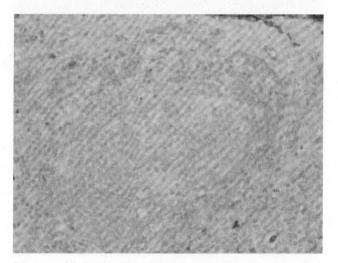

Figure 4.38. **Multicentric Castleman disease involving lymph nodes, kappa immunostain:** Kappa immunostain highlighting absence of kappa expression in the neoplastic plasmablastic cells.

SAMPLE SIGN OUT FOR LYMPH NODES WITH FOLLICULAR REGRESSION

Lymph node, cervical, excision:

• Reactive follicular hyperplasia with focal regressive changes, see comment.

Comment: The lymph node demonstrates preserved architecture with prominent reactive secondary lymphoid follicles. Occasional follicles demonstrate regressive changes reminiscent of hyaline vascular Castleman disease. Additional immunostains (pankeratin, EBER and HHV8) did not demonstrate any metastatic carcinoma cells, EBV-positive cells, or evidence of any HHV8 infected lymphoid cells within the mantle zones. The changes are nonspecific. Additional flow cytometry and molecular studies are not pursued.

Lymph node, cervical, excision:

• HHV8+ multicentric Castleman disease (MCD) in a patient with HIV, see comment.

Comment: The lymph node demonstrates distorted architecture with multiple regressed lymphoid follicles with prominent mantle zones and attenuated germinal centers. There is prominent interfollicular plasmacytosis. Scattered single large plasmablastic cells are seen within the mantle zones of several follicles. Additional immunostains (CD20, CD79a, CD3,

IgG, IgD, IgM, CD30, kappa, lambda, HHV 8) and in situ hybridization for EBV demonstrate that the large plasmablastic cells in the mantle zones are positive for IgM and lambda with HHV8 coinfection. These large cells are negative for CD20, IgG, IgD, and CD30 as well as kappa. The interfollicular areas are notable for polytypic plasma cells along with scattered immunoblasts positive for CD30 and CD79a with scattered small EBV-positive cells. The overall features are in keeping with the above diagnosis.

Diagnostic Checklist for Lymph Nodes Demonstrating Follicular Regression*

1. Is it a single large mass in a patient without HIV with uniform regression all over?
   a. Likely hyaline vascular Castleman disease.
2. Is it a small lymph node with focal regressive features that is draining a carcinoma site?
   a. Likely reactive changes and not hyaline vascular Castleman disease.
3. **Does the patient have multiple enlarged lymph nodes and a history of HIV?**
   a. HIV-related lymphadenopathy or multicentric Castleman disease (perform HHV8).
4. Is the history significant for recurrent lymphadenopathy without much systemic symptoms and focal regression on histology?
   a. Possible IgG4-related lymphadenopathy, performed IgG4 immunostain.

*I typically do not perform IgG4 and IgG at the same time. I add IgG only if IgG4-positive plasma cells are significantly increased.

PROGRESSIVE TRANSFORMATION OF GERMINAL CENTERS

Progressive transformation of germinal centers (PTGC) presents in young and middle-aged patients with recurrent solitary lymph node enlargement, most often in superficial sites. Affected lymph nodes demonstrate variable numbers of reactive secondary follicles, and in addition, there are several other follicles that are nearly two to three times the size of the surrounding normal secondary follicles and are notable for marked expansion of the mantle zones (Figures 4.39-4.43). Follicles demonstrating early involvement by progressive transformation display mantle lymphocytes which often extend into the germinal centers forming toothlike projections apparent on the IgD immunostaining.

Figure 4.39. **Progressive transformation of germinal centers, H&E:** Low-power view showing normal smaller follicles at the bottom with a markedly expanded follicle involved by progressive transformation at the top of the field.

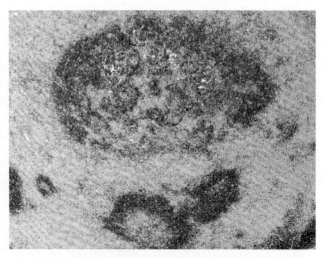

Figure 4.40. **Progressive transformation of germinal centers, IgD immunostain:** IgD immunostain highlights numerous positive cells throughout the follicle involved by progressive transformation in contrast to the follicle in the bottom demonstrating IgD+ cells restricted mostly to mantle zones of secondary lymphoid follicles.

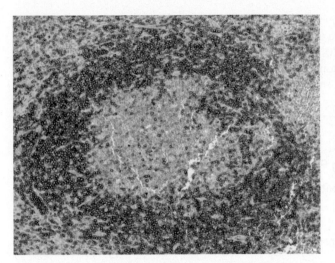

Figure 4.41. **Progressive transformation of germinal centers, IgD immunostain:** Early PTGC demonstrating slight indentation of the mantle zones into the germinal centers on IgD immunostain.

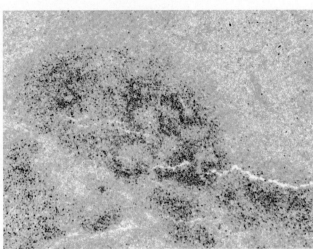

Figure 4.42. **Progressive transformation of germinal centers, CD10 immunostain:** CD10 immunostain at low power demonstrates moth-eaten pattern due to disruption of germinal centers.

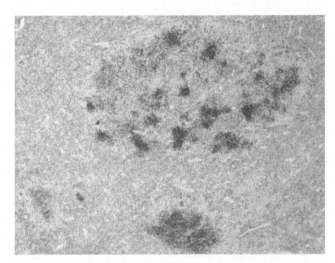

Figure 4.43. **Progressive transformation of germinal centers, PD-1 immunostain:** Numerous PD-1–positive lymphoid cells are often seen within follicles involved by progressive transformation with similar moth-eaten pattern as noted on CD10 immunostain.

In more advanced cases, most of the germinal centers are disrupted by numerous mantle zone lymphocytes and the germinal center/mantle zone borders are entirely disrupted. Frequently, advanced cases are notable for a marked increase in follicular helper T-cells within affected follicles. Some cases of progressive transformation of germinal centers are associated with preceding or subsequent development of nodular lymphocyte–prominent Hodgkin lymphoma, although it is unclear if the presence of PTGC indicates increased risk of subsequent development of nodular lymphocyte–predominant Hodgkin lymphoma.[6]

FAQ: There are numerous BCL2-positive cells within nodular follicular structures corresponding to B-cells; can I make a diagnosis of follicular lymphoma?

Answer: BCL2 is positive in normal T-cells and mantle zone B-cells. Numerous interfollicular T-cells and an influx of mantle zone B-cells into reactive germinal centers can give the impression of CD10, BCL2, and CD20 on the same cells. Therefore, careful examination of CD3 immunostain (corresponding to BCL2-positive T-cells) is necessary before making a diagnosis of follicular lymphoma.

KIMURA DISEASE

Two entities are associated with prominent eosinophilia, namely Kimura disease and angiolymphoid hyperplasia with eosinophilia (ALHE). The former is more common in patients of Asian origin and involves lymph nodes more frequently. The latter entity occurs more commonly in Caucasian population with cutaneous involvement and less frequent lymph node involvement. Nodal involvement by Kimura disease takes the form of variable follicular hyperplasia associated with a prominent infiltrate of eosinophils in the paracortical as well as follicular regions with frequent formation of eosinophilic microabscesses and associated Charcot-Leyden crystals with surrounding giant cell reaction (Figure 4.44). Deposition of eosinophilic material within involved reactive secondary lymphoid follicular germinal centers is also noted (Figure 4.45). Immunostaining for IgE highlights increased deposition within involved follicles (Figure 4.46). Some of these entities may have overlapped with IgG4-related lymphadenopathy inasmuch as increased numbers of IgG4+ plasma cells may be seen in the interfollicular regions with associated sclerosis. Classical Hodgkin lymphoma should be excluded in every case with eosinophilia before considering Kimura lymphadenopathy.

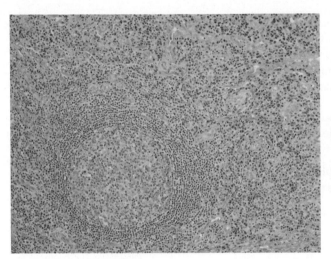

Figure 4.44. Kimura lymphadenopathy, H&E: Lymph node involvement takes the form of reactive follicular hyperplasia with prominent and often striking paracortical infiltrate of eosinophils.

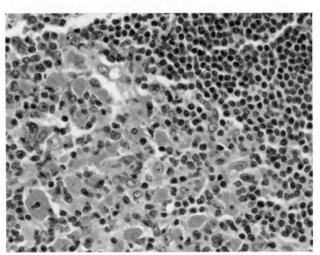

Figure 4.45. Kimura lymphadenopathy, H&E: At higher power, variable follicular regression and hyalinization is often present.

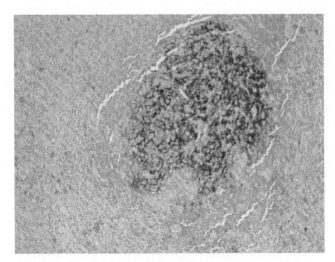

Figure 4.46. Kimura lymphadenopathy, IgE immunostain: Prominent staining for IgE is notable in follicles involved by this process.

ATTENUATED MANTLE ZONES

1. HIV: With progression of disease, lymph nodes involved by HIV demonstrate evidence of follicular lysis after their follicular hyperplasia stage with regression of germinal centers and dissolution of the mantle zones. In some cases, residual disrupted germinal centers without surrounding mantle zone cells may be seen.
2. Common variable immunodeficiency (CVID): Patients with CVID demonstrate frequent follicular hyperplasia with attenuation of the mantle zones (Figure 4.47). There is usually a paucity of plasma cells in the medullary cords. Scattered small EBV-positive cells may be seen in the background related to EBV reactivation in the setting of immunodeficiency.

OTHER INFECTIOUS PROCESSES

TOXOPLASMA

Lymph nodes involved by toxoplasma are notable for prominent follicular hyperplasia, paracortical/perisinusoidal monocytoid B-cell hyperplasia, and characteristic clusters of epithelioid histiocytes with expanded mantle zones of reactive follicles (Figure 4.48). Usually organisms are hard to demonstrate despite an immunostain, and in some cases, trophozoites within macrophages may be detected.

Table of key lymph node compartment-specific entities and useful diagnostic features

Nodal Compartment	Morphologic Features	Stains	Entity to Consider
Follicles	Regressed follicles	HHV8, IgG4	Hyaline vascular Castleman disease; multicentric Castleman disease
	Giant reactive back-to-back follicles	CD10, BCL2	Giant hyperplasia or pediatric follicular lymphoma
	Eosinophilic deposits in germinal centers	IgE	Kimura disease
	Reactive follicles with plasma cells inside follicles and perifollicular granulomas	IgG4	IgG4-related adenopathy
Mantle zone	Histiocytes in mantle zone	Toxoplasma	Toxoplasmosis
	Attenuated mantle zone	IgD	CVID
	Expanded mantle zones within large disrupted follicles	IgD	PTGC, HIV (follicular lysis)
Perifollicular	Several immunoblasts	CD30 and EBER	Reactive EBV-driven immunoblastic proliferation

CVID, common variable immunodeficiency; HIV, human immunodeficiency virus; PTGC, progressive transformation of germinal center.

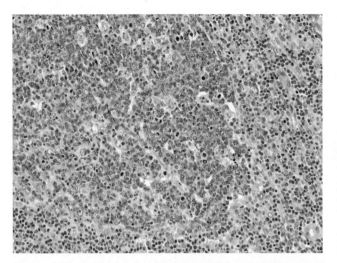

Figure 4.47. **Common variable immunodeficiency, H&E:** Involved lymph nodes show follicular hyperplasia with variable disruption of the light zone/dark zone architecture within the germinal centers along with variable attenuation of the mantle zones as noted in this picture.

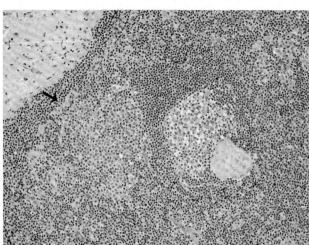

Figure 4.48. **Toxoplasmosis, H&E:** Low-power image showing a small noncaseating epithelioid granuloma within the mantle zone of a reactive secondary lymphoid follicle. Note the presence of a large cluster of monocytoid B-cells (black arrow) outside the follicle to the left.

FAQ: Are monocytoid B-cell expansions typical of toxoplasmosis?

Answer: Reactive monocytoid B-cell expansion in the perisinusoidal areas can be seen in multiple conditions including toxoplasmosis and viral infections (CMV and EBV) as well as in patients with autoimmune conditions. It is not unique to toxoplasmosis.

NEAR MISS CASE 3: CMV Lymphadenitis

A 43-year-old man had localized lymphadenopathy, and an excisional biopsy was performed accordingly. Histologically, there were florid geographic reactive follicles with multifocal perisinusoidal monocytoid B-cell expansion, and initially, interfollicular classical Hodgkin lymphoma, toxoplasma, EBV-related processes, and IgG4-related adenopathy were all considered in the differential. The case was signed out as florid follicular hyperplasia. However, after sign out, examination of the areas with monocytoid B-cell expansion demonstrated large cells with prominent eosinophilic nucleoli/inclusions. An additional cytomegalovirus immunostain was positive leading to an amendment of the final diagnosis to CMV lymphadenitis. CMV lymphadenitis does not have to occur only in an immunocompromised setting and can present as reactive follicular hyperplasia. This case highlights the need to be able to recognize perisinusoidal monocytoid B-cell expansions and to look within these areas carefully for possible CMV inclusions (Figures 4.49-4.52).

PEARLS & PITFALLS

CD30 stain often shows numerous reactive immunoblasts in a perifollicular location. These should be not be confused with Hodgkin cells. Hence, routine CD30 is not recommended.

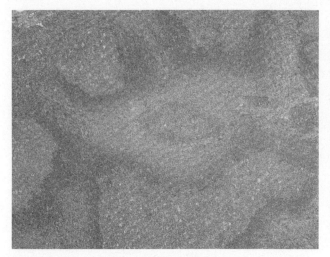

Figure 4.49. **CMV lymphadenitis, H&E:** Prominent reactive follicular hyperplasia noted in CMV lymphadenitis.

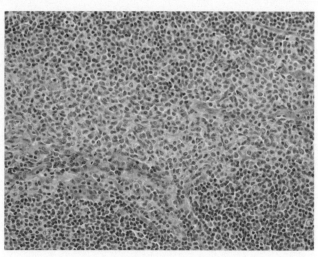

Figure 4.50. **CMV lymphadenitis, H&E:** Prominent reactive follicular hyperplasia noted in CMV lymphadenitis.

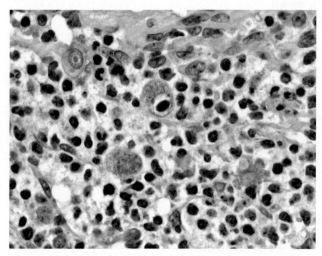

Figure 4.51. **CMV lymphadenitis, H&E:** On closer examination, foci of perisinusoidal monocytoid B-cell expansion is noted, and also, viral inclusions typical of CMV are noted.

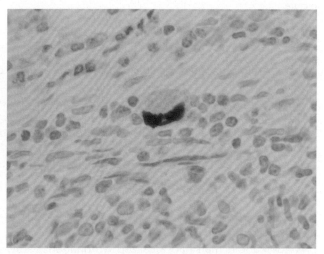

Figure 4.52. **CMV lymphadenitis, CMV immunostain:** This focus of perisinusoidal monocytoid B-cell expansion stains positive with the immunostain for CMV.

Checklist of Preneoplastic and Neoplastic Entities That May Be Lurking Despite Seemingly Preserved Nodal Architecture

1. B-cell processes
   a. Interfollicular classical Hodgkin lymphoma
   b. Marginal zone lymphoma (without follicular colonization)
   c. In situ follicular neoplasia (ISFN)
   d. Is situ mantle cell neoplasia (ISMCN)
      i. Mantle cell lymphoma with mantle zone pattern (Figures 4.53 and 4.54)
2. T-cell processes
   a. Early forms of angioimmunoblastic T-cell lymphoma (perifollicular pattern)
   b. Anaplastic large cell lymphoma with sinusoidal pattern (frequently lurking only in subcapsular sinus) (Figure 4.55)

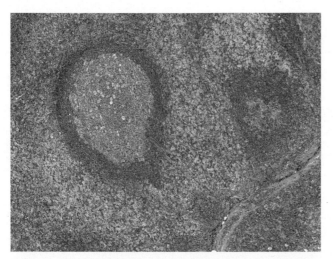

Figure 4.53. Mantle cell lymphoma, H&E: Lymph nodes involved by mantle cell lymphoma with prominent mantle zone pattern show reactive follicular hyperplasia.

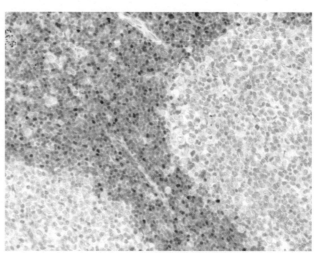

Figure 4.54. Mantle cell lymphoma, Cyclin D1 immunostain: Immunostain for cyclin D1 highlights lymphoma cells within the mantle zones.

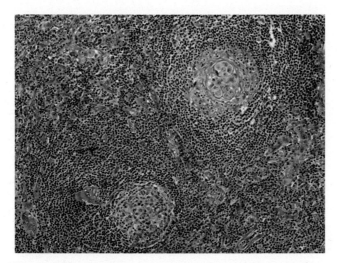

Figure 4.55. Anaplastic large cell lymphoma, H&E: Involvement by anaplastic large cell lymphoma can be rather subtle with predominant isolated sinusoidal involvement in otherwise reactive appearing nodes with secondary lymphoid follicles. Rarely, interfollicular aggregates of anaplastic large cell lymphoma cells may be observed.

References

1. Louissaint A Jr, Schafernak KT, Geyer JT, et al. Pediatric-type nodal follicular lymphoma: a biologically distinct lymphoma with frequent MAPK pathway mutations. *Blood*. 2016;128(8):1093-1100.

2. Nam-Cha SH, San-Millán B, Mollejo M, et al. Light-chain-restricted germinal centres in reactive lymphadenitis: report of eight cases. *Histopathology*. 2008;52:436-444.

3. Cong P, Raffeld M, Teruya-Feldstein J, Sorbara L, Pittaluga S, Jaffe ES. In situ localization of follicular lymphoma: description and analysis by laser capture microdissection. *Blood*. 2002;99(9):3376-3382.

4. Swerdlow SH, Campo E, Harris NL, Jaffe ES, Pileri SA, Stein H. *WHO Classification of Tumours of Haematopoietic and Lymphoid Tissues, Revised*. 4th ed.. Lyon, France: IARC; 2017.

5. Sato Y, Notohara K, Kojima M, Takata K, Masaki Y, Yoshino T. IgG4-related disease: historical overview and pathology of hematological disorders. *Pathol Int*. 2010;60:247-258.

6. Hartmann S, Winkelmann R, Metcalf RA, et al. Immunoarchitectural patterns of progressive transformation of germinal centers with and without nodular lymphocyte-predominant Hodgkin lymphoma. *Hum Pathol*. 2015;46(11):1655-1661.

CHAPTER OUTLINE

The lymph node paracortex is the area between the follicles and medullary cords (Figures 5.1-5.3). In a normal resting lymph node, this area predominantly contains small lymphocytes, with some admixed histiocytes, interdigitating dendritic cells (IDCs), and small vessels (Figure 5.4). The lymphocytes in the paracortex are predominantly T-cells, which are a mixture of CD4 and CD8-positive cells with CD4-positive T-cells predominating (see Chapter 1). The scattered IDCs are highlighted by S100, which is why S100 is a suboptimal stain when screening lymph nodes for metastatic melanoma.

Abnormalities of the paracortex typically include expansion, abnormal vasculature, and the presence of atypical cells. Apparent compression of the paracortex is often seen in lymph nodes that exhibit florid follicular hyperplasia.

PARACORTICAL HYPERPLASIA

The most frequent cause of paracortical expansion encountered in the typical clinical practice is reactive paracortical hyperplasia (Figure 5.5). Paracortical hyperplasia is a nonspecific finding and is often accompanied by a component of follicular hyperplasia. It is frequently encountered in the context of dermatopathic lymphadenopathy and infection, but it can also be seen in association with anticonvulsant drugs and autoimmune conditions. It should also be noted that lymph nodes that are involved by metastatic carcinoma or are draining a site involved by tumor can also show reactive changes, including paracortical and follicular hyperplasia as well as sinus histiocytosis.[1]

The expanded paracortex in paracortical hyperplasia contains the same populations of small T-lymphocytes, histiocytes, and IDCs found in the normal paracortex of resting lymph nodes (Figure 5.6); however, reactive lymphocytes known as immunoblasts are also frequently seen in paracortical hyperplasia (Figure 5.7). Immunoblasts are relatively large B- or T-lymphocytes with conspicuous nucleoli. They express variable CD30 (Figure 5.8) and MUM-1 (Figure 5.9). B-immunoblasts may show partial expression of CD20 (Figure 5.10), and T-immunoblasts may show dim or partial expression of CD3.

PEARLS & PITFALLS

Immunoblasts can be difficult to distinguish from Hodgkin/Reed-Sternberg (H/RS) cells; however, these cell types can usually be differentiated from one another using careful cytomorphologic evaluation and immunostains (Figure 5.11).

The nucleoli of immunoblasts are typically not as large as the nucleoli of H/RS cells, and the nucleoli of H/RS often have a slightly eosinophilic cast (Figure 5.12; also see Chapter 1). Additionally, immunoblasts are almost never binucleate.

While immunoblasts express CD30, the intensity of staining is variable, ranging from very weak to relatively strong. Additionally, immunoblasts are invariably negative for CD15. In contrast, H/RS cells exhibit strong and uniform CD30 expression and may express CD15.

Of note, CD20 and Pax-5 may not be useful for distinguishing B-immunoblasts from H/RS cells. Both immunoblasts and H/RS cells express Pax-5 at lower level of intensity than background small B-cells, and both cell types can also express variable CD20.[2]

DERMATOPATHIC LYMPHADENOPATHY

One of the most common causes of lymphadenopathy encountered in routine clinical practice is dermatopathic lymphadenopathy. Dermatopathic lymphadenopathy is seen in peripheral lymph nodes that drain the skin, and the diagnosis should not be entertained in central lymph nodes. The enlarged nodes often drain an area of skin that is involved by a rash or other pruritic skin disorder, though dermatopathic lymphadenopathy is not only seen in patients with dermatologic disorders.[3] Given its association with rashes, dermatopathic lymphadenopathy is frequently seen in children. Additionally, mildly enlarged axillary lymph nodes in patients with a history of adenocarcinoma of the breast often show mild

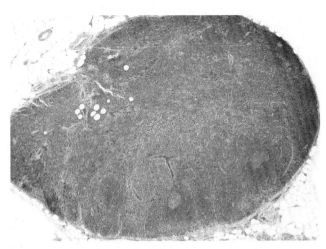

Figure 5.1. A small (3 mm) lymph node with scattered reactive follicles.

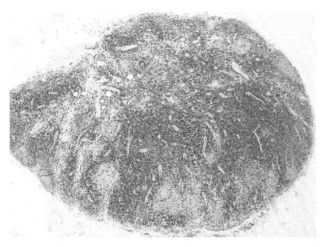

Figure 5.2. The paracortex of the lymph node in Figure 5.1 is located in between follicles and is rich in T-cells (CD3 immunostain).

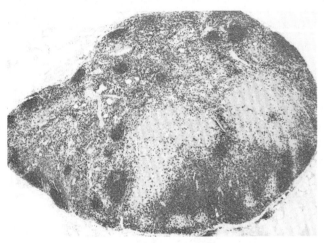

Figure 5.3. B-cells in the lymph node in Figure 5.1 are concentrated in follicles (CD20 immunostain).

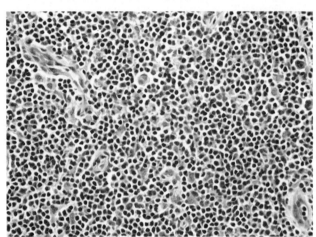

Figure 5.4. The parcortex is composed of a mixture of lymphocytes with a few admixed histiocytes and interdigitating dendritic cells, as well as small vessels.

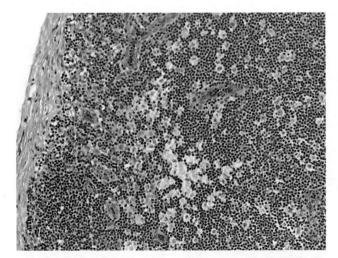

Figure 5.5. Admixed histiocytes can be prominent in paracortical hyperplasia, imparting a "moth-eaten" appearance.

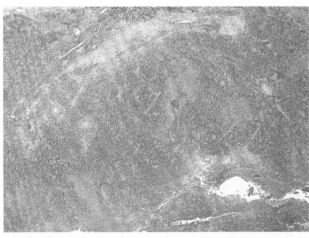

Figure 5.6. Paracortical hyperplasia of unclear etiology in a reactive lymph node. A few clusters of monocytoid lymphocytes are seen.

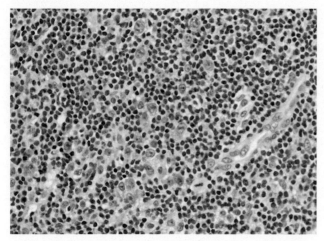

Figure 5.7. In paracortical hyperplasia, there may be frequent immunoblasts. Immunoblasts are large lymphocytes with one or more prominent nucleoli. Mitotic figures can occasionally be seen in the paracortical hyperplasia, as well.

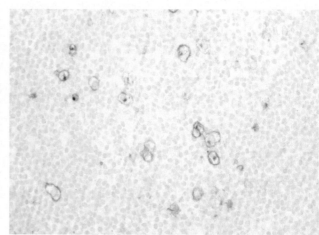

Figure 5.8. Immunoblasts express CD30, often in a membrane and Golgi pattern. Immunoblasts express CD30 at varying levels of intensity unlike the strong and uniform expression of CD30 seen on Hodgkin/Reed-Sternberg cells.

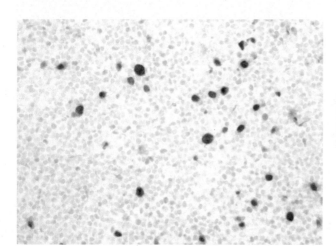

Figure 5.9. Immunoblasts are also highlighted by MUM-1.

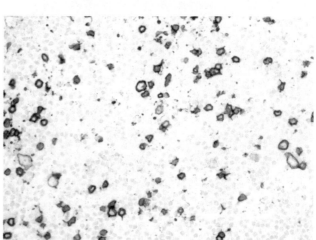

Figure 5.10. Immunoblasts may express variable/dim CD20 (as seen in this image) or CD3, depending on whether they are B- or T-immunoblasts.

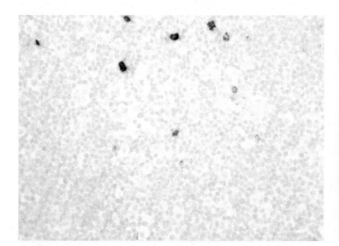

Figure 5.11. In contrast to Hodgkin/Reed-Sternberg cells, immunoblasts are negative for CD15. The scattered CD15+ cells seen in this image are granulocytes.

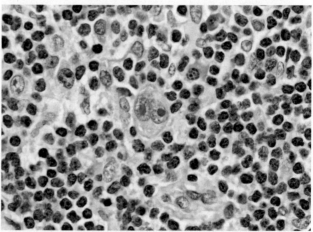

Figure 5.12. A Reed-Sternberg cell. Hodgkin/Reed-Sternberg cells often have larger and slightly more eosinophilic nucleoli than immunoblasts.

dermatopathic changes. Careful examination of these lymph nodes for metastatic disease is critical; however, if the nodes are negative, then it is often comforting for the patient and treatment team if the dermatopathic changes are documented, as it provides an explanation for the clinically worrisome lymphadenopathy.[4]

The histologic findings in dermatopathic lymphadenopathy initially manifest as follicular hyperplasia. Over time, the follicles regress and paracortical hyperplasia dominates (Figures 5.13 and 5.14). Well-developed dermatopathic lymphadenopathy is characterized by increased IDCs and Langerhans cells (LCs), which may form loose clusters (Figure 5.15).[3] The paracortex often contains admixed eosinophils, and the CD4:CD8 ratio is often elevated (>4:1). There are also scattered histiocytes that appear foamy or contain pigment (Figure 5.16). The pigment-laden histiocytes contain melanin and/or hemosiderin; if needed, this can be confirmed using special stains for melanin (Fontana-Masson) or iron.

Immunostains are not required for a diagnosis of dermatopathic lymphadenopathy. If there are significant numbers of pigment-laden histiocytes, then care should be taken when interpreting immunostains, as the melanin and hemosiderin pigments have a brown coloration that may be mistaken for a positive immunostain. The IDCs and LCs are highlighted by S100, and the LCs are positive for CD1a and langerin (Figures 5.17 and 5.18). LCs can be markedly increased in dermatopathic lymphadenopathy, and the increased S100 and CD1a-positive cells should not be mistaken for Langerhans cell histiocytosis (LCH).[5] LCH is typically associated with a pronounced increase of LCs in the sinuses rather than the paracortex, and admixed eosinophils are often prominent. Additionally, the neoplastic LCs may express Cyclin D1 and/or harbor a *BRAF* V600 E mutation.[6]

It is important to note that lymph node involvement by mycosis fungoides (MF; cutaneous T-cell lymphoma) is morphologically indistinguishable from dermatopathic lymphadenopathy.[7] The T-cells in MF may show immunophenotypic abnormalities, such as loss of CD7, which can be detected using immunostains. The most convincing way to prove nodal involvement by MF, however, is to perform T-cell receptor gene rearrangement studies on both the lymph node specimen and a skin biopsy and confirm the presence of the same clonal peak in both specimens. If a portion of the lymph node was submitted for flow cytometric analysis, then an atypical T-cell population can be identified via this modality, as well.

SAMPLE SIGNOUT: Dermatopathic Lymphadenopathy

1. Lymph node (excisional biopsy): Reactive lymph node with paracortical hyperplasia, increased Langerhans cells, and scattered pigment-laden histiocytes, most consistent with dermatopathic lymphadenopathy. See note.

Note: There is no evidence of lymphoma or metastatic carcinoma. Dermatopathic lymphadenopathy is associated with rashes and other skin diseases, and clinical correlation is needed.

INFECTION

Viral Infection

Viral infections are frequently associated with both follicular and paracortical hyperplasia. The relative composition of follicular hyperplasia and paracortical hyperplasia may vary throughout the course of infection.

Epstein-Barr Virus

Acute Epstein-Barr virus (EBV) infection is associated with lymphadenopathy, which also includes other lymphoid tissues including the tonsils and spleen. Lymph node biopsies for acute EBV infection are relatively rare, as the clinical syndrome (infectious mononucleosis) is well described and the diagnosis can be confirmed via laboratory testing. Infectious mononucleosis is most common in adolescents and young adults and is very rare in older adults. The lymph nodes typically show a mixture of follicular and paracortical hyperplasia

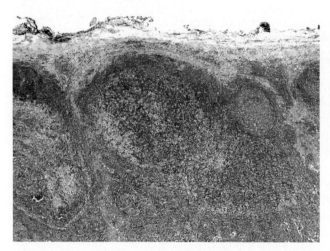

Figure 5.13. An axillary lymph node in a patient with a long-standing rash. There are both follicular and paracortical hyperplasia. The pale areas that expand the paracortex and partially encircle the follicles are composed of a mixture of Langerhans cells and interdigitating dendritic cells.

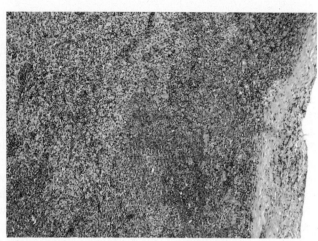

Figure 5.14. Higher-power image of the lymph node involved by dermatopathic lymphadenopathy in Figure 5.13.

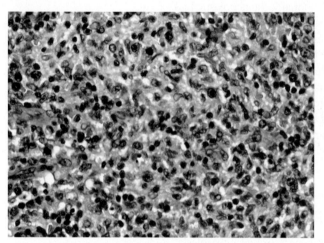

Figure 5.15. A cluster of Langerhans cells and interdigitating dendritic cells in the lymph node in Figures 5.13 and 5.14. These cell types cannot be differentiated from one another on an H&E section. A few subtle pigment-laden histiocytes are present in this image.

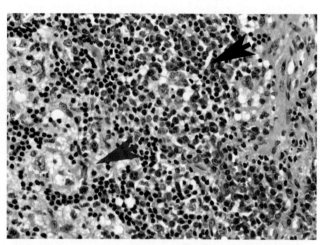

Figure 5.16. Pigment-laden histiocytes (black arrow) and foamy histiocytes (blue arrow) in dermatopathic lymphadenopathy. The pigment-laden histiocytes in dermatopathic lymphadenopathy are most often identified at the periphery of the node.

Figure 5.17. An S100 immunostain marks both the Langerhans cells and interdigitating dendritic cells in dermatopathic lymphadenopathy.

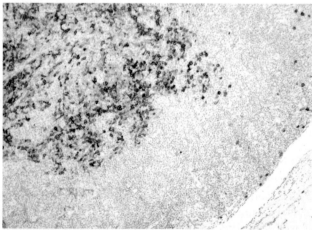

Figure 5.18. A CD1a immunostain marks the Langerhans cells in dermatopathic lymphadenopathy.

(Figure 5.19). Paracortical hyperplasia may predominate, with extension through the lymph node capsule. There is often focal necrosis with many apoptotic cells. Involved lymph nodes may contain many immunoblasts, some of which can be binucleated and mimic the H/RS cells of classical Hodgkin lymphoma (CHL).[8] The cellular background in EBV lymphadenitis does not, however, show the mixed inflammatory infiltrate that is characteristic of CHL.

The pattern of immunohistochemical staining in EBV lymphadenitis is as expected, with the reactive follicles enriched in CD20-positive B-cells (Figure 5.20). The paracortex is enriched in CD3-positive T-cells (Figure 5.21) with frequent CD30-positive immunoblasts (Figure 5.22). The CD4:CD8 ratio is often decreased or inverted in EBV lymphadenitis.[9] The Ki-67 proliferation index is expectedly high in the reactive follicles and is also often increased in the paracortex (Figure 5.23).

Due to the nonspecific nature of the lymph node findings in acute EBV infection, it is difficult to distinguish infectious mononucleosis from other viral causes of lymphadenitis based on morphologic findings alone. *In situ* hybridization (ISH) for Epstein-Barr virus–encoded small RNAs (EBER) is recommended to confirm the diagnosis (Figure 5.24). Immunohistochemical staining for EBV latent membrane protein-1 (EBV-LMP) is also available in many laboratories. While EBV-LMP will mark infected cells, EBER-ISH is preferable as it is far more sensitive than the EBV-LMP immunostain.[10]

PEARLS & PITFALLS

A diagnosis of acute EBV infection should be approached with caution in older adults or patients treated with immunosuppressive drugs, as these patients have an elevated risk of developing an EBV-positive lymphoma. Molecular studies may be helpful in distinguishing between acute EBV infection and an EBV+ lymphoproliferative disorder. Infectious mononucleosis does not characteristically show the clonal immunoglobulin heavy chain (*IGH*) gene rearrangements seen in EBV+ B-cell lymphomas; however, clonal T-cell patterns can be seen in this setting.[11]

A diagnosis of infectious mononucleosis is inappropriate in a patient who has had a transplant, as this is best classified as "post-transplant lymphoproliferative disorder (PTLD), infectious mononucleosis subtype." EBV+ cells can also be seen in reactive lymphoid proliferations in both the nondestructive and destructive subtype of PTLD. Of note, nondestructive PTLD is more often associated with florid follicular hyperplasia and plasmacytic hyperplasia as opposed to paracortical hyperplasia.

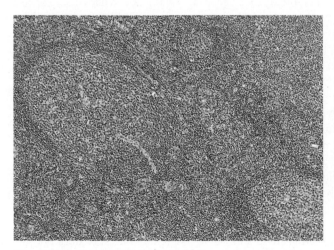

Figure 5.19. Acute EBV infection (infectious mononucleosis) shows follicular and paracortical hyperplasia.

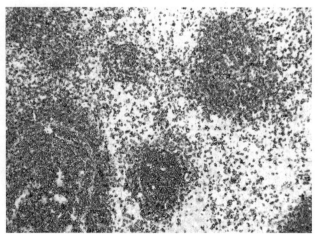

Figure 5.20. A CD20 immunostain marks the B-cells in the reactive follicles in infectious mononucleosis.

KEY FEATURES: Post-Transplant Lymphoproliferative Disorders (PTLD)

Category of PTLD	Subtype	Description	EBV?	Clonal?	Notes
Nondestructive (often seen in children)	Infectious mononucleosis Plasmacytic hyperplasia	Typically seen in patients who were previously EBV-negative but received an organ from an EBV-positive donor (children > adults)	+	No	Lymphoid pro-liferation in a transplant patient **that does not result in tissue destruction**
	Follicular hyperplasia	May regress spontaneously	+/−		
Destructive	Polymorphic	Mass lesion composed of lymphocytes in various stages of maturation (small lymphocytes, immunoblasts, plasma cells)	+/−, most are +	Usually (clonal B-cells)	Mass lesion results in tissue destruc-tion but does not meet criteria for a specific lymphoma
	Monomorphic	Fulfills the criteria for a known aggressive B-cell lymphoma (diffuse B-cell lymphoma, Burkitt lymphoma, plasma cell neoplasm), EBV+ extran-odal marginal zone lym-phoma, T-cell lymphoma, or NK/T-cell lymphomas	+/−	Yes* (B and T-cell lymphomas) *Clone not identified in NK/T-cell lymphomas	Frequently EBV-positive when the lesion devel-ops soon after transplant; less likely to be EBV-positive years after transplant
	Classical Hodgkin lymphoma	Fulfills the criterion for clas-sical Hodgkin lymphoma	+	B-cell clonality may be seen	Unlike garden-variety CHL, the Hodgkin/Reed-Sternberg cells of PTLD-CHL must be CD15+

Cytomegalovirus

Acute cytomegalovirus (CMV) infection is associated with a clinical syndrome similar to acute EBV infection. The lymph node changes are also similar, with follicular and paracortical hyperpla-sia as well as occasional foci of monocytoid cells (Figures 5.25 and 5.26). While large H/RS-like cells can be found in CMV lymphadenitis, there are also scattered immunoblasts containing large eosinophilic intranuclear inclusions that are surrounded by a clear halo (Figures 5.27 and 5.28). Immunostains can be very helpful in the diagnosis of CMV lymphadenitis, as the inclusions are not always readily identified on the H&E stain and normal-appearing cells can also be infected.

Herpes Simplex Virus

Herpes simplex virus (HSV) lymphadenitis shows nonspecific morphologic findings similar to those in EBV and CMV lymphadenitis, though paracortical hyperplasia tends to predom-inate and foci of acute inflammation and necrosis are more prominent in HSV lymphadeni-tis. HSV lymphadenitis is rare and typically occurs in immunocompromised patients. It may also be seen in association with low-grade B-cell lymphomas such as chronic lymphocytic leukemia/small lymphocytic lymphoma (CLL/SLL) (Figure 5.29).[12] Cells infected with HSV show characteristic nuclear changes, including a ground glass appearance with margination of the chromatin (Figure 5.30). The nuclear changes of HSV lymphadenitis are often best identified at the interface between necrotic and viable tissue. Of note, HSV does not just infect lymphocytes but can also infect many cell types including endothelium and epithe-lium.[13] As with EBV and CMV lymphadenitis, an immunostain for HSV is very helpful in identifying and/or confirming the etiology of the lymphadenitis (Figure 5.31).

Human Immunodeficiency Virus

In the era of highly active antiretroviral therapy (HAART), lymph node specimens involved by human immunodeficiency virus (HIV) lymphadenitis are not often seen in routine clinical practice; however, they do occasionally make an appearance.

The initial HIV infection is associated with acute HIV lymphadenitis with nonspecific florid follicular hyperplasia and patches of monocytoid cells. Warthin-Finkeldey-type polykaryocytes can be seen in acute HIV infection; however, these cells are nonspecific and can be seen in other infectious disorders (ie, measles lymphadenitis) or clinical conditions (ie, Kimura lymphadenopathy, systemic lupus lymphadenopathy). Warthin-Finkeldey cells are thought to represent multinucleated follicular dendritic cells (Figure 5.32).[14]

HIV lymphadenopathy can persist for years. Over time, the reactive germinal centers involute, resulting in atretic and fibrosed follicles (Figure 5.33). Both the follicles and paracortex are depleted of lymphocytes, but the paracortex remains expanded with abundant plasma cells and prominent vasculature (Figures 5.34-5.38).[16]

PEARLS & PITFALLS

Clinical history is necessary for a diagnosis of HIV lymphadenopathy, and immunostains directed against HIV are not available in most clinical laboratories. While HIV lymphadenopathy is no longer a frequent diagnosis, patients with HIV are at an increased risk for lymphoproliferative disorders, and close evaluation of lymph nodes in patients with a history of HIV infection is recommended. This includes inspection of the capsule for possible Kaposi sarcoma.

Bacterial Infection

Nonspecific bacterial lymphadenitis is typically associated with microabscess formation or diffuse replacement of the lymph node parenchyma by neutrophils without marked paracortical hyperplasia. A few subtypes of bacterial lymphadenitis have a characteristic morphologic appearance with paracortical involvement.

Syphilitic (Luetic) Lymphadenitis

Syphilitic lymphadenitis, as covered in more detail in Chapter 2, is associated with florid follicular hyperplasia, increased plasma cells, and a markedly thickened capsule; however, the node often also exhibits a component of paracortical hyperplasia with numerous immunoblasts (see Chapter 2 for images).

Cat Scratch Lymphadenitis and Lymphogranuloma Venereum

Two forms of bacterial lymphadenitis characteristically show stellate microabscesses with areas of necrosis: cat scratch lymphadenitis and lymphogranuloma venereum (LGV). Cat scratch lymphadenitis/disease (CSD) is caused by *Bartonella henselae*, and LGV is caused by *Chlamydia trachomatis*. Differentiation between these two entities may be aided by clinical history. CSD is typically associated with a history of a cat scratch in an area drained by the enlarged lymph nodes, whereas LGV is associated with inguinal, femoral, and pelvic lymphadenopathy. Both LGV and CSD can result in lymph node rupture with sinus tract formation.[17,18]

Lymph nodes involved by CSD (see Chapter 9) or LGV show stellate microabscesses with central necrosis (Figure 5.39). The necrotic areas contain neutrophils (Figure 5.40). The surrounding lymphoid tissue exhibits follicular and paracortical hyperplasia (Figures 5.41 and 5.42). Organisms can sometimes be identified on a Warthin-Starry special stain; however, molecular and/or serologic studies may be required for definitive diagnosis.[19-21]

Protozoal Infection

The protozoal lymphadenitis that is commonly seen in routine practice is associated with *Toxoplasma gondii* infection. Like CSD, *Toxoplasma* lymphadenitis has a component of

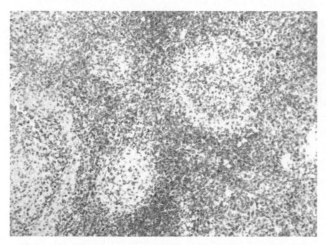

Figure 5.21. The paracortex is largely composed of CD3-positive T-cells in infectious mononucleosis.

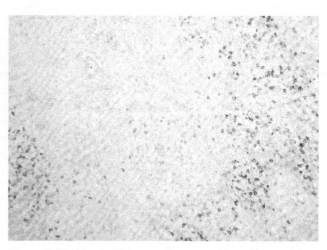

Figure 5.22. Immunoblasts may be increased in infectious mononucleosis. Most of the immunoblasts are in the paracortex, and they express variable CD30.

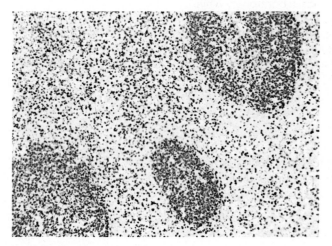

Figure 5.23. The Ki-67 proliferation index is expectedly high in the germinal centers, but it is often increased in the paracortex, as well, in infectious mononucleosis.

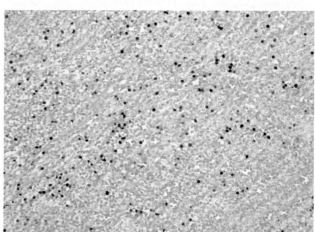

Figure 5.24. *In situ* hybridization for EBV (EBER) marks frequent cells in EBV lymphadenitis.

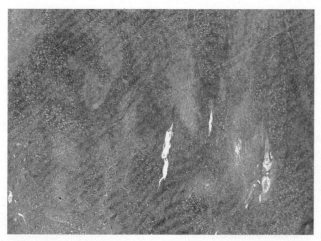

Figure 5.25. Cytomegalovirus lymphadenitis with follicular and paracortical hyperplasia.

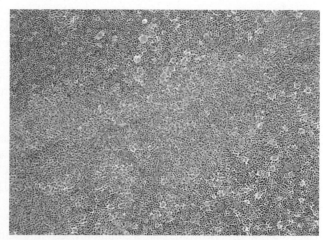

Figure 5.26. Scattered large atypical cells are seen in cytomegalovirus lymphadenitis.

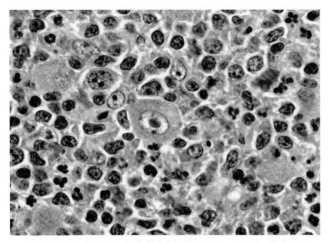

Figure 5.27. Cytomegalovirus (CMV) viral inclusions are very large and eosinophilic. The inclusions are not always obvious, and a CMV immunostain can be helpful for making the diagnosis of CMV lymphadenitis.

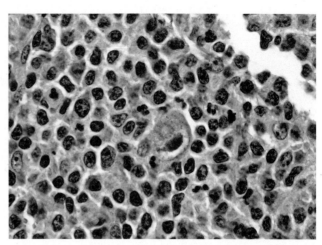

Figure 5.28. Cells with cytomegalovirus viral inclusions may resemble Hodgkin/Reed-Sternberg cells (H/RS), but the inclusions are larger than the prominent nucleoli of H/RS cells (see Figure 5.12).

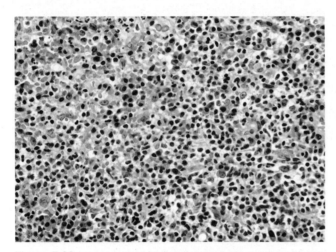

Figure 5.29. Herpes simplex virus lymphadenitis in a lymph node that is also involved by nodal marginal zone lymphoma. There is focal acute inflammation (top left) in this image.

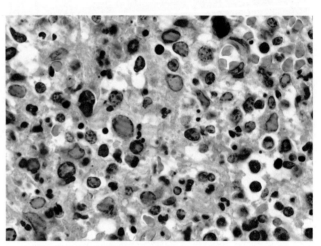

Figure 5.30. Cells infected with herpes simplex virus have glassy nucleoli with marginated chromatin.

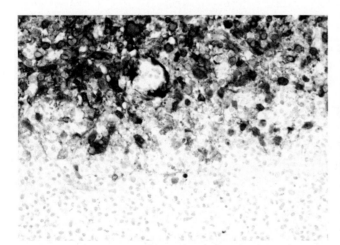

Figure 5.31. Cells exhibiting the characteristic changes of herpes simplex virus (HSV) may be difficult to identify on H&E sections, and an HSV immunostain can be helpful.

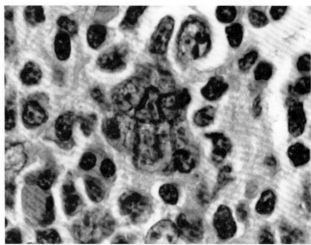

Figure 5.32. Warthin-Finkeldey type cells (center of image) with clustered nuclei are often seen in acute HIV lymphadenitis, but they are not specific for HIV lymphadenopathy.

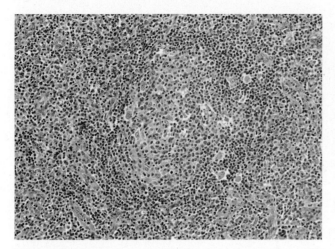

Figure 5.33. An atretic follicle in long-standing HIV lymphadenopathy.

Figure 5.34. The paracortex is expanded in long-standing HIV lymphadenopathy.

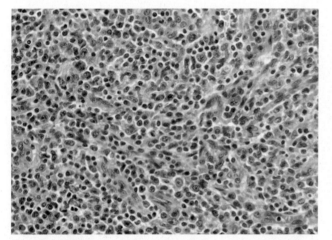

Figure 5.35. A higher-power view of the paracortex illustrates the prominent vasculature and frequent plasma cells seen in HIV lymphadenopathy.

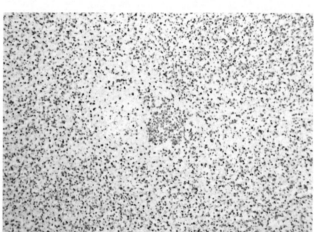

Figure 5.36. A Ki-67 immunostain demonstrates the elevated proliferation index in the paracortex. A germinal center with an appropriately high proliferation index is present at the center of the field. The mantle zone has a relatively low proliferation rate, and the surrounding paracortex has a brisk proliferation index.

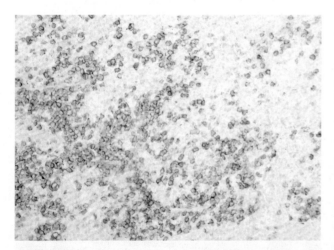

Figure 5.37. The frequent plasma cells seen in long-standing HIV lymphadenopathy are highlighted by a CD138 immunostain.

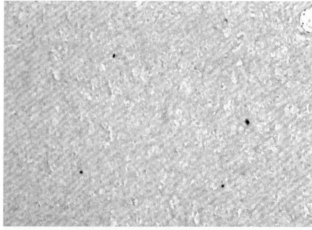

Figure 5.38. Lymph nodes involved by HIV lymphadenopathy frequently contain a few singly scattered EBV-positive cells, as seen in this in situ hybridization for EBV (EBER).[15]

Figure 5.39. An enlarged (4.3 cm) inguinal lymph node in a 22-year-old man. The node shows the stellate microabscesses that are characteristic of lymphogranuloma venereum.

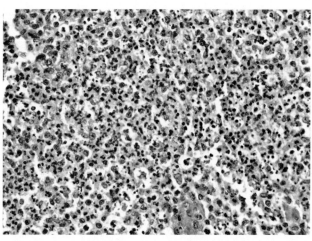

Figure 5.40. High-power view of the center of a stellate abscess in lymphogranuloma venereum.

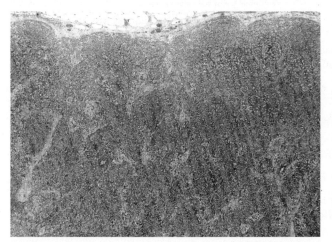

Figure 5.41. Areas of the lymph node that are uninvolved by microabscesses show paracortical hyperplasia in lymphogranuloma venereum.

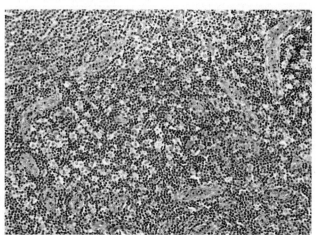

Figure 5.42. Higher-power view of paracortical hyperplasia in lymphogranuloma venereum.

paracortical hyperplasia and is frequently blamed on cats. However, in defense of our feline companions, it should be noted that many *Toxoplasma* infections are thought to result from the ingestion of undercooked meat or accidental ingestion of soil from unwashed produce.[22] *Toxoplasma* is postulated to be the etiologic factor behind a significant proportion of unexplained cervical lymphadenopathy and is frequently associated with posterior cervical lymphadenopathy.[23]

Toxoplasma lymphadenopathy has a characteristic histologic triad of (1) follicular hyperplasia, (2) areas of monocytoid B-cells, and (3) clusters of epithelioid histiocytes that encroach on germinal centers (Figure 5.43). The follicular hyperplasia of *Toxoplasma* lymphadenopathy is often florid, and the germinal centers can form serpiginous shapes. There are also clusters of monocytoid B-cells that are medium in size with clear or pale cytoplasm (Figures 5.44-5.46). The third characteristic finding in *Toxoplasma* lymphadenitis is the distinctive clusters of epithelioid histiocytes (Figure 5.47), which can encroach on germinal centers (Figures 5.48 and 5.49). Many laboratories have a *Toxoplasma* immunostain; however, this stain is often of limited use in the diagnosis of *Toxoplasma* lymphadenitis, and serologic studies may be needed for definitive diagnosis.

FAQ: What are the characteristic anatomic sites of enlarged nodes in common nonneoplastic causes of lymphadenopathy?

Clinical Condition	Location of Lymphadenopathy
Cat scratch disease	Upper extremities > cervical > groin (nodes that drain the site of a prior cat scratch; overlying skin is often erythematous)
Cytomegalovirus	No specific anatomic site
Epstein-Barr virus	Tonsils, cervical lymph nodes, spleen (may also show generalized lymphadenopathy)
Dermatopathic	Peripheral nodes draining the skin including cervical, axillary, and inguinal nodes (not seen in central nodes such as mesenteric or periaortic)
Kikuchi	Usually cervical nodes
Kimura	Head and neck, often near the ear (if the process only involves the dermis and not lymph nodes, then it is best classified as angiolymphoid hyperplasia with eosinophilia)
Lymphogranuloma venereum	Men: inguinal and femoral nodes; women: pelvic and perianal lymph nodes
Sarcoidosis	Mediastinal and hilar; also can be generalized
Sinus histiocytosis with massive lymphadenopathy (Rosai-Dorfman disease)	Cervical lymph nodes (extranodal disease, including soft tissue and central nervous system involvement, is also relatively common)
Syphilis	Inguinal lymph nodes (cervical nodes can also be involved)
Toxoplasma gondii	Cervical nodes (characteristically the posterior cervical nodes)

DRUG-ASSOCIATED LYMPHADENOPATHY

A significant number of drugs are associated with lymphadenopathy, most commonly anticonvulsants including phenytoin and phenobarbital.[24] The lymph node findings are nonspecific with follicular and paracortical hyperplasia; thus, clinical information is crucial for making the diagnosis. Drug-associated lymphadenopathy can be associated with increased eosinophils ("drug rash with eosinophilia and systemic symptoms" or DRESS syndrome).[25]

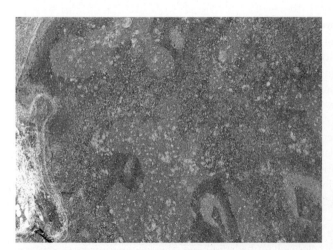

Figure 5.43. An enlarged lymph node exhibiting the characteristic features of *Toxoplasma* lymphadenopathy, including follicular hyperplasia, areas of monocytoid cells, and scattered clusters of epithelioid histiocytes that encroach on germinal centers.

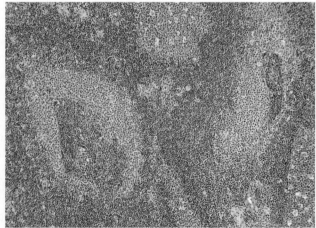

Figure 5.44. Higher-power view of clusters of monocytoid cells in *Toxoplasma* lymphadenopathy.

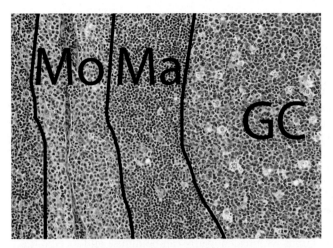

Figure 5.45. Annotated view of a reactive germinal center (GC), the surrounding mantle (Ma), and an area rich in monocytoid cells (Mo) in *Toxoplasma* lymphadenopathy.

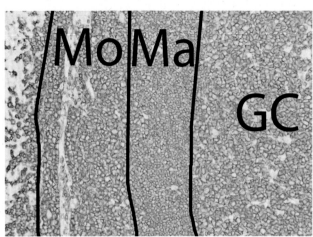

Figure 5.46. A CD20 immunostain corresponding to Figure 5.45 demonstrates that the germinal center, mantle zone, and monocytoid cells are B-cells.

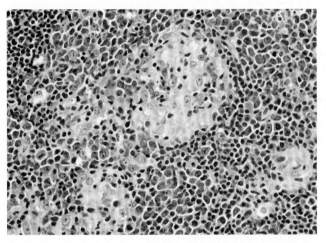

Figure 5.47. High-power view of clusters of epithelioid histiocytes in *Toxoplasma* lymphadenopathy. Well-formed granulomas are not seen.

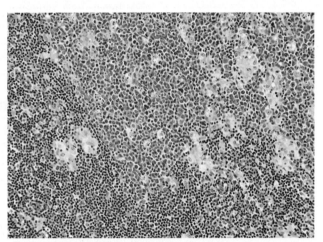

Figure 5.48. Clusters of epithelioid histiocytes encroach on germinal centers in *Toxoplasma* lymphadenopathy.

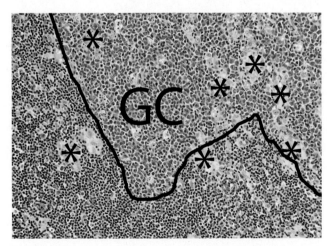

Figure 5.49. An annotated view of Figure 5.48 marks the rough boundary between the germinal center (GC) and mantle zone. Clusters of epithelioid histiocytes are marked by asterisks.

Enlarged lymph nodes in patients treated with anticonvulsant therapy show nonspecific follicular and paracortical hyperplasia (Figures 5.50-5.52). The paracortex contains frequent histiocytes and occasional immunoblasts (Figure 5.53).

AUTOIMMUNE CONDITIONS

Patients with various autoimmune conditions such as systemic lupus erythematosus (SLE), adult onset Still disease, and autoimmune lymphoproliferative syndrome may show lymphadenopathy with paracortical hyperplasia.[25,26]

SYSTEMIC LUPUS ERYTHEMATOSUS LYMPHADENOPATHY

Patients with SLE can present with lymphadenopathy; however, the histologic findings in lymph nodes are variable. Classically, patients with SLE show extensive aneutrophilic necrosis in a Kikuchi-like pattern (see Figures 5.153-5.155); however, lupus lymphadenopathy without necrosis does occur.[27] Lupus lymphadenopathy can be diffuse and metabolically active on imaging studies, raising clinical suspicion for lymphoma. Additionally, patients with SLE may have false positives on rapid plasma regain (RPR) or Venereal Disease Research Laboratory (VDRL) testing, introducing clinical concern for syphilitic lymphadenitis.

The lymph nodes in nonnecrotic lupus lymphadenopathy exhibit follicular and paracortical hyperplasia, often with vascular proliferation and numerous immunoblasts (Figures 5.54-5.58). Warthin-Finkeldey-type cells can be seen in lupus lymphadenopathy as well (Figure 5.59).[28] While the paracortical hyperplasia may appear somewhat atypical, the findings are not those of a lymphoma and the nodes also do not show the markedly thickened capsule of syphilitic lymphadenitis.

ATYPICAL PARACORTICAL HYPERPLASIA

Occasionally, the nodal architecture is largely intact, but the paracortex is expanded and shows worrisome cytomorphologic atypia with a high Ki-67 proliferation index. These cases are difficult and often require a fairly extensive workup. Lymphomas that are associated with atypical paracortical hyperplasia include angioimmunoblastic T-cell lymphoma (Figures 5.60-5.68) and interfollicular classical Hodgkin lymphoma (see Chapter 1, "Near Misses"). If there is no definitive evidence of lymphoma, then a diagnosis of "atypical paracortical hyperplasia" is appropriate, with a note recommending close clinical follow-up.

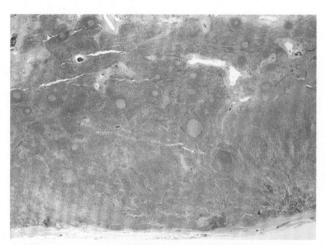

Figure 5.50. Lymphadenopathy in a 7-year-old boy treated with phenobarbital. The lymph node shows follicular and paracortical hyperplasia. An area of particularly pronounced paracortical hyperplasia is seen in the lower right of the image.

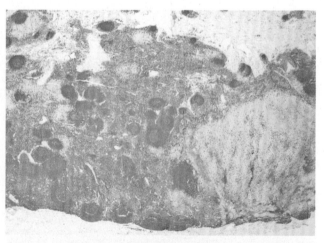

Figure 5.51. CD20 marks the B-cells, which are concentrated in follicles in the lymph node pictured in Figure 5.50.

FAQ: What is the workup of atypical paracortical hyperplasia?

Stains
- Distribution of B- and T-cells: CD20 and CD3
- Proliferation index of paracortex: Ki-67
- Presence or absence of H/RS cells: CD30 and CD15 (MUM-1 can be helpful)
- Characterization of T-cells: CD4, CD8, CD7, CD10/PD-1
- Organization of underlying follicular dendritic cell meshworks: CD21 and/or CD23
- Presence or absence of EBV+ cells: in situ hybridization for EBV (EBER)

Flow cytometry
- Abnormalities in the CD4:CD8 ratio
- Loss of T-cell antigens on mature T-cells (CD2, CD5, and/or CD7)
- CD4+/CD10+ T-cells with loss of CD7
- CD4+ T-cells with loss of surface CD3

Molecular studies
- T-cell receptor (TCR) gene rearrangement studies

Additional information (if available)
- Clinical history, imaging studies, medications

HISTIOCYTIC PROLIFERATIONS

Histiocytes are normal residents of the paracortex, but they can be increased in several conditions. These histiocytes may be present in various patterns, including (1) singly or in small clusters, (2) granulomas, or (3) a diffuse pattern with extensive replacement of the node.

SINGLY/SMALL CLUSTERS

Lipid Lymphadenopathy

Lymph nodes draining the portal system may contain scattered lipid droplets of various sizes. These droplets are found in the interfollicular space but are actually located in the medullary sinuses as opposed to the paracortex (Figure 5.69). Histiocytes engulf the lipid droplets, and multinucleated giant cells are frequent (Figure 5.70).

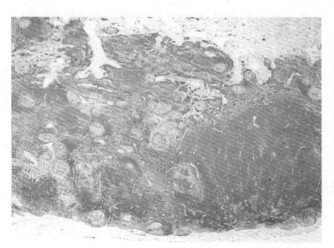

Figure 5.52. CD3 marks the paracortex in the lymph node pictured in Figure 5.50, including the area of paracortical hyperplasia in the lower right of the image.

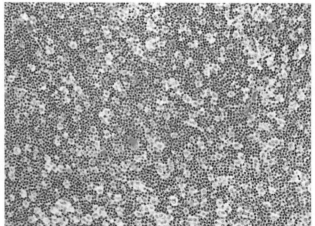

Figure 5.53. Scattered histiocytes impart a "moth-eaten" appearance to the paracortex in a lymph node involved by drug-associated lymphadenopathy. Eosinophils may be increased in drug-associated lymphadenopathy, though they are not increased in this lymph node.

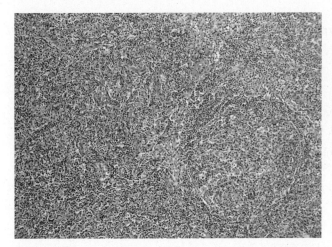

Figure 5.54. An enlarged lymph node with follicular and paracortical hyperplasia in a 26-year-old man with systemic lupus erythematosus.

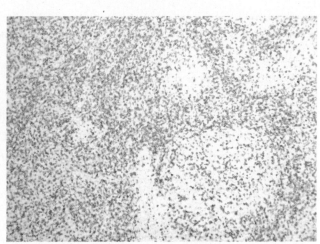

Figure 5.55. CD3 marks the T-cells, which are concentrated in the somewhat expanded paracortex in the lymph node in Figure 5.54.

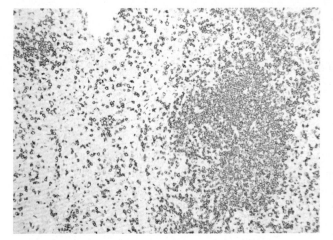

Figure 5.56. CD20 marks the B-cells in the lymph node in Figure 5.54.

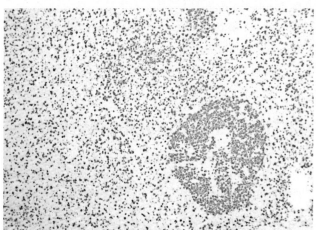

Figure 5.57. An immunostain for Ki-67 shows that the proliferation index is increased in both the follicles and the paracortex in the lymph node in Figure 5.54.

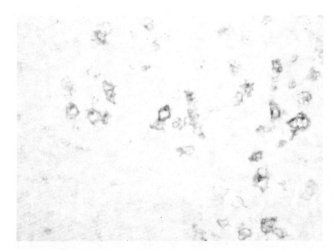

Figure 5.58. Scattered CD30+ immunoblasts can be seen in the paracortex in lupus lymphadenopathy.

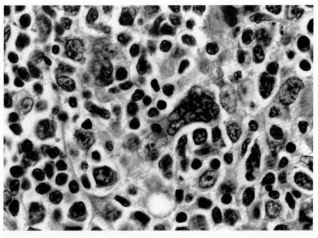

Figure 5.59. Warthin-Finkeldey-type giant cells are not restricted to viral lymphadenopathy and can also be seen in lupus lymphadenopathy.

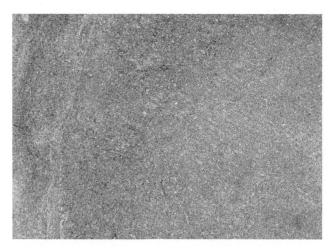

Figure 5.60. The paracortex often shows an atypical pattern of expansion in angioimmunoblastic T-cell lymphoma.

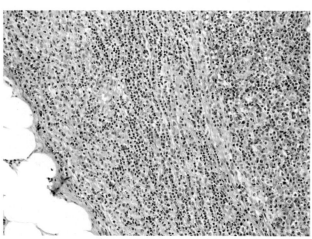

Figure 5.61. The atypical lymphoid infiltrate may extend through the capsule into the perinodal adipose tissue in angioimmunoblastic T-cell lymphoma.

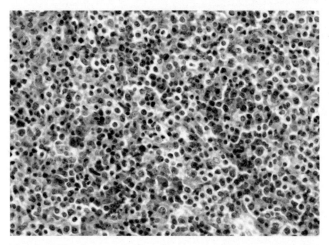

Figure 5.62. The lymphocytes in angioimmunoblastic T-cells lymphoma are small- to medium-sized cells, which often have clear cytoplasm. There are occasional admixed eosinophils, plasma cells, and immunoblasts.

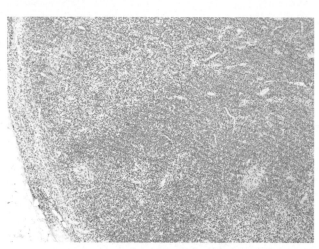

Figure 5.63. CD3 marks the atypical paracortical expansion in the angioimmunoblastic T-cell lymphoma shown in Figure 5.60.

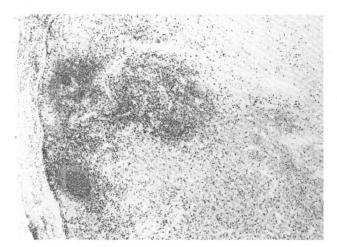

Figure 5.64. CD20 marks residual follicles in the angioimmunoblastic T-cell lymphoma shown in Figure 5.60.

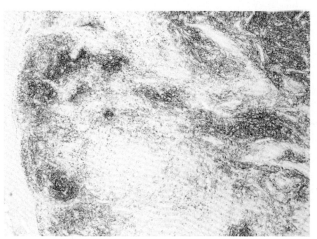

Figure 5.65. CD23 highlights expanded follicular dendritic cell meshworks in the angioimmunoblastic T-cell lymphoma shown in Figure 5.60. In angioimmunoblastic T-cell lymphoma, these meshworks are not limited to areas underlying follicles and are also present in surrounding vessels and in areas that lack B-cells. This is particularly pronounced in the upper right corner of the image (compare with the CD3 and CD20 immunostain images).

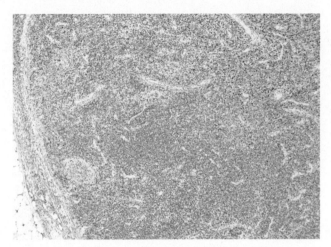

Figure 5.66. The neoplastic T-cells in angioimmunoblastic T-cell lymphoma are CD4-positive (lymphoma pictured in Figure 5.60).

Figure 5.67. The neoplastic CD4+ T-cells in angioimmunoblastic T-cell lymphoma characteristically show significant loss of CD7, which is not seen in reactive paracortical hyperplasia (lymphoma pictured in Figure 5.60).

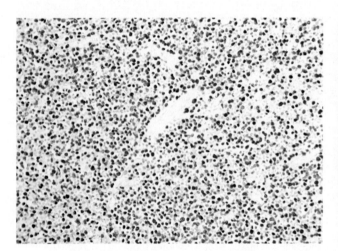

Figure 5.68. The Ki-67 proliferation index in angioimmunoblastic T-cell lymphoma is typically high.

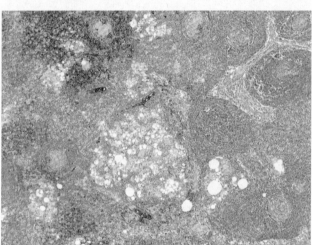

Figure 5.69. A portal node in a woman with cholelithiasis. Numerous lipid droplets are seen in the interfollicular space.

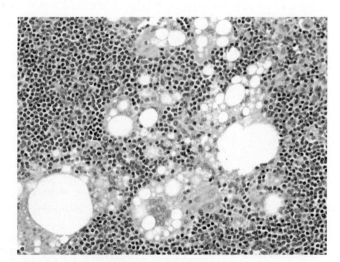

Figure 5.70. Many of the droplets have been engulfed by multi-nucleated giant cells.

Tattoo Powder

Tattoo powder can also be seen within histiocytes. Tattoo powder has a chunkier texture than hemosiderin or melanin and is nonrefractile (Figures 5.71-5.73). Tattoo powder is often identified in peripheral nodes that drain the skin. It can also be seen in lymph nodes that are sampled during colectomies when the original site of the tumor was marked with tattoo powder by the endoscopist.

Toxoplasma Lymphadenopathy

As noted in a previous section, *Toxoplasma* lymphadenopathy shows characteristic clusters of epithelioid histiocytes that are scattered throughout the paracortex and encroach on the germinal centers (Figures 5.74 and 5.75; see also Figures 5.43-5.49).

GRANULOMAS

Sarcoid Lymphadenopathy

Sarcoidosis is characterized by noncaseating granulomatous inflammation within lymph nodes and other tissues and is often associated with lymphadenopathy (Figure 5.76). The granulomas are well formed with crisp edges and are often tightly packed (Figure 5.77). The granulomas may contain multinucleated giant cells (Figure 5.78), and occasional histiocytes may contain cytoplasmic inclusions called asteroid bodies (Figure 5.79). While asteroid bodies are often associated with sarcoid, they are nonspecific and can also be seen in other conditions.[29] Degenerative changes and focal necrosis (but not caseous necrosis) may be seen in the center of the granulomas in sarcoid lymphadenopathy (Figure 5.80). Fibrosis may surround the granulomas later in the course of disease.

Immunostains and special stains do not play a large role in the diagnosis of sarcoid lymphadenopathy; however, due to the presence of the granulomas, special stains for microorganisms (fungi and acid-fast bacilli [AFB]) are recommended. The CD4:CD8 ratio of the background T-cells is often elevated in well-developed sarcoid lymphadenopathy.[30]

SAMPLE SIGNOUT: Sarcoid Lymphadenopathy

1. Lymph node (excisional biopsy): Lymph node with noncaseating granulomatous inflammation. See note.

Note: Special stains for microorganisms (AFB, Grocott-Gomori methenamine silver [GMS]) are negative. In the appropriate clinical context, these findings are compatible with sarcoidosis lymphadenopathy.

Mycobacterium Tuberculosis

Hilar lymph nodes in patients with tuberculosis can show granulomatous inflammation. The granulomas often show caseous necrosis and may be surrounded by fibrosis (see Chapter 9). The mycobacteria can be identified using various special stains for AFB. An auramine-rhodamine fluorescent dye is more sensitive than the typical special stains, but an immunofluorescence microscope is needed to interpret the stain.[31]

IgG4-Related Lymphadenopathy

As covered in Chapter 2, IgG4-related lymphadenopathy may contain distinctive granulomas that curve around reactive germinal centers (Figure 5.81, also see Chapter 1). These granulomas often contain admixed eosinophils.

EXTENSIVE/DIFFUSE

Histiocytic Lymphadenopathy Associated With Joint Replacement ("Particle Disease")

Patients with metal joint prostheses can exhibit an inflammatory reaction against particles generated by wear and tear on the prosthesis.[32] This reaction typically results in enlarged

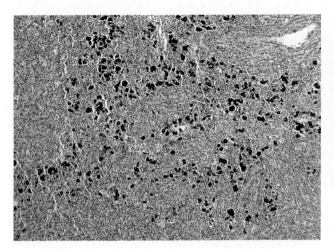

Figure 5.71. Low-power view of tattoo powder in histiocytes.

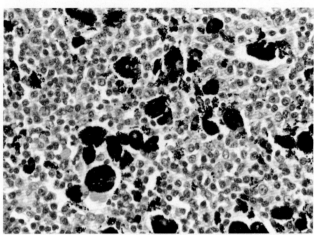

Figure 5.72. High-power view of tattoo power in histiocytes illustrating the chunky, granular texture.

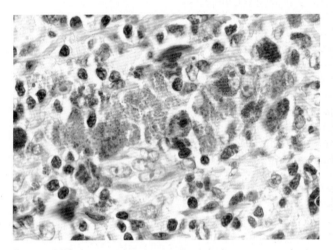

Figure 5.73. Hemosiderin and melanin in histiocytes in dermatopathic lymphadenopathy. Both are granular, but hemosiderin is somewhat chunkier with a golden brown color. Hemosiderin is refractile, whereas melanin is nonrefractile.

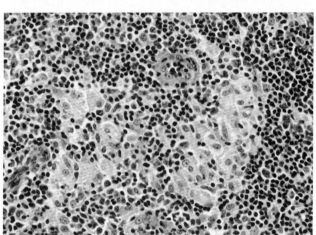

Figure 5.74. Clusters of epithelioid histiocytes in *Toxoplasma* lymphadenopathy.

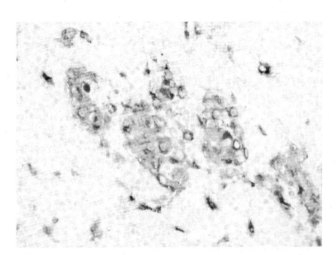

Figure 5.75. The clusters of epithelioid histiocytes in *Toxoplasma* lymphadenopathy are highlighted by a CD68 immunostain.

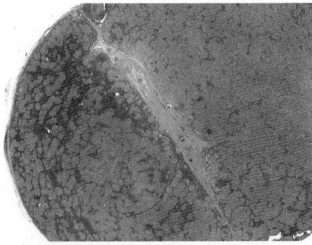

Figure 5.76. Low-power view of a hilar lymph node involved by sarcoidosis.

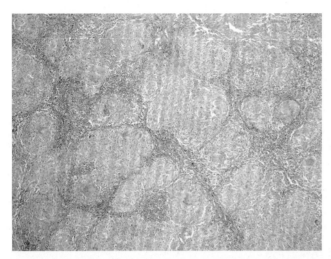

Figure 5.77. The granulomas in sarcoidosis are well-formed and often tightly packed and may be surrounded by fibrosis.

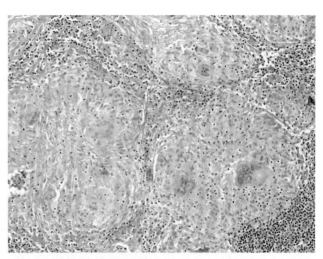

Figure 5.78. The granulomas of sarcoid lymphadenopathy often contain multinucleated giant cells.

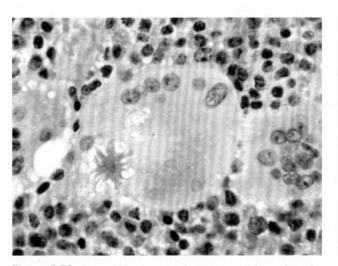

Figure 5.79. Asteroid bodies may be present in the multinucleated giant cells of sarcoid lymphadenopathy, but they are not specific for sarcoidosis.

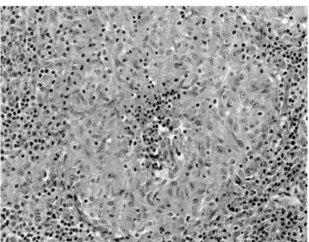

Figure 5.80. While the granulomas in sarcoid lymphadenopathy do not show caseous necrosis, necrotic foci can occasionally be identified.

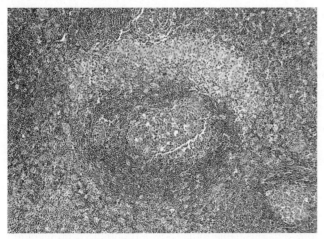

Figure 5.81. Lymphadenopathy associated with increased IgG4+ plasma cells often shows distinctive granulomas that curve around reactive follicles. The granulomas usually contain admixed eosinophils.

regional lymph nodes that drain the area of the prosthesis. These nodes demonstrate sheets and cords of foamy histiocytes that contain debris, including metal fragments and polarizable material (Figures 5.82-5.85).

Hemophagocytic Lymphohistiocytosis

Patients with hemophagocytic lymphohistiocytosis (HLH, hemophagocytic syndrome) can show a marked increase in histiocytes within lymph nodes (Figures 5.86 and 5.87). These histiocytes may or may not exhibit hemophagocytosis (Figures 5.88 and 5.89).[33] Unlike sinus histiocytosis with massive lymphadenopathy (SHML or Rosai-Dorfman disease), in which the histiocytes contain intact cells, the histiocytes in HLH contain a mixture of intact cells and cellular debris (Figure 5.90). Additionally, the increased histiocytes in HLH are not limited to the sinuses. It should be noted that the diagnosis of HLH is based on clinical criteria, and while lymph node (and bone marrow) findings are supportive, correlation with numerous other clinical and laboratory criteria are necessary for a definitive diagnosis.

Atypical Mycobacterial Infection

Atypical mycobacterial infections in immunocompromised patients can result in spindle cell pseudotumor, in which the lymph node is partially or completely replaced by spindled histiocytes that have engulfed mycobacterial organisms. This lesion can mimic a soft-tissue tumor, but special stains for AFB are diagnostic (Figures 5.91-5.96).[34]

VASCULAR CHANGES

The small vessels within lymph nodes are part of the paracortex. Vessels are frequently increased in paracortical hyperplasia, but can also show a marked increase or other abnormalities in specific conditions.

VASCULAR PROLIFERATION

Castleman Lymphadenopathy, Hyaline Vascular Variant

The hyaline vascular variant of Castleman disease (HV-CD) typically presents as a large mass involving a lymph node or lymph node group. HV-CD often involves the mediastinum, but can occur at other locations as well.[35] HV-CD is usually localized to a focal anatomic location, which is referred to as "unicentric disease." The mass may be detected incidentally or the patient may have symptoms related to the mass itself, but systemic symptoms are rare in the hyaline vascular variant. Interestingly, HV-CD has been postulated to be a precursor of follicular dendritic cell sarcoma.[36]

Interfollicular changes in HV-CD include a marked vascular proliferation (Figures 5.97 and 5.98). Some of the vessels may show sclerosis (Figure 5.99). The background cells in the interfollicular area are small lymphocytes with admixed eosinophils, plasma cells, and immunoblasts; however, sheets of plasma cells are not seen (Figures 5.100 and 5.101). The interfollicular area may also contain nodules of plasmacytoid dendritic cells (Figures 5.102-5.105). These nodules often have interspersed tingible body macrophages but have a low Ki-67 proliferation index (Figure 5.106). The scattered atypical follicles are the hallmark of HV-CD. They are typically atretic with occasional penetrating vessels. The mantle zones show a characteristic concentric distribution and may contain more than one germinal center (Figure 5.107). Of note, the HHV-8+ subtype of the plasma cell variant of Castleman lymphadenopathy (HHV+ PC-CD; discussed below) can also show increased vascularity within the interfollicular areas.

Angiomyomatous Hamartoma

Occasionally, lymphadenopathy results from abnormal vasculature or vascular tumors.[37] Lymph nodes involved by angiomyomatous hamartoma show a pronounced proliferation of haphazardly arranged, variably sized, thick-walled blood vessels in a background of collagen, hemorrhage, adipose tissue, and areas of benign smooth muscle proliferation (Figure 5.108).[38] Neither nuclear atypia nor mitotic activity is readily identified. Islands of residual

Figure 5.82. Patients with joint replacements can show extensive replacement of the node by foamy histiocytes.

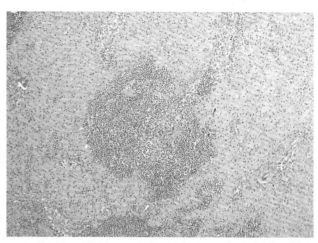

Figure 5.83. Higher power view of histiocytes surrounding a follicle and replacing the paracortex in a patient with a joint replacement.

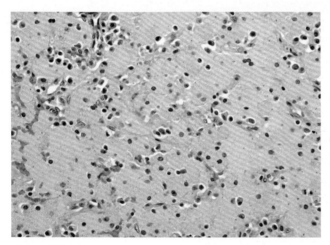

Figure 5.84. The histiocytes in "particle disease" have abundant pale cytoplasm.

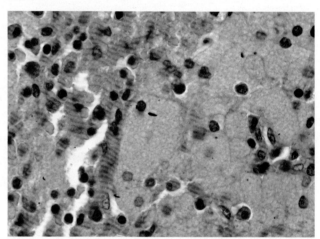

Figure 5.85. Small fragments of metal can occasionally be seen in particle disease (center), and the debris is often polarizable.

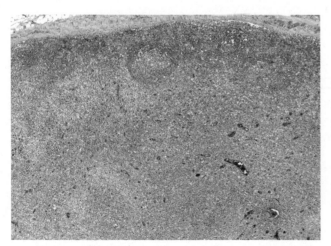

Figure 5.86. An enlarged lymph node in a patient with hemophagocytic lymphohistiocytosis shows a proliferation of histiocytes that expand the paracortex.

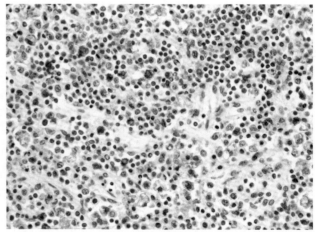

Figure 5.87. The histiocytes are highlighted by a CD68 immunostain.

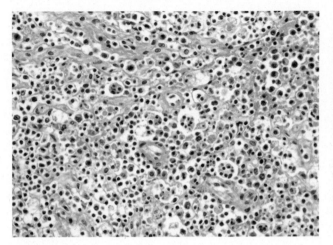

Figure 5.88. The histiocytes in the lymph nodes of patients with hemophagocytic lymphohistiocytosis frequently demonstrate hemophagocytosis.

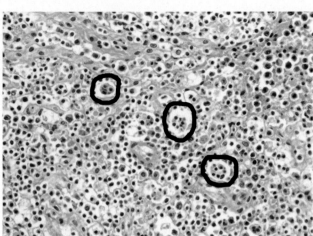

Figure 5.89. Annotated image (Figure 5.88) with several of the hemophagocytic histiocytes highlighted.

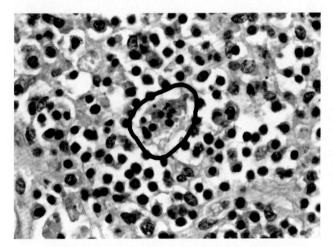

Figure 5.90. A high-power view of a hemophagocytic histiocyte. In contrast to Rosai-Dorfman disease, the material engulfed by the histiocytes in hemophagocytic lymphohistiocytosis is degraded, and cellular debris is seen in the histiocytes.

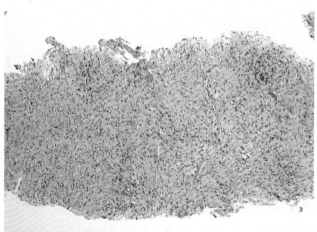

Figure 5.91. A 60-year-old man with HIV presented with retroperitoneal lymphadenopathy, and a core biopsy showed that the node was largely replaced by spindled cells.

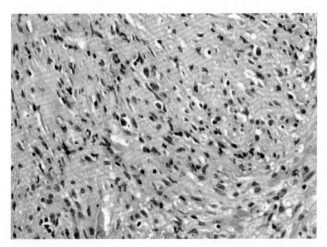

Figure 5.92. Higher power view of the spindled cells in Figure 5.91.

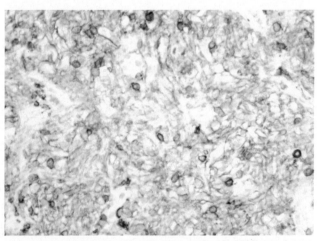

Figure 5.93. The spindled cells in the lesion in Figure 5.91 express dim CD45, indicating that the atypical cells are hematolymphoid.

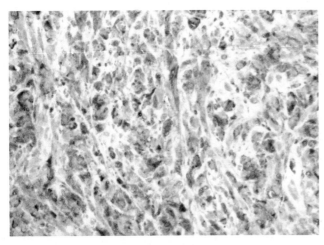

Figure 5.94. The spindled cells in the lesion in Figure 5.91 are highlighted by CD68.

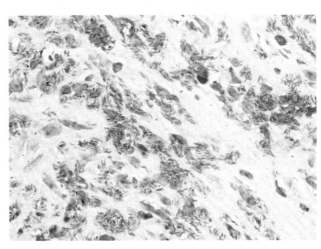

Figure 5.95. An acid-fast bacilli (AFB) special stain demonstrates that the histiocytes are packed with AFB+ atypical mycobacteria.

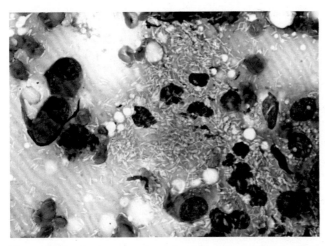

Figure 5.96. Touch preparations of spindle cell pseudotumors may help to identify the organisms, which are not stained by a Wright-Giemsa stain.

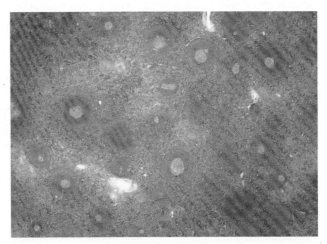

Figure 5.97. An enlarged lymph node involved by the hyaline vascular variant of Castleman lymphadenopathy shows expansion of the interfollicular areas with a pronounced vascular proliferation.

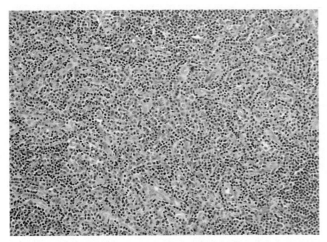

Figure 5.98. High-power view of the interfollicular vascular proliferation in the hyaline vascular variant of Castleman lymphadenopathy.

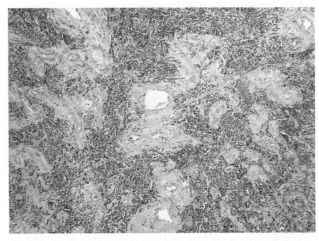

Figure 5.99. Vessels in the hyaline vascular variant of Castleman lymphadenopathy can show sclerosis.

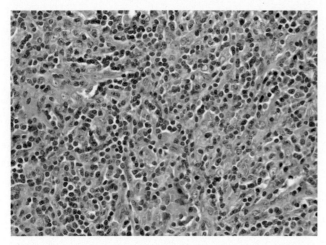

Figure 5.100. The cells in the interfollicular area of the hyaline vascular variant of Castleman lymphadenopathy are a mixture of small lymphocytes, plasma cells, immunoblasts, and eosinophils.

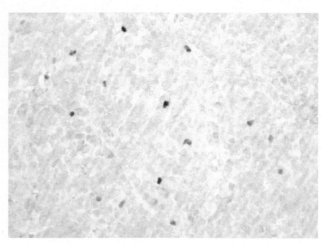

Figure 5.101. The interfollicular areas of the hyaline vascular variant of Castleman lymphadenopathy may contain scattered TdT+ cells. Scattered TdT+ cells can also be seen in follicular dendritic cell sarcoma, which may occur in association with or following HV-CD.

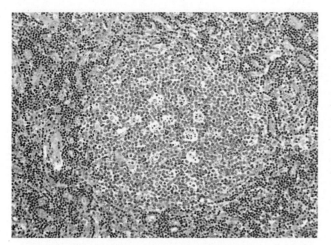

Figure 5.102. Nodules of plasmacytoid dendritic cells may be seen in the hyaline vascular variant of Castleman lymphadenopathy.

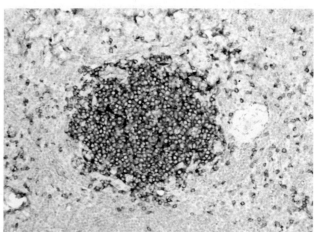

Figure 5.103. CD123 highlights the nodules of plasmacytoid dendritic cells. These cells are also positive for TCL-1 (TCL-1 immunostain not shown).

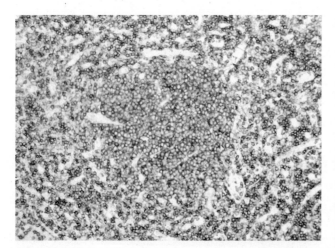

Figure 5.104. The nodules of plasmacytoid dendritic cells are CD4-positive.

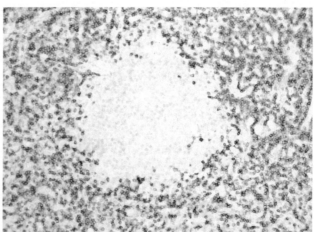

Figure 5.105. The nodules of plasmacytoid dendritic cells are CD3-negative.

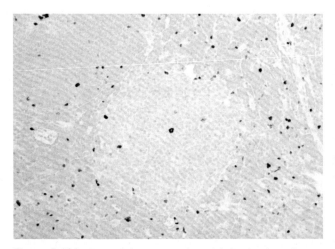

Figure 5.106. Despite the scattered tingible body macrophages, the nodules of plasmacytoid dendritic cells in the hyaline vascular variant of Castleman lymphadenopathy have a low Ki-67 proliferation index.

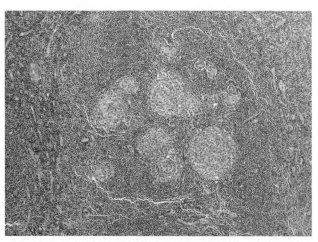

Figure 5.107. One mantle zone may contain multiple germinal centers in the hyaline vascular variant of Castleman lymphadenopathy. This is often referred to as "twinning" when one mantle zone contains two atretic germinal centers. The follicle in this image, however, appears to be having higher order multiples.

normal lymph node are present between the increased vasculatures (Figure 5.109). The vessels are highlighted by immunostains for ERG (Figure 5.110) and CD34, and HHV-8 and HMB45 immunostains are negative.

ABNORMALITIES OF VESSEL WALLS

Amyloid and Light Chain Deposition

Both amyloid and light chains can show widespread deposition; however, both have a tendency to involve vessel walls. The involved vessels appear somewhat thickened or disrupted by the deposition of amorphous eosinophilic material.

Amyloid is readily identified by its characteristic salmon pink staining with a Congo red special stain and apple green birefringence under polarized light (Figure 5.111). Amyloid deposition can be seen in a localized pattern in association with marginal zone lymphoma or in a systemic pattern in association with a plasma cell neoplasm. Amyloidosis is often, but not always, associated with lambda light chain–positive neoplasms.

Light chain deposition disease, on the other hand, is more strongly correlated with kappa light chain expression by the associated neoplasm. As with amyloidosis, light chain deposition can be localized or systemic.[39,40] The light chain may deposit as eosinophilic cords within the vessels (Figure 5.112) and can incite a vigorous foreign body giant cell response (Figure 5.113). The light chain deposits are not highlighted by a Congo red stain. Mass spectroscopy of the tissue may be required for definitive diagnosis.

Mantle Cell Lymphoma

Mantle cell lymphoma often shows hyalinized vessel walls (Figure 5.114).

EXPANSION/INFILTRATION OF THE PARACORTEX BY UNEXPECTED CELLS

Occasionally, a lymph node contains scattered follicles, but the paracortex is no longer composed of a polymorphous mixture of mature lymphocytes, immunoblasts, and histiocytes. Instead, the paracortex is expanded or replaced by a proliferation of one cell type or by cells that are not typically found in the paracortex. These "unauthorized" cells can, of course, include metastatic carcinoma and melanoma; however, lymph node involvement by nonhematolymphoid neoplasms is not covered in this section.

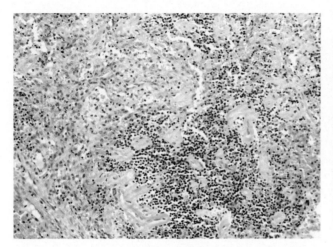

Figure 5.108. This lymph node contains a proliferation of thick-walled blood vessels and areas of smooth muscle proliferation, which are characteristics of angiomyomatous hamartoma.

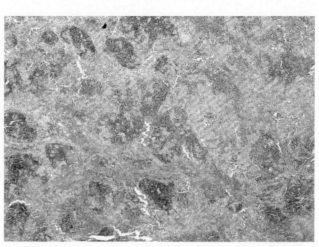

Figure 5.109. A low-power view of a lymph node involved by angiomyomatous hamartoma, showing the residual islands of lymphoid tissue. These islands are often most prominent at the periphery of the node.

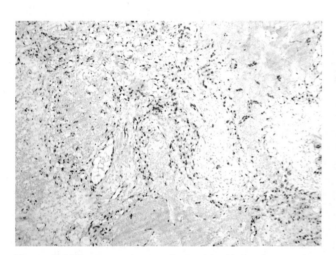

Figure 5.110. An immunostain for ERG highlights the vessels in angiomyomatous hamartoma.

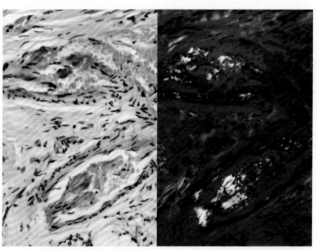

Figure 5.111. Amyloid deposition often involves vessels walls. The left side of the image is a Congo red stain, with salmon pink staining of the amyloid. The right side of the image shows the Congo red stain under polarized light; the amyloid demonstrates apple green birefringence.

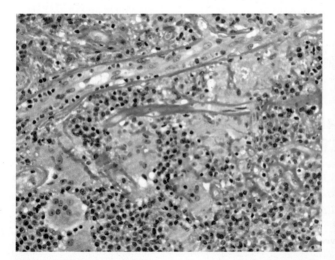

Figure 5.112. Eosinophilic material deposited along vessels in light chain deposition disease.

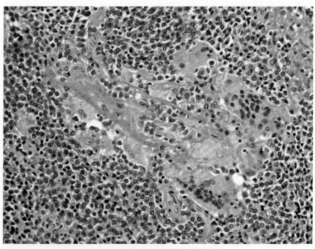

Figure 5.113. The deposits of light chains are often associated with a foreign body giant cell response.

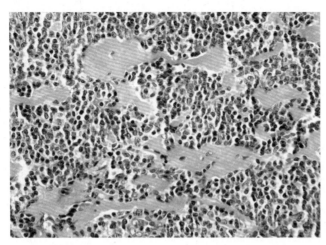

Figure 5.114. Vessels in mantle cell lymphoma are frequently hyalinized.

ATYPICAL LYMPHOCYTES/LYMPHOMAS

Both aggressive and low-grade lymphomas can involve lymph nodes in an interfollicular pattern, sparing scattered follicles. This is occasionally seen in CLL/SLL and mantle cell lymphoma (Figures 5.115-5.121).[41] Aggressive lymphomas less frequently show this distribution, as the rapidly proliferating neoplastic cells tend to grow quickly, obliterating the nodal architecture. An interfollicular pattern is, however, occasionally seen in aggressive neoplasms, particularly with peripheral T-cell lymphomas and lymphoblastic lymphomas (Figures 5.122-5.128).

Classical Hodgkin lymphoma can also show an unusual interfollicular distribution (Figures 5.129-5.133), as covered in more detail in Chapter 1 ("Near Misses").

PLASMA CELLS

Castleman Lymphadenopathy, Plasma Cell Variant

In addition to the HV-CD (discussed above), there is also a plasma cell variant of Castleman disease (PC-CD).[35] PC-CD comes in several flavors: unicentric versus multicentric and HHV-8-positive versus HHV-8-negative. The further subclassification of PC-CD can be somewhat confusing. In brief, there are two clinical conditions associated with PC-CD: unicentric and multicentric disease. As with HV-CD, unicentric disease refers to localized disease, whereas patients with multicentric disease have widespread adenopathy and systemic symptoms. Multicentric PC-CD is often, but not invariably, associated with HHV-8-positive disease. Distinguishing between unicentric and multicentric disease requires clinical correlation, and distinguishing between HHV-8-positive versus HHV-8-negative disease requires an HHV-8 immunostain.

The sinuses in all forms of PC-CD are typically patent, and there is a marked expansion of the interfollicular region and medullary cords by sheets of plasma cells. The follicles in PC-CD also tend to show some of the changes that are seen in HV-CD, though to a lesser degree. The histologic findings in the HHV-8-positive (Figures 5.133-5.137) and HHV-8-negative (Figures 5.138-5.140) subtypes of PC-CD are similar. The HHV-8-positive variant of PC-CD tends to show some features of HV-CD, including interfollicular vascular proliferation and follicular changes, neither of which is pronounced in the HHV-8-negative variant. However, as noted above, it is necessary to do an HHV-8 immunostain to differentiate between HHV-8-positive and HHV-8-negative PC-CD.

HHV-8-positive PC-CD contains scattered HHV-8+ cells in the mantle zone, some of which are large plasmablasts (Figure 5.141). Additionally, HHV-8 can sometimes stain follicular dendritic cell meshworks within the follicles (Figure 5.142). The interfollicular plasma cells may express a mixture of kappa and lambda light chains in both HHV-8-negative and HHV-8-positive PC-CD (Figure 5.143). However, the HHV-8-positive plasmablasts in HHV-8+ PC-CD are often lambda-positive, and the plasma cells in HHV-8-positive PC-CD are infrequently lambda light chain-restricted.[42]

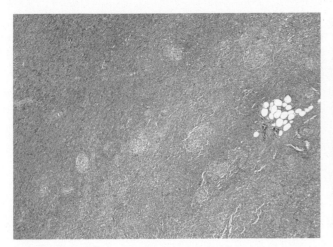

Figure 5.115. Expansion of the interfollicular space by small lymphocytes in mantle cell lymphoma, with sparing of scattered germinal centers.

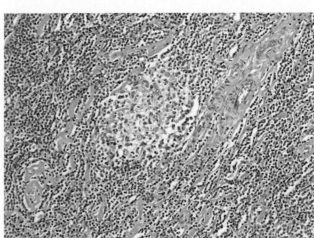

Figure 5.116. A higher power view of a germinal center with surrounding monotonous small lymphocytes in Figure 5.115. The hyalinized vessels often seen in mantle cell lymphoma are also seen in this image.

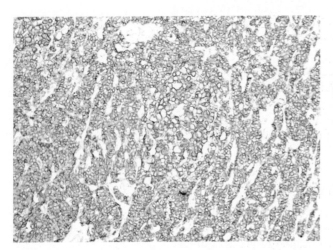

Figure 5.117. A CD20 immunostain of the follicle in Figure 5.116. The cells in the germinal center are slightly larger than the surrounding lymphocytes.

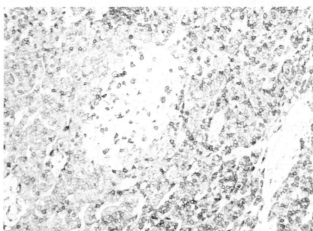

Figure 5.118. CD5 is dimly expressed on the interfollicular small B-cells in Figures 5.116 and 5.117. The small lymphocytes that express relatively bright CD5 are residual normal T-cells.

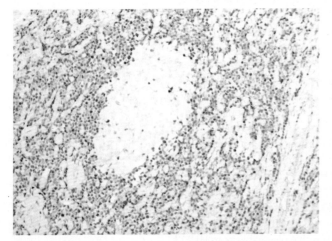

Figure 5.119. The interfollicular small B-cells in Figures 5.116-5.118 are positive for Cyclin D1, confirming the diagnosis of mantle cell lymphoma.

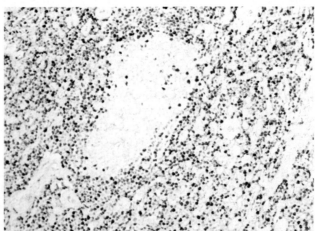

Figure 5.120. The interfollicular small B-cells in Figures 5.116-5.119 are also positive for Sox-11, as is frequently seen in mantle cell lymphoma.

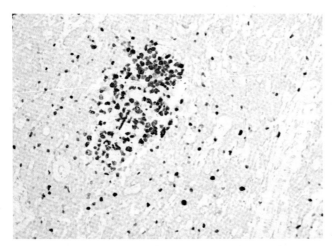

Figure 5.121. The mantle cell lymphoma cells in Figures 5.116-5.120 have a low Ki-67 proliferation index, although the proliferation index within the residual germinal center is appropriately high.

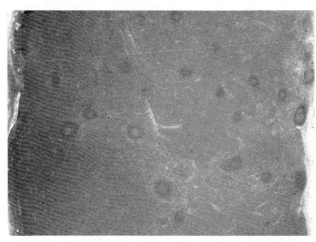

Figure 5.122. Expansion of the interfollicular space by lymphoblasts in nodal involvement by T-lymphoblastic lymphoma.

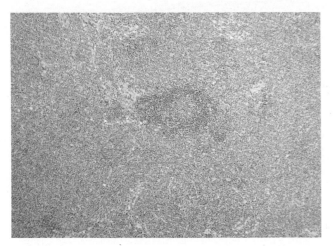

Figure 5.123. A higher power view of the atypical infiltrate that expands the paracortex in Figure 5.122.

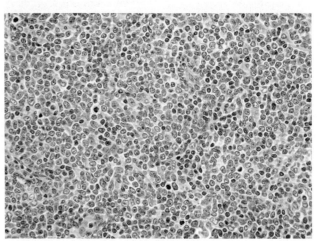

Figure 5.124. The atypical interfollicular cells in Figure 5.122 have fine chromatin and occasional mitotic figures are seen.

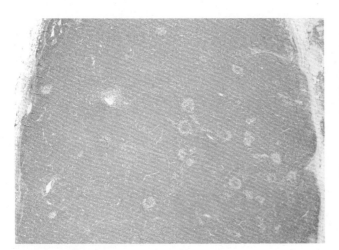

Figure 5.125. An immunostain for CD3 highlights the atypical cells that expand the interfollicular areas in the lymph node in Figure 5.122.

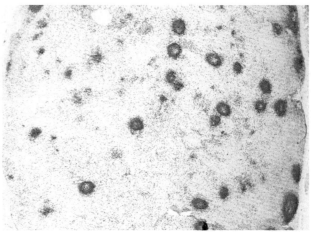

Figure 5.126. CD20 marks residual follicles in Figure 5.122.

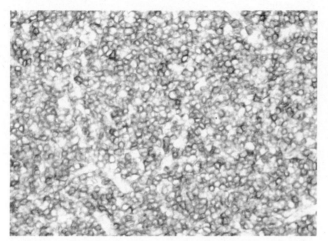

Figure 5.127. An immunostain for CD7 demonstrates that the atypical T-cell infiltrate shows relatively bright expression of CD7, which would be unusual for a mature T-cell lymphoma.

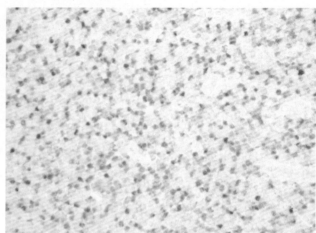

Figure 5.128. The atypical T-cells are positive for TdT, confirming a diagnosis of nodal infiltration by T-lymphoblastic lymphoma.

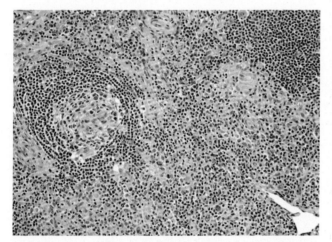

Figure 5.129. A cervical lymph node in a 46-year-old woman showed a mixed inflammatory infiltrate in between follicles.

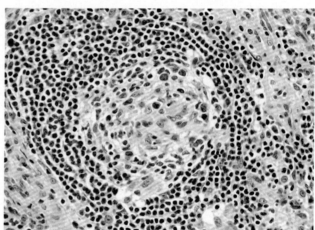

Figure 5.130. Some of the follicles show Castleman-like changes, which has been associated with interfollicular classical Hodgkin lymphoma.

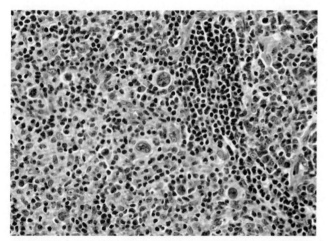

Figure 5.131. A higher power view of the interfollicular areas in the lymph node in Figure 5.129 shows a mixture of small lymphocytes, eosinophils, histiocytes, plasma cells, and large atypical cells with prominent nucleoli.

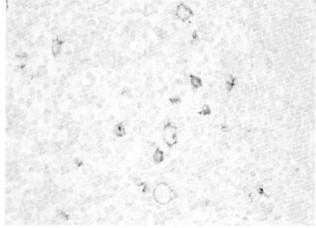

Figure 5.132. A CD30 immunostain highlights the atypical cells in Figure 5.131.

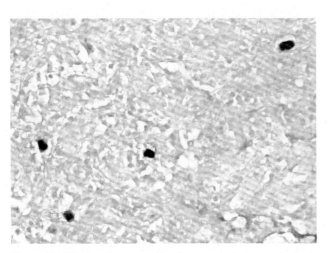

Figure 5.133. The large atypical cells in Figure 5.131 are also highlighted by an in situ hybridization for EBV (EBER), confirming the diagnosis of classical Hodgkin lymphoma.

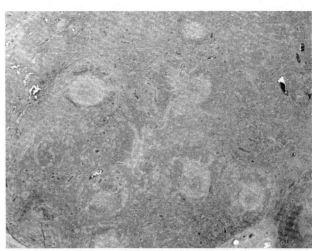

Figure 5.134. The HHV-8+ plasma cell variant of Castleman disease shows an expansion of the paracortex with increased vasculature.

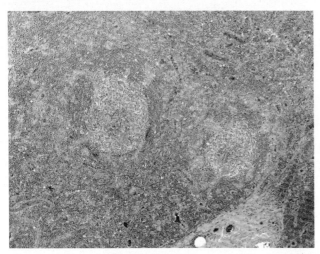

Figure 5.135. A higher power view of a lymph node involved by HHV-8+ Castleman disease. The follicles show some features of the hyaline vascular variant of Castleman disease, including layered mantle zones and somewhat atretic follicles with penetrating vessels.

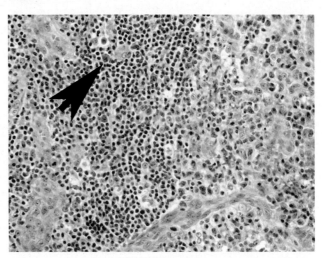

Figure 5.136. The mantle zone of follicles in HHV-8+ Castleman disease often contain scattered large immunoblasts or plasmablasts (arrow).

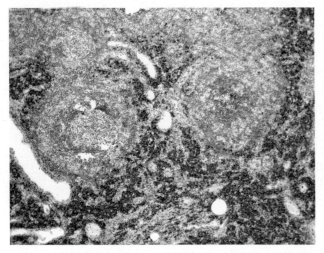

Figure 5.137. CD138 marks the increased interfollicular plasma cells in the HHV-8+ plasma cell variant of Castleman lymphadenopathy.

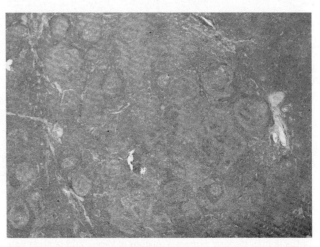

Figure 5.138. The HHV-8-negative plasma cell variant of Castleman disease shows an expansion of the paracortex. This case also contains numerous follicles.

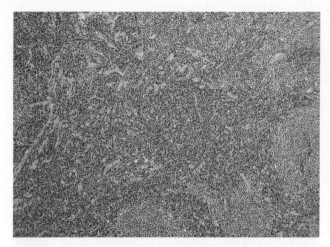

Figure 5.139. A higher power view of the interfollicular area of the HHV-8-negative plasma cell variant of Castleman disease in Figure 5.138. Plasma cells are markedly increased.

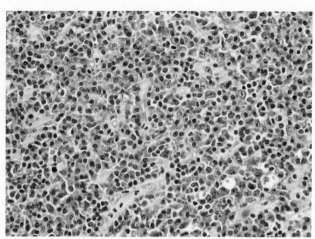

Figure 5.140. The plasma cells in the HHV-8-negative plasma cell variant of Castleman disease are morphologically unremarkable.

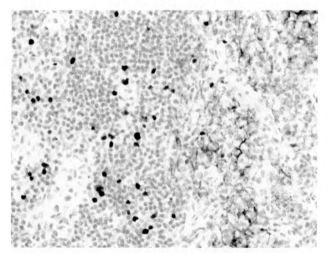

Figure 5.141. HHV-8 stains scattered cells in the HHV-8+ plasma cell variant of Castleman disease. These cells are concentrated in the mantle zone (left side of the image), but can also be seen in between follicles. HHV-8 often stains the large plasmablasts in the mantle.

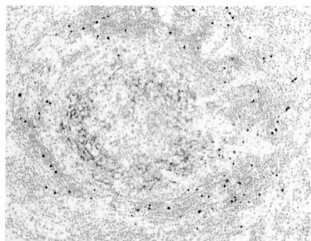

Figure 5.142. HHV-8 can also stain the follicular dendritic meshworks in the HHV-8+ plasma cell variant of Castleman disease.

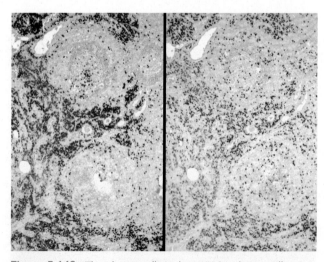

Figure 5.143. The plasma cells in the HHV-8+ plasma cell variant of Castleman disease express a mixture of kappa and lambda light chains (in situ hybridization for kappa light chain on the left and lambda light chain on the right). The plasmablasts in the mantle zone disproportionately express lambda light chain.

KEY FEATURES: Castleman Lymphadenopathy

Subtype	HHV-8?	Unicentric (Localized)	Multicentric (Involves Multiple Regions)	Systemic Symptoms	Notes
Hyaline vascular variant	–	Usually	Rare	Rare	Most common form of Castleman disease; associated with follicular dendritic cell sarcoma
Plasma cell variant	–	Sometimes	Sometimes	Frequent	May be associated with POEMS syndrome (poly-neuropathy, organomegaly, endocrinopathy, monoclonal gammopathy, skin changes)
	+	Rare	Frequent	Frequent	May be seen in HIV- and HIV+ patients

Rheumatoid Lymphadenopathy

Patients with rheumatoid arthritis (RA) often have lymphadenopathy at some point in the course of the disease.[24] Involved lymph nodes are enlarged with intact nodal architecture. They typically show follicular hyperplasia without paracortical hyperplasia, but interfollicular plasma cells are increased (Figures 5.144-5.146). Clinical correlation is critical for making this diagnosis. Additionally, patients with RA are often treated with immunosuppressive agents, and careful evaluation for involvement by an iatrogenic immunodeficiency-associated lymphoproliferative disorder is recommended.[43]

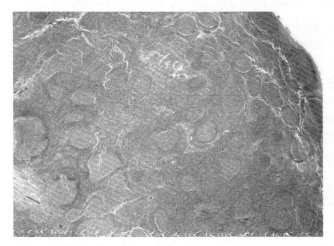

Figure 5.144. This enlarged lymph node from a 58-year-old woman shows the common features of rheumatoid lymphadenopathy, namely follicular hyperplasia and interfollicular plasmacytosis without prominent paracortical hyperplasia.

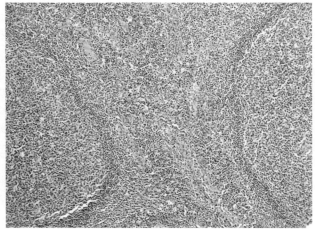

Figure 5.145. Plasma cells are increased in between the reactive follicles.

CHECKLIST: Lymph Nodes With Increased Plasma Cells

HIV lymphadenopathy	Increased plasma cells in long-standing HIV lymphadenopathy
Kaposi sarcoma	HHV-8+ vascular proliferation with increased interfollicular plasma cells
Rheumatoid lymphadenopathy	Florid follicular hyperplasia with increased interfollicular plasma cells
Castleman lymphadenopathy, plasma cell variant	HHV-8-positive or HHV-8-negative Can be seen in association with POEMS syndrome (polyneuropathy, organomegaly, endocrinopathy, monoclonal gammopathy, skin changes)
Involvement by a plasma cell neoplasm	CD138+ plasma cells are monoclonal and are phenotypically abnormal (ie, aberrant expression of CD56, CD117, Cyclin D1, CD20)
Marginal zone lymphoma with extensive plasma cell differentiation	Plasma cells often show limited or variable expression of CD138, usually associated with a population of clonal mature B-cells

SPINDLED CELLS
Mastocytosis

Systemic mastocytosis (SM) can show lymph node involvement, with partial replacement of the paracortex.[44] The mast cells are spindled, and there are typically admixed eosinophils (Figures 5.147 and 5.148). Normal mast cells express CD117 (bright), mast cell tryptase, and calretinin. The mast cells in SM express one or more of these markers (Figures 5.149 and 5.150), but typically show immunophenotypic abnormalities as well, including aberrant expression of CD2, CD25 (Figure 5.151), and/or CD30; loss of mast cell tryptase expression; and variation in the intensity of CD117 expression (Figure 5.152).[45] SM is associated with an activating point mutation at codon 816 in the KIT gene, which can be confirmed via molecular studies on formalin-fixed and paraffin-embedded tissue.

CHECKLIST: Conditions Associated With Eosinophils in Lymph Nodes

Dermatopathic lymphadenopathy
IgG4-related lymphadenopathy
Kimura lymphadenopathy
Drug-associated lymphadenopathy
Castleman disease, hyaline vascular variant
Classical Hodgkin lymphoma
Angioimmunoblastic T-cell lymphoma
Peripheral T-cell lymphoma, NOS
Myeloid sarcoma
Myeloid/lymphoid neoplasms with eosinophilia and gene rearrangements (*PDGFRA, PDGFRB, FGFR1*)
Systemic mastocytosis
Langerhans cell histiocytosis

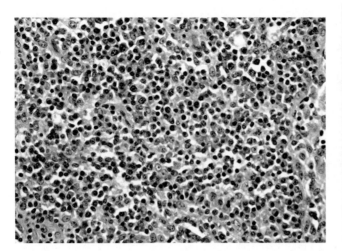

Figure 5.146. The interfollicular plasma cells are morphologically unremarkable and are polytypic (kappa and lambda immunostains not shown).

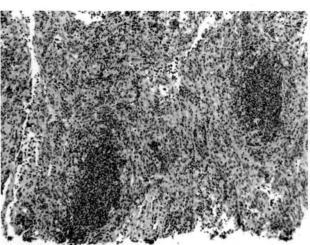

Figure 5.147. A core biopsy of an enlarged precaval node in a 45-year-old man with lymphadenopathy, splenomegaly, diarrhea, nausea, chronic back pain, a maculopapular rash throughout the body, skin hyperpigmentation, and night sweats. The interfollicular areas contain a proliferation of pale, spindled cells.

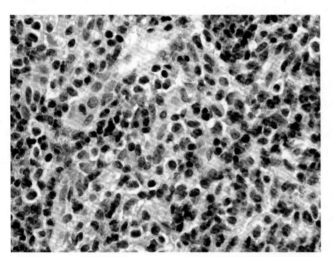

Figure 5.148. A higher power view of the biopsy in Figure 5.147 shows that the interfollicular areas contain numerous admixed eosinophils.

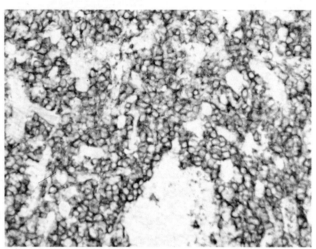

Figure 5.149. The atypical cells in between the follicles in Figure 5.147 express bright CD117.

Figure 5.150. The atypical cells in between the follicles in Figure 5.147 express calretinin.

Figure 5.151. The atypical mast cells in Figure 5.147 express aberrant CD25. Abnormal mast cells can also express aberrant CD2 or CD30.

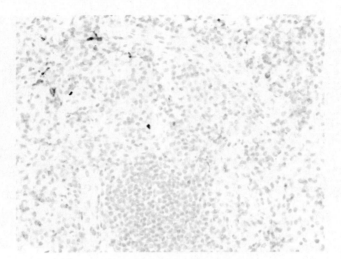

Figure 5.152. The atypical mast cells in Figure 5.147 show complete loss of mast cell tryptase. Rare normal mast cells are highlighted by the stain. The finding indicates that this patient may not show the increased tryptase characteristic of systemic mastocytosis.

NECROSIS

Kikuchi lymphadenitis and systemic lupus lymphadenitis are virtually indistinguishable morphologically. Kikuchi lymphadenitis tends to affect young women and often involves cervical nodes.

The histiocytic necrotizing lymphadenitis seen in both of these entities often shows a paracortical distribution (Figures 5.153 and 5.154). The necrotic areas entirely lack neutrophils ("aneutrophilic necrosis"; Figure 5.155). The presence of any neutrophils should prompt investigation for other causes of necrosis, including stains for microorganisms. Additionally, granulomas and giant cells are not typically seen in Kikuchi lymphadenitis.

SAMPLE SIGNOUT: Kikuchi and/or Systemic Lupus Erythematosus Lymphadenopathy

1. Lymph node (excisional biopsy): Histiocytic necrotizing lymphadenitis. See note.

Note: There is no morphologic or immunophenotypic evidence of lymphoma in the submitted material. The findings of patchy aneutrophilic necrosis with abundant admixed histiocytes, immunoblasts, and plasmacytoid dendritic cells are consistent with both systemic lupus lymphadenitis and Kikuchi lymphadenopathy. The morphologic and immunophenotypic findings in these two conditions are similar, and clinical correlation is needed.

NEAR MISSES

HAMAZAKI-WESENBERG BODIES IN SARCOIDOSIS LYMPHADENOPATHY

Sarcoidosis frequently involves hilar lymph nodes. The involved nodes contain nonnecrotizing granulomas, which can raise the possibility of mycobacterial or fungal infection. Occasionally, small golden brown extracellular ovoid structures that may mimic budding yeast are seen (Figures 5.156 and 5.157)[46]. These bodies are not present within the granulomas. Like many fungi, these bodies are highlighted by both GMS (Figure 5.158) and periodic acid-Schiff stains; however, unlike most fungi, these ovoid bodies are also positive on a Fontana-Masson stain (Figure 5.159).

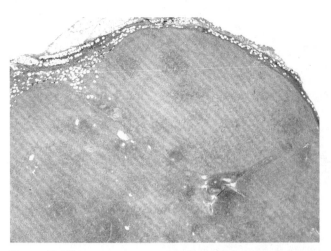

Figure 5.153. An enlarged cervical lymph node in a 28-year-old woman shows extensive necrosis involving the paracortical areas.

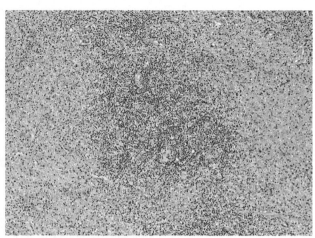

Figure 5.154. A higher power view of the lymph node in Figure 5.153 demonstrates that the necrosis spares occasional follicles.

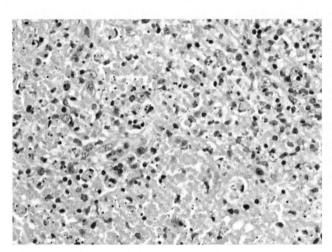

Figure 5.155. The necrosis entirely lacks neutrophils ("aneutrophilic necrosis") and there are occasional admixed histiocytes with C-shaped nuclei. This pattern is characteristic of both Kikuchi and Lupus lymphadenopathy.

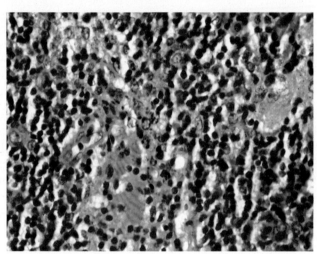

Figure 5.156. A lymph node in a patient with sarcoidosis shows small golden brown ovid bodies, some of which appear to be budding.

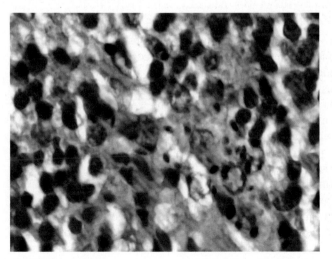

Figure 5.157. A higher power view of the Hamazaki-Wesenberg bodies in Figure 5.156.

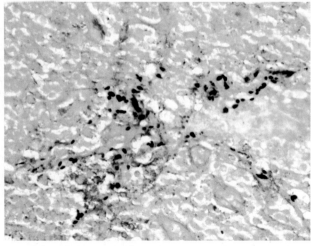

Figure 5.158. The Hamazaki-Wesenberg bodies in Figure 5.156 are highlighted on a fungal stain (GMS).

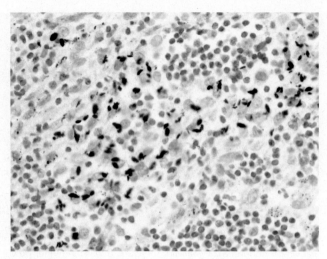

Figure 5.159. The Hamazaki-Wesenberg bodies in Figure 5.156 are also highlighted by a Fontana-Masson stain.

It is important to recognize that these represent Hamazaki-Wesenberg bodies and are not fungal forms. Hamazaki-Wesenberg bodies are frequently seen in sarcoidosis, but occasionally can be seen in other conditions as well.

INDOLENT T-LYMPHOBLASTIC PROLIFERATION

In rare cases, the paracortex (or interfollicular areas of the tonsils and adenoids) may be expanded by a proliferation of polyclonal immature T-cell precursors. These T-lymphoblasts have a cortical thymocyte-like phenotype and are CD4/CD8 double-positive cells that co-express immature markers including CD99 and TdT. Thymic epithelium is absent, the immature T-cells do not show cytomorphologic or immunophenotypic abnormalities, and the immature T-cell proliferation does not efface the nodal architecture (Figures 5.160-5.170). Bone marrow involvement is absent.

These expansions of T-cell precursors are indolent T-lymphoblastic proliferations (iT-LBP).[47] iT-LBP can be seen as an isolated finding or in association with Castleman disease, angioimmunoblastic T-cell lymphoma, or metastatic carcinoma. It is difficult to make this diagnosis in the absence of clinical information. Molecular studies are of particular value, as iT-LBP exhibits a polyclonal pattern on T-cell receptor gene rearrangement studies, whereas CD4+/CD8+ T-lymphoblastic lymphoma will show a clonal pattern.

LYMPH NODE INVOLVEMENT BY MYELOID/LYMPHOID NEOPLASMS WITH *PDGFRA* REARRANGEMENT

Clinical correlation can be critically important in making the most accurate diagnosis in lymph node pathology. An enlarged lymph node in a middle-aged woman showed atypical immature T-cells with an abnormal phenotype expanding the paracortex (Figures 5.171-5.178). Admixed eosinophils were rare; however, the patient was noted to have a pronounced eosinophilia (Figure 5.179). Bone marrow evaluation was performed in order to evaluate for marrow involvement by T-lymphoblastic leukemia/lymphoma. The marrow was markedly hypercellular with a myeloid predominance and increased eosinophils; however, there was no evidence of involvement by T-lymphoblastic leukemia (Figures 5.180 and 5.181). The lymph node specimen was submitted for fluorescence in situ hybridization (FISH) studies, which identified a *FIP1L1-PDGFRA-KIT* locus rearrangement in 76% of analyzed cells. FISH studies were negative for *PDGFRB* and *FGFR1* rearrangements.

This case illustrates the critical nature of clinical information. The eosinophilia and bone marrow findings ensured that a diagnosis of "involvement by myeloid/lymphoid neoplasm with *PDGFRA* rearrangement" was rendered on the lymph node.[48] This diagnosis has significant clinical ramifications as tyrosine kinase inhibitors are utilized in the treatment of this entity, but are not routinely used in the treatment of typical T-lymphoblastic leukemia/lymphomas.

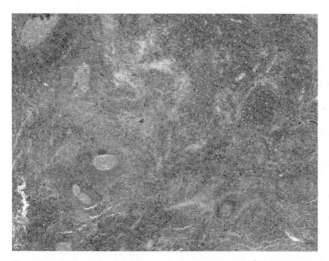

Figure 5.160. An enlarged cervical lymph node in a 22-year-old woman with a 6-year history of cervical lymphadenopathy shows expansion of the paracortex.

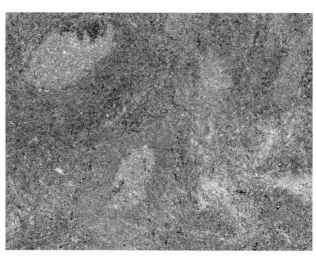

Figure 5.161. The lymph node in Figure 5.160 contains intact follicles.

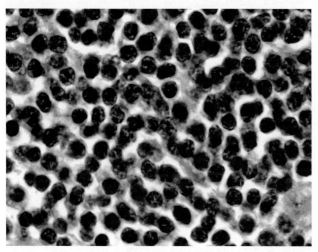

Figure 5.162. The cells that expand the paracortex in the lymph node in Figure 5.160 are small lymphocytes that do not show morphologic atypia (compare with the interfollicular lymphocytes in Figure 5.125).

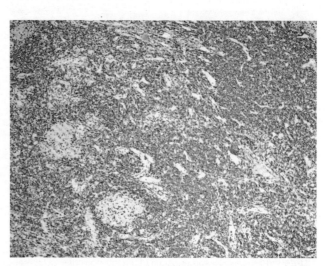

Figure 5.163. An immunostain for CD3 on the lymph node in Figure 5.160 shows that the paracortex predominantly contains CD3+ T-cells.

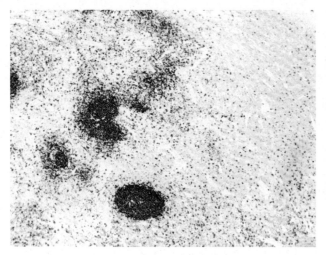

Figure 5.164. An immunostain for CD20 on the lymph node in Figure 5.160 highlights the B-cells, which are concentrated in intact follicles.

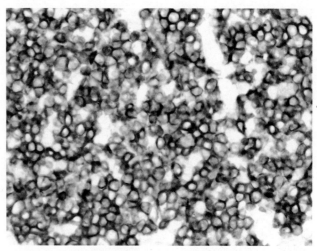

Figure 5.165. High-power view of CD3 immunostain in Figure 5.163.

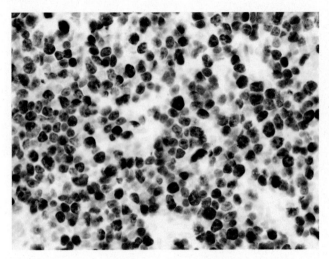

Figure 5.166. The interfollicular CD3+ cells in Figure 5.165 have an unusually high Ki-67 proliferation index.

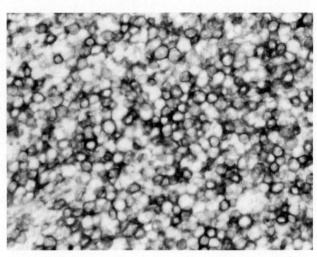

Figure 5.167. A CD4 immunostain of the interfollicular CD3+ cells in Figure 5.165.

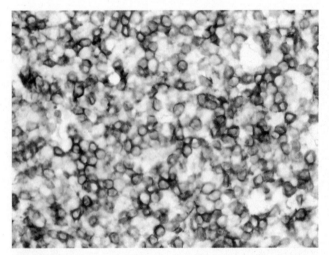

Figure 5.168. A CD8 immunostain of the interfollicular CD3+ cells in Figure 5.165 is also positive in many of the cells, compatible with CD4/CD8 double-positive T-cells.

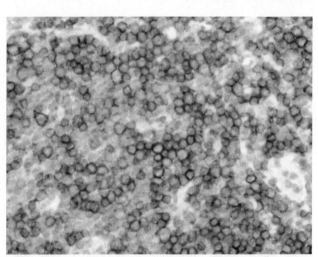

Figure 5.169. The interfollicular CD3+ cells in Figure 5.165 are positive for CD99.

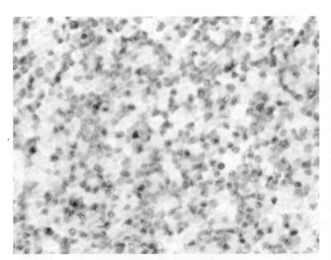

Figure 5.170. The interfollicular CD3+ cells in Figure 5.165 also express TdT, confirming an immature phenotype.

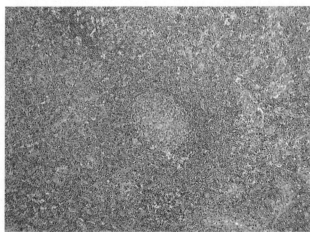

Figure 5.171. An enlarged inguinal lymph node in a 66-year-old woman shows expansion of the paracortex by small- to medium-sized lymphocytes.

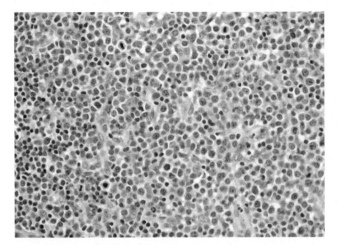

Figure 5.172. The interfollicular lymphocytes in Figure 5.171 have fine chromatin and are slightly larger than mature lymphocytes (compare with a few residual mantle zone lymphocytes in the lower left-hand corner of the image). Rare admixed eosinophils are seen.

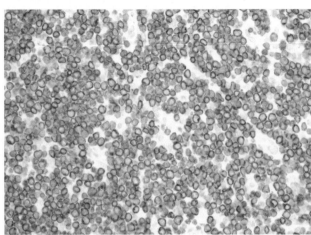

Figure 5.173. The interfollicular lymphocytes in Figure 5.172 are positive for CD3.

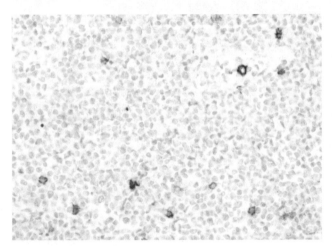

Figure 5.174. CD20 is negative on the atypical interfollicular lymphocytes in Figure 5.172.

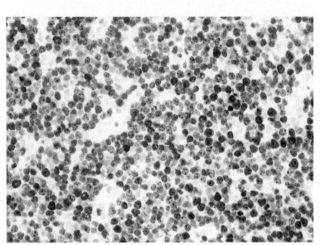

Figure 5.175. The interfollicular lymphocytes in Figure 5.172 have a very high Ki-67 proliferation index.

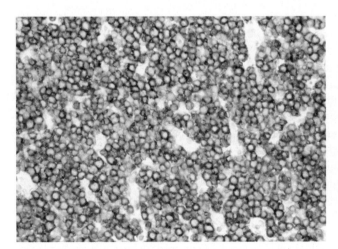

Figure 5.176. The interfollicular lymphocytes in Figure 5.172 express strong CD7. The expression of CD7 is often diminished or absent in mature T-cell neoplasms.

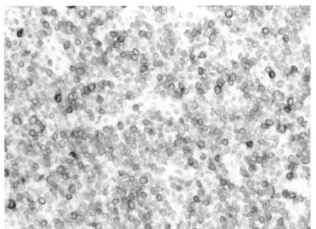

Figure 5.177. The interfollicular lymphocytes in Figure 5.172 express dim CD79a. While CD79a is typically considered to be a B-cell/plasma cell neoplasm, it is also rarely expressed on T-lymphoblastic leukemia/lymphomas.

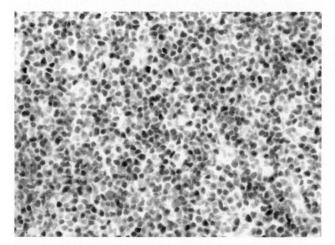

Figure 5.178. The interfollicular lymphocytes in Figure 5.172 are positive for TdT.

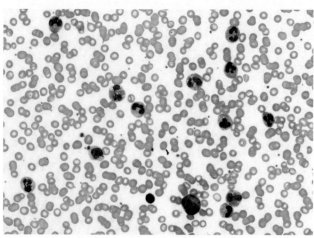

Figure 5.179. The patient whose lymph node is pictured in Figure 5.171 was noted to have a pronounced eosinophilia, as seen in her peripheral blood smear.

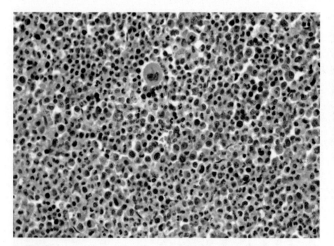

Figure 5.180. A bone marrow biopsy from this patient showed a markedly hypercellular marrow with a myeloid predominance and increased eosinophils. There was no evidence of involvement by T-lymphoblastic leukemia/lymphoma.

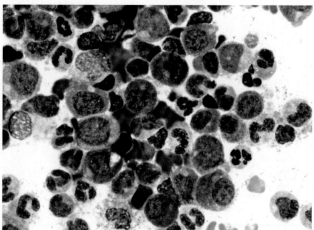

Figure 5.181. The corresponding aspirate from the biopsy in Figure 5.180 confirms the myeloid predominance with abundant eosinophils and eosinophil precursors. Blasts are not increased.

References

1. Ioachim HL, Mediros LJ. *Tumor-reactive lymphadenopathy.* In: *Ioachim's Lymph Node Pathology.* 4th ed. Philadelphia, PA: Wolters Kluwer/Lippincott Williams & Wilkins; 2009:243-247.

2. Weiss LM. Atypical phenotypes in classical Hodgkin lymphoma. *Surg Pathol Clin.* 2013;6(4):729-742.

3. Garces S, Yin CC, Miranda RN, et al. Clinical, histopathologic, and immunoarchitectural features of dermatopathic lymphadenopathy: an update. *Mod Pathol.* 2020;33(6):1104-1121.

4. Rocco N, Della Corte GA, Rispoli C, et al. Axillary masses in a woman with a history of breast cancer: dermatopathic lymphadenopathy. *Int J Surg.* 2014;12(suppl 2):S40-S43.

5. Ravindran A, Goyal G, Failing JJ, Go RS, Rech KL. Florid dermatopathic lymphadenopathy – A morphological mimic of Langerhans cell histiocytosis. *Clin Case Rep.* 2018;6(8):1637-1638.

6. Shanmugam V, Craig JW, Hornick JL, Morgan EA, Pinkus GS, Pozdnyakova O. Cyclin D1 is expressed in neoplastic cells of Langerhans cell histiocytosis but not reactive Langerhans cell proliferations. *Am J Surg Pathol.* 2017;41(10):1390-1396.

7. Burke JS, Colby TV. Dermatopathic lymphadenopathy. Comparison of cases associated and unassociated with mycosis fungoides. *Am J Surg Pathol.* 1981;5:343-352.

8. Kutok JL, Wang F. Spectrum of Epstein-Barr virus–associated diseases. *Annu Rev Pathol.* 2006;1:375-404.

9. Barros MHM, Vera-Lozada G, Segges P, Hassan R, Niedobitek G. Revisiting the tissue micro-environment of infectious mononucleosis: identification of EBV infection in T cells and deep characterization of immune profiles. *Front Immunol*. 2019;10:146.

10. Hamilton-Dutoit SJ, Pallesen G. Detection of Epstein-Barr virus small RNAs in routine paraffin sections using non-isotopic RNA/RNA in situ hybridization. *Histopathology*. 1994;25:101-111.

11. Siliézar MM, Muñoz CC, Solano-Iturri JD, et al. Spontaneously ruptured spleen samples in patients with infectious mononucleosis: analysis of histology and lymphoid subpopulations. *Am J Clin Pathol*. 2018;150(4):310-317.

12. Hodgson YA, Jones SG, Knight H, Sovani V, Fox CP. Herpes Simplex necrotic lymphadenitis masquerading as Richter's transformation in treatment-naive patients with chronic lymphocytic leukemia. *J Hematol*. 2019;8(2):79-82.

13. Heldwein EE, Krummenacher C. Entry of herpesviruses into mammalian cells. *Cell Mol Life Sci*. 2008;65(11):1653-1668.

14. Orenstein JM. The Warthin-Finkeldey-type giant cell in HIV infection, what is it? *Ultrastruct Pathol*. 1998;22(4):293-303.

15. Kalungi S, Wabinga H, Bostad L. Reactive lymphadenopathy in Ugandan patients and its relationship to EBV and HIV infection. *APMIS*. 2009;117:302-307.

16. Barrionuevo-Cornejo C, Dueñas-Hancco D. Lymphadenopathies in human immunodeficiency virus infection. *Semin Diagn Pathol*. 2018;35(1):84-91.

17. O'Byrne P, MacPherson P, DeLaplante S, Metz G, Bourgault A. Approach to lymphogranuloma venereum. *Can Fam Physician*. 2016;62(7):554-558.

18. Carithers HA. Cat-scratch disease. An overview based on a study of 1,200 patients. *Am J Dis Child*. 1985;139:1124-1133.

19. Peng J, Fan Z, Zheng H, Lu J, Zhan Y. Combined application of immunohistochemistry and Warthin-Starry silver stain on the pathologic diagnosis of cat scratch disease. *Appl Immunohistochem Mol Morphol*. 2020.

20. Allizond V, Costa C, Sidoti F, et al. Serological and molecular detection of Bartonella henselae in specimens from patients with suspected cat scratch disease in Italy: a comparative study. *PLoS One*. 2019;14(2):e0211945.

21. Martin IM, Alexander SA, Ison CA, Macdonald N, McCarthy K, Ward H. Diagnosis of lymphogranuloma venereum from biopsy samples. *Gut*. 2006;55(10):1522-1523.

22. Montoya JG, Liesenfeld O. Toxoplasmosis. *Lancet*. 2004;363(9425):1965-1976.

23. Krick JA, Remington JS. Toxoplasmosis in the adult – An overview. *N Engl J Med*. 1978;298(10):550-553.

24. Gru AA, O'Malley DP. Autoimmune and medication-induced lymphadenopathies. *Semin Diagn Pathol*. 2018;35(1):34-43.

25. Saltzstein SL, Ackerman LV. Lymphadenopathy induced by anticonvulsant drugs and mimicking clinically pathologically malignant lymphomas. *Cancer*. 1959;12:164-182.

26. Jeon YK, Paik JH, Park SS, et al. Spectrum of lymph node pathology in adult onset Still's disease; analysis of 12 patients with one follow up biopsy. *J Clin Pathol*. 2004;57(10):1052-1056.

27. Kojima M, Motoori T, Asano S, Nakamura S. Histological diversity of reactive and atypical proliferative lymph node lesions in systemic lupus erythematosus patients. *Pathol Res Pract*. 2007;203(6):423-431.

28. Kubota K, Tamura J, Kurabayashi H, Yanagisawa T, Shirakura T, Mori S. Warthin-Finkeldey-like giant cells in a patient with systemic lupus erythematosus. *Hum Pathol*. 1988;19(11):1358-1359.

29. Jorns JM, Knoepp SM. Asteroid bodies in lymph node cytology: infrequently seen and still mysterious. *Diagn Cytopathol*. 2011;39:35-36.

30. Akao K, Minezawa T, Yamamoto N, et al. Flow cytometric analysis of lymphocyte profiles in mediastinal lymphadenopathy of sarcoidosis. *PLoS One*. 2018;13(11):e0206972.

31. Annam V, Kulkarni MH, Puranik RB. Comparison of the modified fluorescent method and conventional Ziehl-Neelsen method in the detection of acidfast bacilli in lymphnode aspirates. *Cytojournal*. 2009;6:13.

32. O'Connell JX, Rosenberg AE. Histiocytic lymphadenitis associated with a large joint prosthesis. *Am J Clin Pathol*. 1993;99(3):314-316.

33. Jaffe ES. Histiocytoses of lymph nodes: biology and differential diagnosis. *Semin Diagn Pathol*. 1988;5(4):376-390.

34. Wood C, Nickoloff BJ, Todes-Taylor NR. Pseudotumor resulting from atypical mycobacterial infection: a "histoid" variety of Mycobacterium avium-intracellulare complex infection. *Am J Clin Pathol*. 1985;83(4):524-527.

35. Wang W, Medeiros LJ. Castleman disease. *Surg Pathol Clin*. 2019;12(3):849-863.

36. Chan AC, Chan KW, Chan JK, Au WY, Ho WK, Ng WM. Development of follicular dendritic cell sarcoma in hyaline-vascular Castleman's disease of the nasopharynx: tracing its evolution by sequential biopsies. *Histopathology*. 2001;38(6):510-518.

37. Chan JK, Frizzera G, Fletcher CD, Rosai J. Primary vascular tumors of lymph nodes other than Kaposi's sarcoma: analysis of 39 cases and delineation of two new entities. *Am J Surg Pathol*. 1992;16:335-350.

38. Moh M, Sangoi AR, Rabban JT. Angiomyomatous hamartoma of lymph nodes, revisited: clinicopathologic study of 21 cases, emphasizing its distinction from lymphangioleiomyomatosis of lymph nodes. *Hum Pathol*. 2017;68:175-183.

39. Ronco PM, Alyanakian MA, Mougenot B, Aucouturier P. Light chain deposition disease: a model of glomerulosclerosis defined at the molecular level. *J Am Soc Nephrol*. 2001;12(7):1558-1565.

40. Baqir M, Moua T, White D, Yi ES, Ryu JH. Pulmonary nodular and cystic light chain deposition disease: a retrospective review of 10 cases. *Respir Med*. 2020;164:105896.

41. Gupta D, Lim MS, Medeiros LJ, Elenitoba-Johnson KS. Small lymphocytic lymphoma with perifollicular, marginal zone, or interfollicular distribution. *Mod Pathol*. 2000;13(11):1161-1166.

42. Dupin N, Diss T, Kellam P, et al. HHV-8 is associated with a plasmablastic variant of Castleman disease that is linked to HHV-8-positive plasmablastic lymphoma. *Blood*. 2000;95:1406-1412.

43. Kojima M, Motoori T, Nakamura S. Benign, atypical and malignant lymphoproliferative disorders in rheumatoid arthritis patients. *Biomed Pharmacother*. 2006;60(10):663-672.

44. Doyle LA, Hornick JL. Pathology of extramedullary mastocytosis. *Immunol Allergy Clin North Am*. 2014;34(2):323-339.

45. Sotlar K, Cerny-Reiterer S, Petat-Dutter K, et al. Aberrant expression of CD30 in neoplastic mast cells in high-grade mastocytosis. *Mod Pathol*. 2011;24(4):585-595.

46. Ro JY, Luna MA, Mackay B, Ramos O. Yellow-brown (Hamazaki-Wesenberg) bodies mimicking fungal yeasts. *Arch Pathol Lab Med*. 1987;111(6):555-559.

47. Ohgami RS, Arber DA, Zehnder JL, Natkunam Y, Warnke RA. Indolent T-lymphoblastic proliferation (iT-LBP): a review of clinical and pathologic features and distinction from malignant T-lymphoblastic lymphoma. *Adv Anat Pathol*. 2013;20(3):137-140.

48. Swerdlow SH, Campo E, Harris NL, et al. *Myeloid/lymphoid neoplasms with PDGFRA rearrangement*. In: *WHO Classification of Tumours of Haematopoietic and Lymphoid Tissues*. Lyon, France: IARC Press; 2017:73-75.

OBLITERATED NODULAR PATTERN

6

CHAPTER OUTLINE

INTRODUCTION

There are very few entities that exhibit diffuse nodular pattern of effacement in the lymph node. However, some of these can be tricky, and a thorough knowledge of all reactive nodular entities is necessary before entertaining the possibility of lymphoma entities in cases with nodular pattern of effaced architecture. A key feature as it relates to knowing the geographic landmarks in the lymph node involves knowing if the nodular areas correspond to underlying lymphoid follicles.

Last but not the least, the one thing that this chapter will not focus on is a formal description of each of the nodular lymphoma entities with detailed histology and the immunophenotype in a textbook format. But rather, this will only discuss approach based on patterns and useful diagnostic features that allow one to get to the right diagnosis. The reader is referred to the WHO 2016 and several other excellent textbooks that discuss these entities in detail.

LIST OF ENTITIES TO CONSIDER IN CASES WITH NODULAR PATTERN

1. **Hodgkin lymphoma**
   a. Nodular lymphocyte-predominant Hodgkin lymphoma (NLPHL)
   b. Nodular lymphocyte-rich classical Hodgkin lymphoma (cHL)
   c. Interfollicular mixed cellularity cHL with reactive regressed/nodular lymphoid follicles
2. **Non-Hodgkin lymphoma entities**
   a. B-cell entities
      i. Follicular lymphoma (FL)
      ii. Mantle cell lymphoma (MCL)
      iii. Small lymphocytic lymphoma (SLL)
   b. T-cell entities
      i. Follicular T-cell lymphoma (follicular and perifollicular patterns)
3. **Castleman disease (CD)–associated lymphoid proliferations**
   a. Hyaline vascular CD
   b. Multicentric Castleman disease (MCD)
      i. Human herpesvirus (HHV)8-associated MCD
      ii. HHV8 negative idiopathic MCD (iMCD)

CHECKLIST: Checklist of Histologic Features to Look for in Cases With Seemingly Nodular Pattern of Effacement:

1. Quality of nodularity
   a. Mottled nodular versus diffuse nodular pattern (NLPHL/cHL vs others)
   b. Definite nodular versus vaguely nodular (Figures 6.1-6.10)
2. Obliteration of the lymph node sinuses (frequently noted in FL)
3. Obliteration of the subcapsular sinuses (frequently noted in angioimmunoblastic T-cell lymphoma; Figure 6.11)
4. Extension of nodular structures beyond the confines of the lymph node into the perinodal adipose tissues (constant feature in FL as well as marginal zone lymphoma [MZL])
5. Partial involvement in seemingly reactive node
6. Atypical Hodgkin-like cells and their location (may be seen in HL [Figures 6.12 and 6.13] and follicular variant of peripheral T-cell lymphoma [F-PTCL])
7. Peri/parafollicular cuffs of atypical lymphoid cells (seen in MZL, chronic lymphocytic leukemia [CLL], and F-PTCL cases with perifollicular pattern of T-cells; Figures 6.14-6.18)

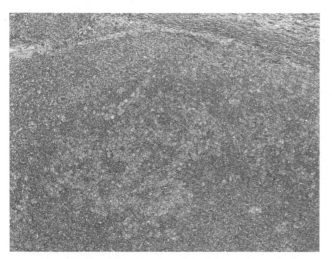

Figure 6.1. Nodular lymphocyte-predominant Hodgkin lymphoma (NLPHL): First flavor of mottled nodular lymphoid proliferation with multiple clusters of pale staining cells.

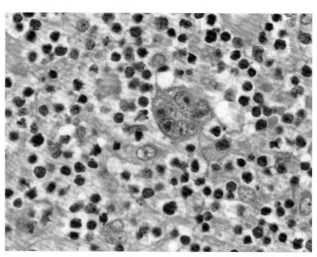

Figure 6.2. Nodular lymphocyte-predominant Hodgkin lymphoma (NLPHL): High-power magnification identifies scattered large atypical lymphoid cells morphologically compatible with lymphocytic and histiocytic (L&H)/lymphocyte-predominant (LP) cells with convoluted nuclear contours and multiple small nucleoli present in the background of lymphocytes.

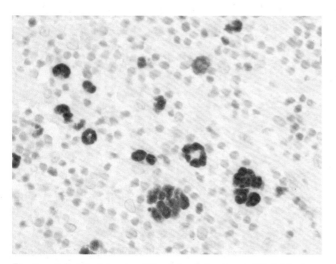

Figure 6.3. Nodular lymphocyte-predominant Hodgkin lymphoma (NLPHL): OCT2 immunostain highlights all abnormal cells in NLPHL. Compared to PAX5, OCT2 is much better stain for identifying scarce LP cells. Also, note the scarcity of small B-cells in the background in this case consistent with a variant pattern rich in T-cells which is associated with adverse outcome.

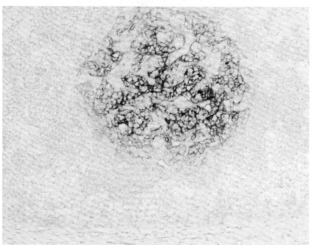

Figure 6.4. Nodular lymphocyte-predominant Hodgkin lymphoma (NLPHL): Expanded disrupted dendritic cell meshworks in NLPHL on CD21 immunostain. This is not necessarily a useful feature in distinguishing from follicular lymphoma (FL) and marginal zone lymphoma (MZL), but its near-total absence should raise the possibility of early transformation to T-cell/histiocyte-rich B-cell lymphoma (T/HRBCL) in NLPHL cases.

FOLLICULAR LYMPHOMA

SOME HISTOLOGIC VARIATIONS THAT REPRESENT PITFALLS IN THE DIAGNOSIS OF FOLLICULAR LYMPHOMA

1. Partial involvement by FL—Look at the whole section including all slides at low power since cases with very focal and partial involvement always stand out better at low power.
2. Small-sized follicles of varying sizes—While textbook teaching tells us that FL always shows large closely packed nearly equal-sized follicles without distinct mantle cuffs (Figures 6.19-6.23), small follicles and cases with distinct mantle cuffs are seen pretty often, and hence, one must be aware of these histologic variations (Figures 6.24-6.26).

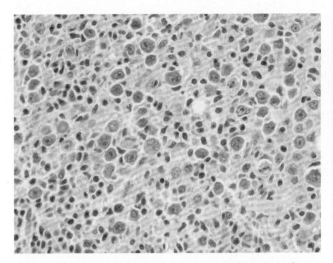

Figure 6.5. Diffuse large B-cell lymphoma (DLBCL) transformation in marrow of patient in Figures 6.1-6.4 with nodular lymphocyte-predominant Hodgkin lymphoma (NLPHL): Bone marrow involvement in the same case as above with sheets of large B-cells indicative of transformation at the same time.

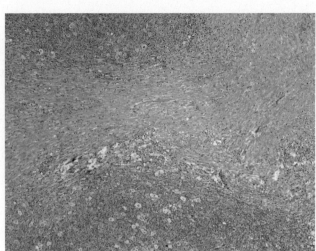

Figure 6.6. Classical Hodgkin lymphoma (cHL): The second flavor of mottled nodular lymphoid proliferation comprising multiple scattered mottled nodular structures with prominent broad bands of compartmentalizing sclerosis replacing the nodal architecture.

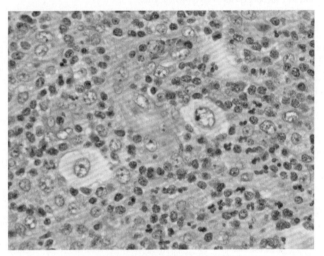

Figure 6.7. Classical Hodgkin lymphoma (cHL): Higher power depicts scattered lacunar cells (Hodgkin/Reed-Sternberg cells) present in the background rich in lymphocytes, eosinophils, and histiocytes, characteristic of nodular sclerosis cHL.

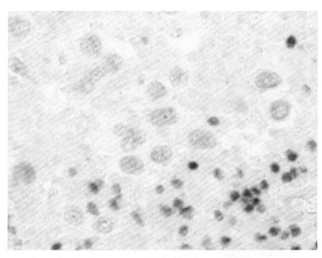

Figure 6.8. Classical Hodgkin lymphoma (cHL): PAX5 immunostain highlights the Hodgkin cells with weak staining with strong expression in surrounding normal B-cells to the bottom right.

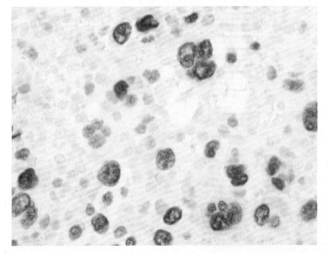

Figure 6.9. Classical Hodgkin lymphoma (cHL): The Hodgkin cells consistently express MUM1, and this is a useful feature when Hodgkin cells are scarce.

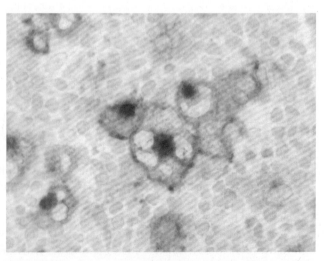

Figure 6.10. Classical Hodgkin lymphoma (cHL): CD30 immunostain positivity confirms cHL with membrane and cytoplasmic staining with Golgi accentuation.

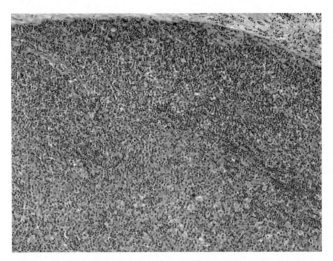

Figure 6.11. **Angioimmunoblastic T-cell lymphoma:** There is nodal effacement with obliteration of the subcapsular sinus.

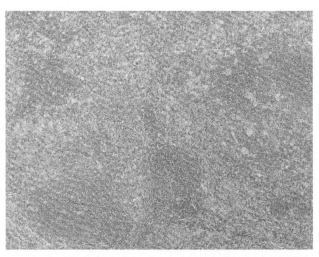

Figure 6.12. **Interfollicular classical Hodgkin lymphoma (cHL):** Scattered nodular structures consistent with primary follicles are present.

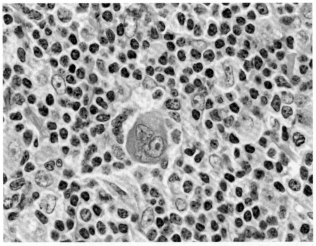

Figure 6.13. **Interfollicular classical Hodgkin lymphoma (cHL):** However, at higher power, scattered Hodgkin cells are easily visualized and could be missed if one does not pay careful attention. The cells exhibited typical phenotype, positive for CD30 and CD15 with weak PAX5 staining. This case was initially called marginal zone lymphoma based on some increase in interfollicular B-cells and a B-cell clone by PCR.

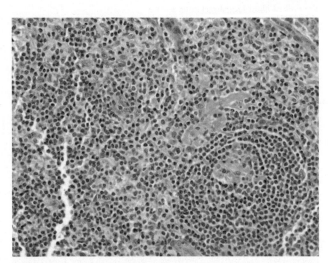

Figure 6.14. **Angioimmunoblastic T-cell lymphoma, pattern 2:** The H&E image in low power demonstrates small diminutive Castleman-like regressed follicles in some areas, with other areas showing nodular collections of small lymphoid cells morphologically compatible with primary follicles that are notable for a circumferential cuff of clear lymphoid cells.

3. Along these lines, really small microfollicles with expanded mantles reminiscent of hyaline vascular Castleman disease may be seen in FL.[1] This is a difficult pitfall unless the expression of CD10 and BCL-2 being colocalized to the same cells is determined (using appropriate immunostains since one might not do any immunostains if the primary diagnostic consideration is hyaline vascular Castleman disease; Figures 6.27-6.32). This patient had extensive lymphadenopathy with significant systemic symptoms, a finding incompatible with hyaline vascular Castleman disease, and hence, additional stains were performed in this case allowing the appropriate diagnosis.

4. Rare follicular lymphoma cases show centrocytes with abundant pale pink cytoplasm imparting the appearance of a histiocytic neoplasm or large cells; with the result such cases often end up upgraded to grade 3b. Examination of the nuclear characteristics with folded nuclei and clumped chromatin is critical in avoiding this pitfall (Figures 6.33-6.36). These cases often are mistaken for other neoplasm like granular cell tumors on H&E since the cytoplasmic borders are indistinct. This case was a duodenal FL with this cytomorphology.

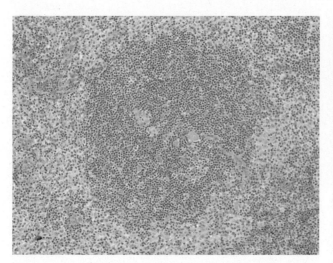

Figure 6.15. Angioimmunoblastic T-cell lymphoma, pattern 2: The H&E image in high power demonstrates small diminutive Castleman-like regressed follicles in some areas with other areas showing nodular collections of small lymphoid cells morphologically compatible with primary follicles that are notable for a circumferential cuff of clear lymphoid cells.

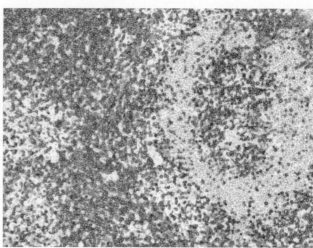

Figure 6.16. Angioimmunoblastic T-cell lymphoma, pattern 2: CD3 immunostain highlights a perifollicular cuff of CD3 positive T-cells.

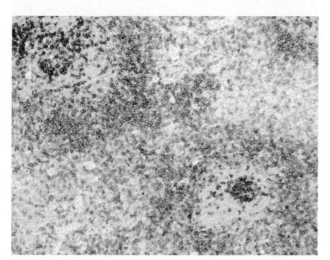

Figure 6.17. Angioimmunoblastic T-cell lymphoma, pattern 2: PD-1 immunostain highlights increased numbers of germinal center follicular helper T-cells, and in addition, note that the perifollicular cuff of CD3 positive lymphoid cells are positive for PD-1, confirming an abnormal pattern of staining consistent with angioimmunoblastic T-cell lymphoma, so-called pattern 2.

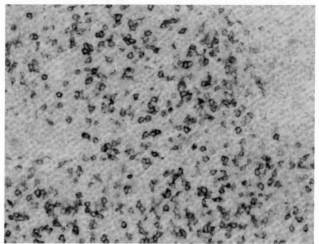

Figure 6.18. Angioimmunoblastic T-cell lymphoma, pattern 2: Variable numbers of CD10 positive lymphoid cells consistent with follicular helper T-cells are also noted within these follicular structures. Cases of pattern 1 typically demonstrate reactive follicular hyperplasia, while cases of pattern 3 demonstrate obliterated lymphoid architecture and morphologically compatible typical hypervascular angioimmunoblastic T-cell lymphoma. Cases comprising patterns 1 and 2 are often dismissed as reactive hyperplasia or hyaline vascular Castleman disease.

KEY FEATURES of the Various Cells Within the Follicular Compartment

- Centroblasts: large cells with convoluted nuclear contours and coarse chromatin and multiple peripheral small nucleoli

- Centrocytes: small, medium, or sometimes large cleaved cells with elongated nuclei and inconspicuous nucleoli

- Tingible body macrophages: large cells with single round or folded nuclei and single small nucleoli with abundant debris-filled cytoplasm

- Follicular dendritic cell: single or doublet nuclei with thin nuclear membranes and empty chromatin and small indistinct nucleoli

- Rare in follicles but useful to look for:
  - Immunoblast: large cells, prominent eosinophilic nucleoli, and moderate amount of amphophilic cytoplasm—typically at the periphery
  - Plasma cell: mature plasma cell, may be observed in autoimmune conditions
  - T-cells: small round lymphocytes at the periphery consistent with follicular helper T-cells (TFH) serve as internal reference for size

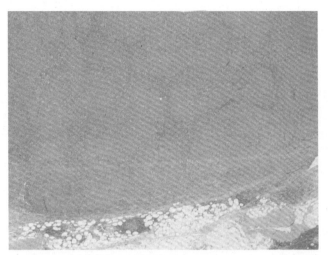

Figure 6.19. **Typical follicular lymphoma (FL):** FL involving the entire lymph node with multiple closely packed expansile nodular follicular structures with indistinct mantle cuffs. Also, note the small nodular microfollicular structures in the perinodal adipose tissues. Frequently there is extranodal extension, which is a useful feature in cases with partial involvement by FL.

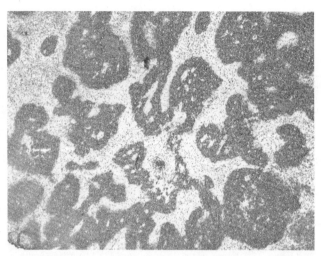

Figure 6.20. **Typical follicular lymphoma (FL) CD20:** Follicles are positive for CD20, highlighting serpiginous follicles. Also note the increase in extrafollicular CD20 positive B-cells corresponding to extrafollicular extension of lymphoma cells, which is frequent in FL.

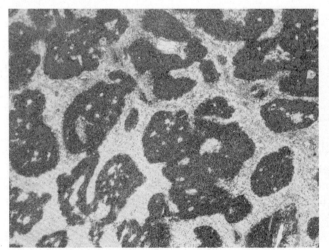

Figure 6.21. **Typical follicular lymphoma (FL) CD10:** Follicles are positive for CD10.

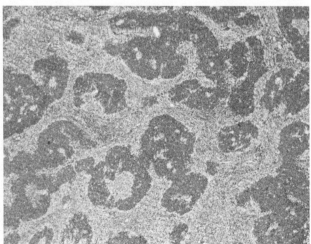

Figure 6.22. **Typical follicular lymphoma (FL):** BCL-2 immunostain highlights all neoplastic follicles, indicating coexpression of CD10 as well as BCL-2. Also note that the interfollicular T-cells are additionally positive for BCL-2. Comparison of the CD20 and BCL-2 immunostain allows inference that the extrafollicular excess of BCL-2 positive cells relative to CD20 is accounted for by T-cells.

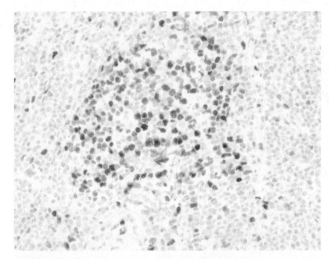

Figure 6.23. **Typical follicular lymphoma (FL):** Ki-67 highlights increased numbers of proliferating cells within the nodules with a nodular staining pattern.

Figure 6.24. **Follicular lymphoma (FL) with micronodular architecture.** This is a lymph node from a 39-year-old asymptomatic man with a 4.8-cm inguinal mass. Rarely, FL might demonstrate multiple diminutive pale follicular structures resembling noncaseating granulomas at low power.

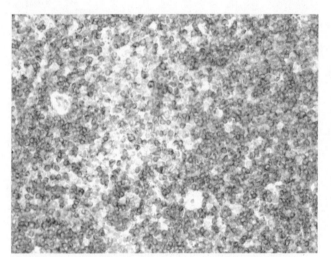

Figure 6.25. **Follicular lymphoma (FL) with micronodular architecture:** CD10 is positive in the lymphoma cells.

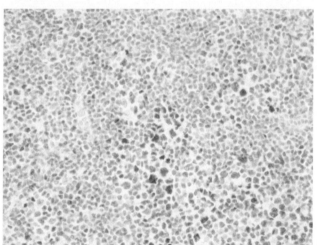

Figure 6.26. **Follicular lymphoma (FL) with micronodular architecture:** BCL-6 is positive in the lymphoma cells within the micronodules (additionally positive for CD20 in this case) confirming a diagnosis of FL. Additional FISH studies demonstrated underlying t(14;18) translocation.

GRADING AND FOLLICULAR LYMPHOMA

The current WHO 2016 recommends the following grades of FL based on the numbers of centroblasts: Grade 1 to 2, grade 3a, and grade 3b variant; grade 1 to 2 exhibit less than 15 centroblasts per high-power field, while grade 3a contains >15 centroblasts per high-power field and grade 3b contains sheets of centroblasts.[2]

While the distinction of grades 1 to 2 versus 3a is often difficult and can be poor to reproduce grading, the clinical relevance of this distinction is less important if the patient is asymptomatic. However, the diagnosis of grade 3b is clinically equal to diffuse large B-cell lymphoma and requires treatment regardless of symptoms in most cases. That said, regardless of the grade of FL, it is necessary to look in the extrafollicular areas for potential clusters of large B-cells on CD20 to assess for possible large cell transformation focally (Figures 6.37-6.39).

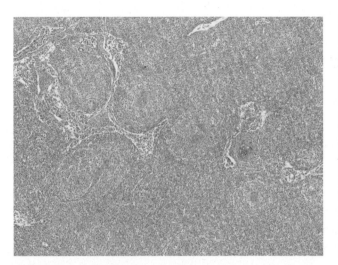

Figure 6.27. **Follicular lymphoma (FL), grade 3a with hyaline vascular Castleman disease–like cytomorphology:** Low-power image with closely packed lymphoid follicles.

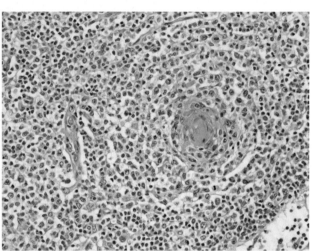

Figure 6.28. **Follicular lymphoma (FL), grade 3a with hyaline vascular Castleman disease–like cytomorphology:** Higher power shows Castleman-like regressed lymphoid follicles with vascularized germinal centers and concentric rings of mantle cuffs.

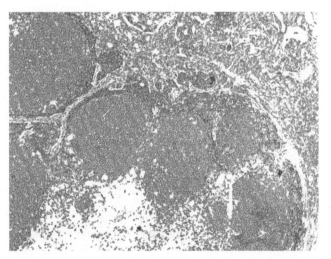

Figure 6.29. **Follicular lymphoma (FL), grade 3a with hyaline vascular Castleman disease–like cytomorphology:** The nodules are diffusely positive for CD20 confirming B-cell origin.

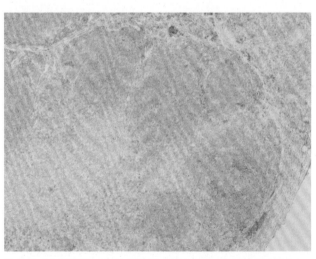

Figure 6.30. **Follicular lymphoma (FL), grade 3a with hyaline vascular Castleman disease–like cytomorphology:** The CD20+ nodules coexpress CD10.

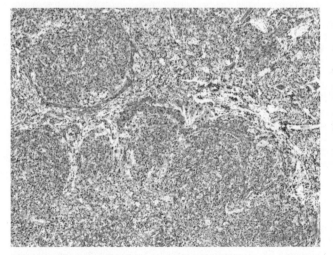

Figure 6.31. **Follicular lymphoma (FL), grade 3a with hyaline vascular Castleman disease–like cytomorphology:** The follicular B-cells coexpress BCL-2 confirming neoplastic follicular center B-cell origin.

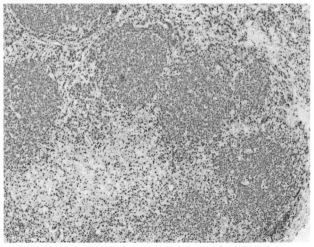

Figure 6.32. **Follicular lymphoma (FL), grade 3a with hyaline vascular Castleman disease–like cytomorphology:** The follicles are uniformly positive for Ki-67, indicative of aggressive biology.

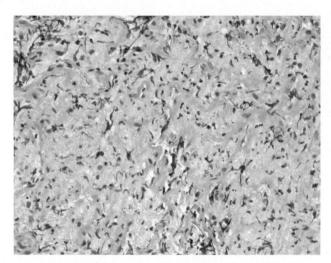

Figure 6.33. Follicular lymphoma (FL) with atypical centrocytes with abundant pink cytoplasm: Low- and high-power H&E depicting clusters of bland nuclei and delicate sclerosis.

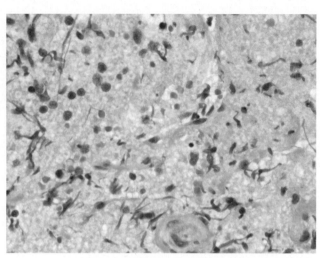

Figure 6.34. Follicular lymphoma (FL) with atypical centrocytes with abundant pink cytoplasm: High-power H&E depicting cells containing abundant foamy pink cytoplasm and delicate sclerosis. Obvious lymphoid cytomorphology is not apparent.

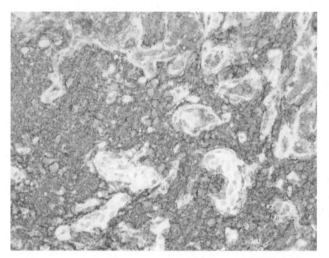

Figure 6.35. Follicular lymphoma (FL) with atypical centrocytes with abundant pink cytoplasm: However, CD20 is positive in these cells confirming neoplastic B-cell origin.

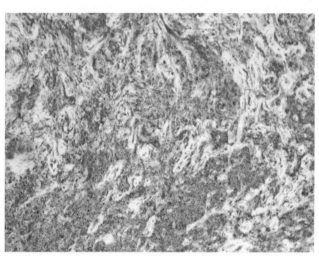

Figure 6.36. Follicular lymphoma (FL) with atypical centrocytes with abundant pink cytoplasm: BCL-2 is both positive in these cells confirming neoplastic B-cell consistent with FL phenotype.

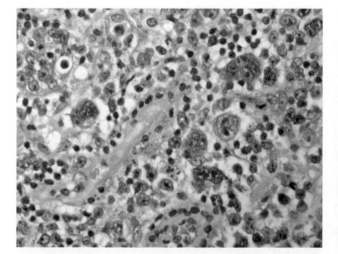

Figure 6.37. Transformed follicular lymphoma (FL) with scattered interfollicular large Hodgkin-like cells: H&E image shows interfollicular areas in a FL patient with Hodgkin-like cells. These cases may sometimes be misconstrued as composite lymphoma.

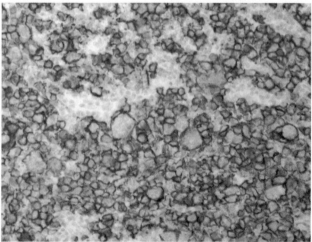

Figure 6.38. Transformed follicular lymphoma (FL) with scattered interfollicular large Hodgkin-like cells: The interfollicular small B-cells represent the FL component on CD20, while the large cells are also strongly positive for CD20.

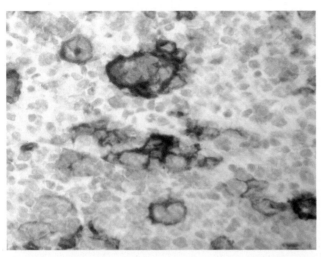

Figure 6.39. **Transformed follicular lymphoma (FL) with scattered interfollicular large Hodgkin-like cells:** These cells are also positive for CD30. Close attention must be paid to the interfollicular areas to look for the transformed component. Hodgkin-like cells may be seen in a variety of conditions including transformed FL, diffuse large B-cell lymphoma, Epstein-Barr virus (EBV) positive large cell lymphomas, as well as T-cell lymphomas. Therefore, a diagnosis of composite lymphoma should not be rendered on such cases.

UNCONVENTIONAL WISDOM RELATING TO FL GRADING

When it comes to FL grading, I must admit that I often use unconventional rules not written in the books but work well nonetheless as long as I pay attention to the clinical context. One of them is to not actually count the number of centroblasts. My typical approach and rationale for which I follow these are detailed below.

1. Perform a low-power scan of all slides that have lymphoma and focus on follicles that appear to have increased numbers of large cells based on the low-power scan before going at high-power to grade such follicles.
2. Ideally, centroblasts would be distributed equally throughout the follicles but in real life, this is not the case, and often, proliferative centroblasts marginalize toward the periphery of lymphoma follicles and one would end up upgrading most cases to grade 3a in what is otherwise grade 1 to 2.

PEARLS & PITFALLS

One should know to distinguish follicular dendritic cells (FDCs) from centroblasts. The former typically occur as doublets with distinct nuclear membrane and single small nucleoli, whereas the latter are folded large cells with multiple peripheral nucleoli. Counting FDCs as centroblasts frequently leads to overgrading as grade 3a.

3. If there seems to be more "large cells" histologically, ask the question "Are there small cells mixed and if these small guys look centrocytic?" If the answer is yes to both these questions, you are still at grade 3a and not 3b (Figures 6.40 and 6.41). Most cases of pediatric-type FL, however, exhibit grade 3 cytomorphology, and this is a pitfall that frequently becomes hard to distinguish from reactive hyperplasia (Figures 6.42 and 6.43). These follicles lacked BCL-2 with immunostaining profile of reactive secondary follicles but showed evidence of B-cell clone by molecular studies, consistent with pediatric-type FL. The line between florid and reactive giant follicular hyperplasia versus pediatric-type FL is often thin, and one must use judgment and molecular studies as necessary to arrive with the diagnosis.

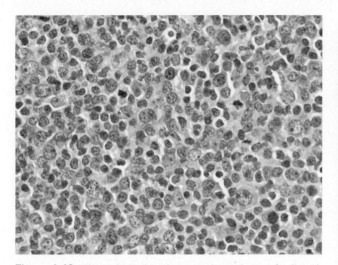

Figure 6.40. **FL grade 3a:** Mostly a mixed population of cells with scattered small lymphoid cells and centroblasts.

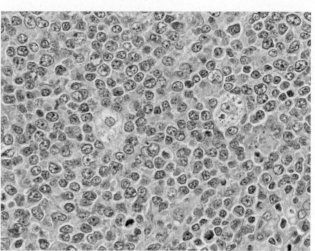

Figure 6.41. **FL grade 3b:** Sheets of centroblasts predominate, allowing designation as grade 3b.

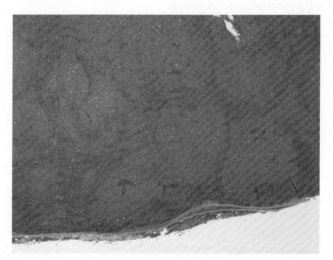

Figure 6.42. **Pediatric-type follicular lymphoma (FL):** H&E image demonstrating multiple closely packed monotonous and expanded follicular structures with tingible body macrophages. Note geographic irregular monotonous follicles on the top and the right side.

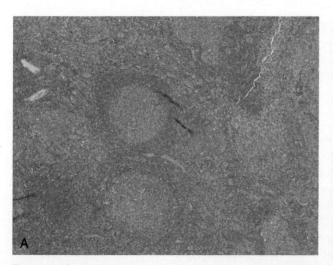

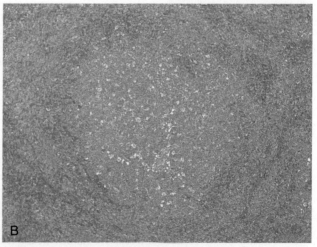

Figure 6.43. **Pediatric-type follicular lymphoma (FL): A** and **B,** H&E images of higher power show that these follicles exhibit variably attenuated mantle cuffs with disruption of the light zone/dark zone distinction and contain scattered tingible body macrophages.

CLL typically shows proliferation centers that are pale and impart a nodular appearance, while MCL is often nodular with scattered single histiocytes with centrocytic or blastoid cytomorphology. Hence the distinction of these entities is not really difficult in most cases (Figures 6.44-6.46).

CHECKLIST: Checklist for FL Grading and Reporting

☐ Check PET/CT to see if any other node is more PET avid than the one biopsied.

☐ Confirm if proliferation is diffuse or nodular (diffuse proliferations are not graded the same way).

☐ Confirm absence of sheets of centroblasts (exclude grade 3b/diffuse large B-cell lymphoma).

☐ Examine if centroblasts are easily visible (if yes, grade 3a).

☐ If core biopsy, are there enough follicles for reliable grading? If yes, report grade.

☐ Look at clinical/radiologic details to decide on recommendation for excision biopsy based on PET/CT results.

Figure 6.44. **Small lymphocytic lymphoma (SLL):** Low-power H&E image demonstrating effaced architecture with scattered ill-defined pale nodular structures, comprising sheets of small lymphoid cells with compact nuclear chromatin.

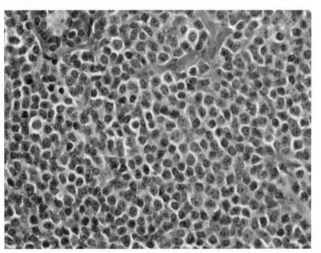

Figure 6.45. **Small lymphocytic lymphoma (SLL):** High-power H&E image shows monotonous small lymphoid cells with compact chromatin typical of SLL.

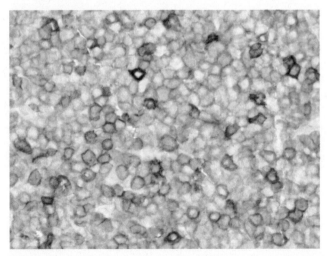

Figure 6.46. **Small lymphocytic lymphoma (SLL):** CD5 immunostain shows biphasic pattern with scattered CD5 bright T-cells, while the chronic lymphocytic leukemia (CLL) cells in the background express dim CD5.

FAQ: I have a morphologically reactive lymph node with a small clonal B-cell population by flow. Should I get PCR for B-cell clonality in such cases?

Floridly reactive germinal centers can occasionally harbor small clonal populations, and hence, routine PCR for B-cell clonality should not be performed if there is not sufficient morphologic support. The only exception is in cases with pediatric-type follicular lymphoma morphology.

IMMUNOSTAINS AND APPROACH IN NODULAR PROLIFERATIONS

My standard immunostaining panel in cases with nodular architecture without any Hodgkin-like cells includes CD20, CD3, CD5, CD10, BCL-6, BCL-2, and Ki-67 in all cases with definite nodular cytomorphology. I reserve cyclin D1, SOX11, and LEF1 as a second-tier panel in CD10 negative cases. In CD10 negative cases that express CD5 with vague nodular pattern, I will add cyclin D1, SOX11, and LEF1 since nodal MCLs are positive for cyclin D1 and SOX11 while only CLL is positive for LEF1.[3] This step-wise approach is necessary only in about 30% of cases where you cannot determine if it is nodular or diffuse. In most cases, one can reliably distinguish FL, CLL, and MCL even with just an H&E.

Typically, FL coexpresses CD10, BCL-6, and BCL-2. Extrafollicular extension by FL cells is typical, and this latter component is usually dim/negative for CD10 and/or BCL-6. Rare cases, however, may be CD10 and/or BCL-2 negative including high-grade FLs (Figures 6.47-6.49) or pediatric FL, which is BCL-2 negative.[2] The latter cases are especially difficult to distinguish from floridly reactive secondary follicles, and hence molecular studies for clonal gene rearrangement or pathogenic mutations implicated in FL are essential for arriving at the diagnosis.[4]

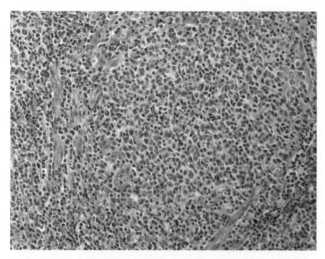

Figure 6.47. **CD10 negative follicular lymphoma (FL):** H&E image depicting a FL, grade 3a with increased centroblasts.

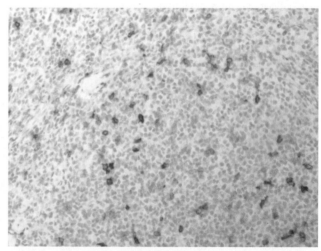

Figure 6.48. **CD10 negative follicular lymphoma (FL):** CD10 is largely negative in these follicular B-cells. Scattered single CD10+ lymphoid cells correspond to follicular helper T-cells, which express CD10.

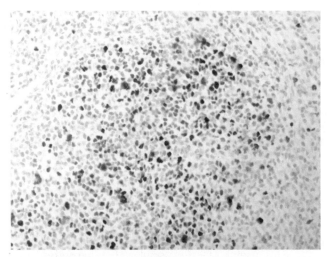

Figure 6.49. **CD10 negative follicular lymphoma (FL):** The lymphoma cells are positive for BCL-6, however, confirming germinal center origin.

CHECKLIST: Checklist for Ordering Immunohistochemistry in Follicular Proliferations

☐ Most proliferations appearing reactive—No lymphoma-specific stains ordered

☐ Monotonous and nodular, the minimum panel—CD20, CD5, CD10, BCL-6, BCL-2, and Ki-67

☐ If it is CD10 negative, add cyclin D1, ZAP-70, and LEF1 (for MCL and SLL)

☐ Additional CD30, IgD, and PD1 become relevant once FL, SLL, and MCL are excluded.

PEARLS & PITFALLS

The immunohistochemistry panel I use is sometimes smaller if flow cytometry has been performed corroborating CD5 or CD10 expression on clonal B-cells. Nevertheless, negative CD5 on flow with positive immunohistochemistry (IHC) is seen frequently since the clones used are different in flow and IHC and hence repeating stains is recommended if morphologic suspicion is high. Likewise, CD19 by IHC may become negative in large B-cell lymphoproliferations, but flow testing may be positive, and this becomes relevant prior to CD19 CAR-T-cell therapy.

KEY FEATURES of Common Useful Immunostains in Nodular Lymphomas and What to Look for in These Stains

Stains	FL	CLL	MCL	cHL/NLPHL
CD20	Stains neoplastic follicles and also stains extra-follicular component (in lymphoma; very useful feature in BCL-2 negative cases)	Dim CD20 expression is apparent	Positive in lymphoma cells	cHL variable; NLPHL strong
CD10	Stains strongly in neoplastic follicles (dim in extra-follicular component)	Negative	Negative	Not useful

Stains	FL	CLL	MCL	cHL/NLPHL
BCL-6	Stains strongly in neoplastic follicles (dim-negative in extrafollicular component)	Negative	Negative	Not useful
BCL-2	Positive in neoplastic follicles (make sure that visually $N_{BCL-2} >> N_{CD3}$ inside seemingly neoplastic follicles, so you know that excess BCL-2 is likely accounted for by B-cells)	Positive (does not help in diagnosis)	Positive (does not help in diagnosis)	Not useful. Mantle zone and T-cells stains
CD3	Necessary for above reason as BCL-2	Not really useful	Not really useful	May see rosettes around Hodgkin/ LP cells in sneaky cases
CD5	Not more useful than CD5 in FL	Dim CD5 in CLL with bright T-cells	Dim CD5 in MCL compared to background T-cells (see Figures 6.50-6.56)	Not useful; will highlight rosettes
Ki-67	Useful in bumping to grade 3a if you are on the fence although rare low-grade FL can show high proliferation	Picks growth centers and may help with pushing to focal transformation	>30% is bad. Need to do all the time[a]	

[a]Along these lines, p53 IHC and molecular studies for TP53 mutation is also critical upfront in MCL.

PEARLS & PITFALLS

I will use CD5 in lieu of CD3 in small cell lymphoproliferations since CD5 can inform about T-cells as well as neoplastic B-cells easily.

FAQ: CD5 was negative by flow cytometry, but morphologically this looks like small lymphocytic lymphoma. Should I repeat CD5 by immunohistochemistry in such cases?

Yes. Sometimes the clones for CD5 and CD10 are different for flow cytometry and immunohistochemistry and hence false-negative studies may be picked by the other clone, and hence, it is a good idea to repeat by immunohistochemistry if either CD5 or CD10 is negative on initial flow cytometry.

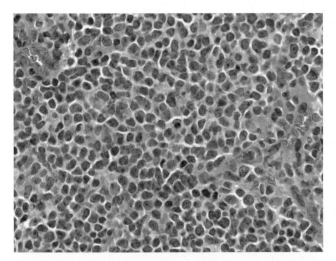

Figure 6.50. **Mantle cell lymphoma (MCL):** May demonstrate vaguely nodular pattern and shows diffuse infiltrate of medium-sized blastoid cells with dispersed nuclear chromatin.

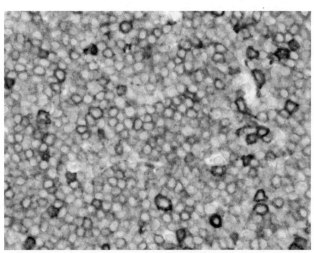

Figure 6.51. **Mantle cell lymphoma (MCL):** CD5 immunostain is positive in the lymphoma cells, while scattered T-cells demonstrate moderate to bright CD5 expression.

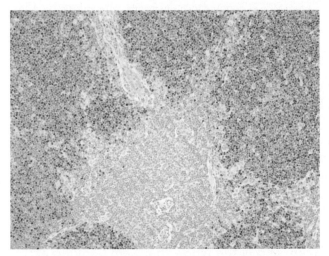

Figure 6.52. **Cyclin D1-/SOX11+ mantle cell lymphoma (MCL):** The lymphoma cells are SOX11 positive here. Lymphoblastic processes and Burkitt lymphoma may also express SOX11.

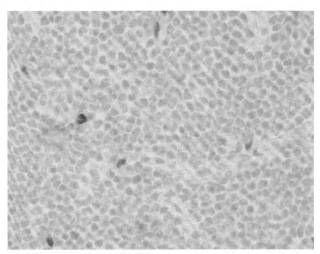

Figure 6.53. **Cyclin D1 negative mantle cell lymphoma (MCL):** cyclin D1 is negative (scattered histiocytes are positive, internal control). Nodal MCLs are often SOX11+ and cyclin D1+, while a proportion of leukemic MCLs are indolent and SOX11 negative frequently.

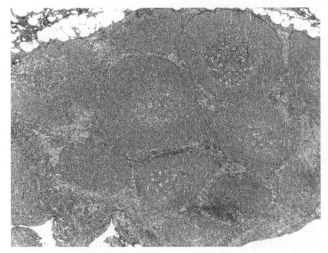

Figure 6.54. **Mantle cell lymphoma (MCL), mantle zone pattern:** Low-power H&E demonstrating nodular architecture with expanded mantle cuffs in seemingly reactive follicles.

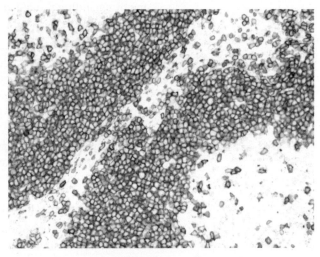

Figure 6.55. **Mantle cell lymphoma (MCL), mantle zone pattern:** CD5 is positive in the mantle zones.

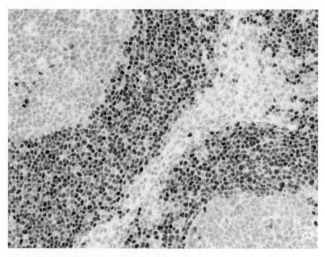

Figure 6.56. **Mantle cell lymphoma (MCL), mantle zone pattern:** SOX11 highlights mantle zones, diffusely confirming the diagnosis of MCL. The thickness of mantle zone involvement and numbers of follicles involved are significantly higher in cases with mantle zone pattern MCL as opposed to in situ mantle cell neoplasia.

SCENARIOS AND CLINICAL DETAILS THAT DETERMINE HOW YOU LOOK AT AND SIGN OUT SOME FOLLICULAR LYMPHOMA CASES

Is This Widespread Disease Based on CT Scan?

In such cases, clinicians are likely to treat, and hence the grading would become critical. It is not a bad idea in these cases to make sure you get another colleague to independently agree with your assigned grade and put in a consensus statement about having procured a concurrence on grade.

Have They Done a PET Scan, and Is the Node that I am Looking at the Most PET Avid Node?

If the biopsied node is not PET avid and there is another node that is more PET avid, a Sample comment I typically put in includes: **"Although the diagnostic features are in keeping with follicular lymphoma, biopsy of the PET avid node is critical for confirming or excluding transformation prior to therapy."**

Cases Comprising Core Biopsies With or Without Crush Artifacts

- Retroperitoneal lymph node/deep site core biopsies: If morphology looks typical and PET scan does not show any other lymph node with more PET avid areas, I typically commit to a diagnosis of FL and do not recommend excision since excision biopsies at the sites are not feasible.

- Axillary lymph node/superficial/accessible site core biopsies: Even if the morphology looks typical and PET scan does not show any of the lymph node with more PET avid areas, I strongly recommend performing excision biopsy.

- **Sample final diagnosis blurbs for these superficial sites include:**
- **"CD10+ B-cell lymphoma, consistent with follicular lymphoma grade 1 to 2; recommend excision biopsy for assessing possible transformed areas."**

SAMPLE COMPLETE REPORT WITH NOTES ON REPORT STRUCTURE AND APPROPRIATE ORDER OF ELEMENTS IN BOLD AND PARENTHESES

Lymph node, site, needle core biopsy:

- Follicular lymphoma, grade 1 to 2, see comment.

Comment: Sections from the core biopsy demonstrate multiple needle cores demonstrating multiple closely packed expansile monotonous follicular structures. These follicular structures comprise predominantly centrocytes with increased numbers of centroblasts and some of the follicles, compatible with follicular lymphoma, grade 3a. No areas of large cell transformation are noted. (**Always mention details of transformation.**)

Additional immunostains performed including CD20, CD3, CD5, CD10, BCL-6, BCL-2, and Ki-67 (**Stains performed**). These demonstrate the neoplastic follicular structures to be positive for CD20 (**lineage defining stain first**) with a significant interfollicular component. These are additionally positive for CD10, BCL-6, and BCL-2 (**additional qualifying stains**). These follicles have a low proliferation on Ki-67 (10%; **prognostic stain**). CD3 and CD5 as well as BCL-2 additionally highlight internodular T cells (**stains positive in the background cells**).

PITFALL CASES OF NODULAR PROLIFERATIONS

PITFALL CASE 1: NODAL MARGINAL ZONE LYMPHOMA WITH FOLLICULAR COLONIZATION

Although not included in the nodular big list, MZL with extensive follicular colonization can resemble FL (Figures 6.57-6.62). The disrupted follicular pattern on CD10, BCL-6, and Ki-67 in colonized follicles and excess interfollicular B-cells is usually the only clue. Flow cytometry identified clonal B-cells lacking CD5 and CD10, consistent with nodal marginal zone lymphoma (NMZL). In the absence of a distinct light chain–restricted plasmacytic component, such follicular colonization is a very useful feature in diagnosing NMZL that lacks significant interfollicular component.

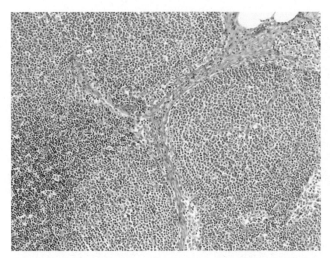

Figure 6.57. Nodal marginal zone lymphoma (NMZL) with extensive follicular colonization mimicking nodular lymphoma: The lymph node architecture is replaced by multiple nodular aggregates of small lymphoid cells reminiscent of primary follicles. There is intervening sclerosis without much interfollicular lymphoid tissue.

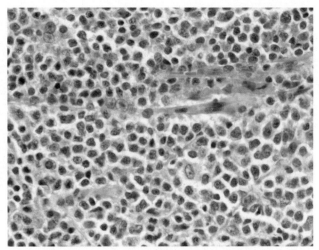

Figure 6.58. Nodal marginal zone lymphoma (NMZL) with extensive follicular colonization mimicking nodular lymphoma: At higher power, the lymphoid cells exhibit monocytoid cytomorphology with scant to moderate amount of clear cytoplasm and centrocytic nuclei.

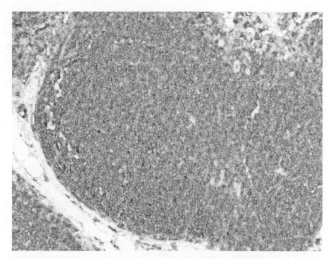

Figure 6.59. **Nodal marginal zone lymphoma (NMZL) with extensive follicular colonization mimicking nodular lymphoma:** The nodules are strongly positive for CD20.

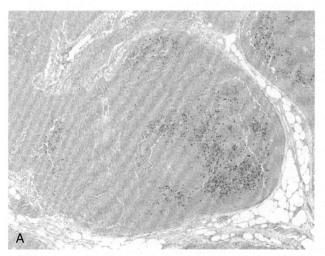

A

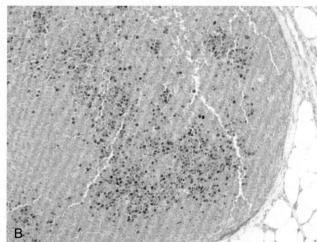

B

Figure 6.60. **Nodal marginal zone lymphoma (NMZL) with extensive follicular colonization mimicking nodular lymphoma:** A and B, BCL-6 immunostain at low power and high power within the nodules demonstrates disrupted moth-eaten pattern but does not recapitulate immunoarchitectural pattern of either normal primary or secondary lymphoid follicles, thereby indicating colonization of germinal center by BCL-6 negative malignant lymphoid cells.

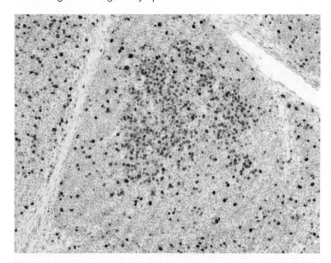

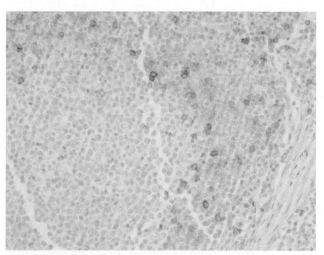

Figure 6.61. Nodal marginal zone lymphoma (NMZL) with extensive follicular colonization mimicking nodular lymphoma: Ki-67 likewise demonstrates similar "moth-eaten" pattern as BCL-6, and the positive cells correspond to residual proliferative germinal center B-cells including centroblastic, while the Ki-67 negative lymphoid cells within the follicles correspond to the colonizing lymphoid component.

Figure 6.62. Nodal marginal zone lymphoma (NMZL) with extensive follicular colonization mimicking nodular lymphoma: IgD immunostain highlights very few mantle zone B-lymphocytes surrounding the follicular structures indicative of markedly disrupted and attenuated mantle cuffs secondary to colonization by marginal zone lymphoma cells.

PTGC-like lymphomas: Along these lines, both NMZL, pediatric type and NLPHL with focal involvement as well as follicular T-cell lymphoma all show extensive nodular PTGC (progressive transformation of germinal center) areas representing significant pitfall entities in diagnosis.

Additional kappa/lambda in situ hybridization is useful in identifying light chain–restricted plasmacytic component in NMZL, and confirmation with PCR or flow may be necessary in such cases that do not show a light chain restricted plasmacytic component by IHC.

In this regard, TFH cells express CD10 and BCL-6 in nodular areas, and careful attention must be paid to know if these cells are B-cells or T-cells since this phenotype may cause confusion with FL. Neoplastic TFH cells express PD-1 and often lose BCL-2, while FL cells will express BCL-2 and are negative for PD-1. Flow cytometry will also be useful in determining CD3/CD10 coexpressing cells seen in TFH-lymphoproliferations.[5]

FAQ: Are there other nodular conditions besides classical Hodgkin lymphoma which express CD30?

Yes. There are several conditions. Variably weak CD30 may be expressed in nodular lymphocyte-predominant Hodgkin lymphoma, T-cell/histiocyte-rich large B-cell lymphoma, and scattered Hodgkin-like cells of peripheral T-cell lymphoma of TFH elevation with scattered Hodgkin-like cells. In addition, numerous reactive interfollicular immunoblasts can be present in any lymphoma and hence correlation with all other stains as well as morphology is critical to avoid misdiagnosis as classical Hodgkin lymphoma solely based on large CD30 positive cells.

Castleman-like lymphomas: FL and cHL may show Castleman-like regressed follicles and hence careful examination using immunostains is necessary. CD30 stains immunoblasts too, so one has to be extra careful before calling out a Castleman-like lymphoproliferation as cHL solely based on a few CD30+ cells. Additional weak CD79a, PAX5, and/or EBER expression restricted to the large Hodgkin-like cells is necessary in such cases to call something as cHL. If in doubt, additional EBER and HHV8 are both useful in cases where true multicentric Castleman disease is a consideration. Also, in seemingly nodular Castleman–like proliferations, one must also pay attention for secondary malignancies like follicular dendritic cell sarcomas, which may coexist in these cases.

PITFALL CASE 2: GERMINOTROPIC LYMPHOPROLIFERATIVE DISORDER, EBV+/HHV8+

Another pitfall case along these lines is the germinotropic lymphoproliferative disorder that may be dismissed as reactive hyperplasia or FL grade 3b in some instances (Figures 6.63-6.65).[6,7]

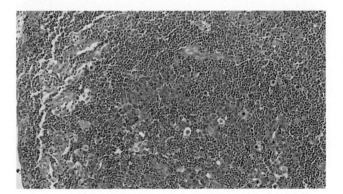

Figure 6.63. Human herpesvirus (HHV)8+/Epstein-Barr virus (EBV)+ germinotropic lymphoproliferative disorder: This is a 35-year-old man with asymptomatic neck lymphadenopathy without evidence of HIV. Initial lymph node biopsies were considered to be reactive follicular hyperplasia with focal Castleman–like features. However, subsequent lymph node biopsy demonstrated occasional atypical lymphoid follicles. H&E image demonstrating scattered nodular lymphoid follicles with clusters of large plasmablastic lymphoid cells.

PITFALL CASE 3: FOLLICULAR VARIANT OF PERIPHERAL T-CELL LYMPHOMA (FIGURES 6.66-6.70)

This node demonstrated seemingly nodular architecture reminiscent of FL with slightly more T-cells inside the nodules. Superficially, the presence of nodular CD20 positive small B cells with coexpression of CD10 and BCL-2 may be construed as FL. However, closer examination reveals that the numbers of BCL-2 positive cells outnumber CD20 positive B cells and help inferring that the T-cells are positive for BCL-2, CD10, CD4, and PD1.[2] This case highlights the importance of the need to compare the numbers of positive cells on each of the stains so one can match up which specific compartment (B-cell vs T-cells) is positive for each of the markers based on the spatial distribution and numbers of positive cells. See (Figure 6.71) for an approach all nodular proliferations.

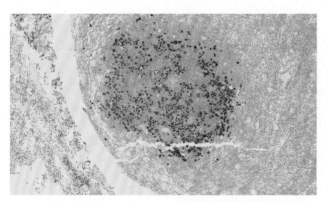

Figure 6.64. Human herpesvirus (HHV)8+/Epstein-Barr virus (EBV)+ germinotropic lymphoproliferative disorder: These lymphoid cells are positive for HHV8.

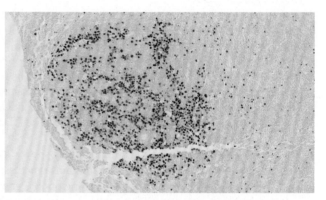

Figure 6.65. Human herpesvirus (HHV)8+/Epstein-Barr virus (EBV)+ germinotropic lymphoproliferative disorder: There is coexpression of EBER, and they were negative for CD20. Both features (co-infection by HHV8/EBV) and lack of CD20 are typical of this entity.

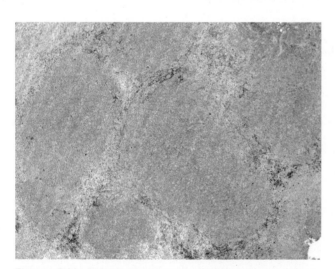

Figure 6.66. Follicular variant of peripheral T-cell lymphoma (F-PTCL): Low-power H&E image demonstrating nodular architecture with closely packed monotonous follicular structures with a mottled appearance.

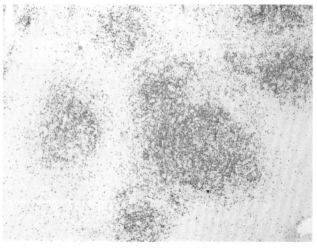

Figure 6.67. Follicular variant of peripheral T-cell lymphoma (F-PTCL): CD20 immunostain demonstrating clusters of small B-cells within the nodules.

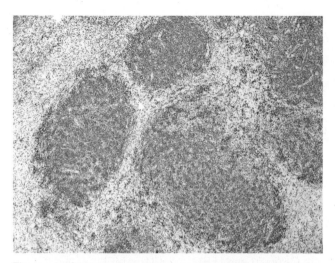

Figure 6.68. Follicular variant of peripheral T-cell lymphoma (F-PTCL): CD3 immunostain highlighting numerous T-cells within the nodules. Note that the numbers of T-cells outnumber the numbers of B cells depicted in Figure 6.67.

Figure 6.69. Follicular variant of peripheral T-cell lymphoma (F-PTCL): CD7 immunostain shows that most of the cells within the nodules are negative for CD7, consistent with aberrant T cells supporting a T-cell neoplasm.

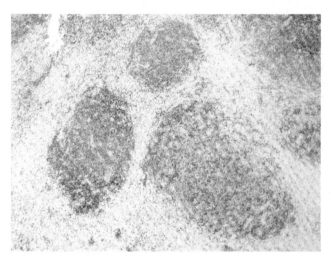

Figure 6.70. Follicular variant of peripheral T-cell lymphoma (F-PTCL): Follicular helper T-cell marker, PD-1 highlights numerous positive lymphoid cells within the follicles matching the numbers of CD3 positive cells confirming involvement by F-PTCL. The cells were additionally positive for CD10.

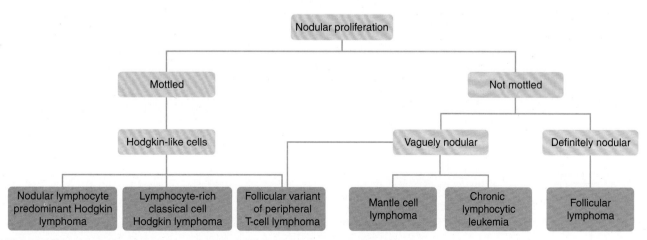

Figure 6.71. Simple flowchart for my approach to all nodular lymphoid proliferations.

KEY FEATURES of Some Nodular Proliferations and Most critical Immunostain Features Useful in Corroborating the Diagnosis

Pattern	Immunostains	Diagnosis
Nodular with few large atypical cells inside nodules	CD20 and OCT2	NLPHL, variant pattern NPHL
Nodular without large cells	CD10/BCL-2	FL grade 1-2
Nodular with cluster of plasmablastic cells	EBV/HHV8	Germinotropic LPD
Nodular with T-cell predominance	Perifollicular PD1 clusters	Follicular T-cell lymphoma
Nodular with sheets of CD10— large B-cells	Ki-67, HGAL	FL grade 3b
Vaguely nodular with CD5 coexpression	Cyclin D1 and LEF1	CLL vs MCL

References

1. Siddiqi IN, Brynes RK, Wang E. B-cell lymphoma with hyaline vascular Castleman disease-like features: a clinicopathologic study. *Am J Clin Pathol.* 2011;135:901-914.

2. Swerdlow SH, Campo E, Harris NL, et al, eds. *WHO Classification of Tumours of Haematopoietic and Lymphoid Tissues.* Revised 4th ed. Lyons: IARC; 2017.

3. Tandon B, Peterson L, Gao J, et al. Nuclear overexpression of lymphoid-enhancer-binding factor 1 identifies chronic lymphocytic leukemia/small lymphocytic lymphoma in small B-cell lymphomas. *Mod Pathol.* 2011;24:1433-1443.

4. Louissaint A Jr, Ackerman AM, Dias-Santagata D, et al. Pediatric-type nodal follicular lymphoma: an indolent clonal proliferation in children and adults with high proliferation index and no BCL2 rearrangement. *Blood.* 2012;120:2395-2404.

5. Alikhan M, Song JY, Sohani AR, et al. Peripheral T-cell lymphomas of follicular helper T-cell type frequently display an aberrant CD3-/dimCD4+ population by flow cytometry: an important clue to the diagnosis of a Hodgkin lymphoma mimic. *Mod Pathol.* 2016;29(10):1173-1182.

6. Chadburn A, Said J, Gratzinger D, et al. HHV8/KSHV-Positive lymphoproliferative disorders and the spectrum of plasmablastic and plasma cell neoplasms: 2015 SH/EAHP Workshop Report-Part 3. *Am J Clin Pathol.* 2017;147:171-187.

7. Du MQ, Diss TC, Liu H, et al. KSHV- and EBV-associated germinotropic lymphoproliferative disorder. *Blood.* 2002;100:3415-3418.

CHAPTER OUTLINE

This chapter focuses on the lymphomas that efface the nodal architecture. Generally, only neoplastic processes will have this effect on the architecture. At low magnification, the typical normal landmarks that are present in a reactive node are not present, such as follicles and paracortex. Also, sinuses will be compressed or absent. There are a variety of lymphomas and diseases that can show this pattern in the lymph node, and we will discuss and show examples of the more common types.

B-CELL LYMPHOMAS

SMALL LYMPHOCYTIC LYMPHOMA AND RICHTER SYNDROME

In small lymphocytic lymphoma (SLL), there is diffuse effacement of the architecture and the infiltrate is composed of small lymphocytes with round nuclear contours, scant cytoplasm, and condensed chromatin (Figure 7.1). These are B-cells staining with CD20 and CD5 as well as CD23 (Figures 7.2-7.5). There are paler areas with a vaguely nodular pattern called proliferation centers that are characteristic at low magnification (Figures 7.6 and 7.7) and

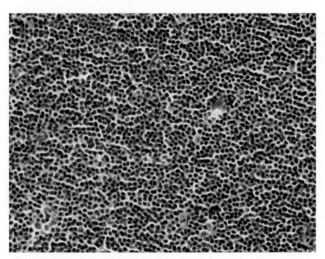

Figure 7.1. SLL: Medium magnification showing monotonous cells that are round with coarse chromatin.

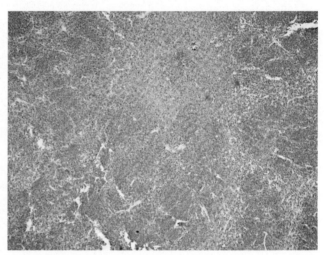

Figure 7.2. SLL: CD20 is diffusely positive.

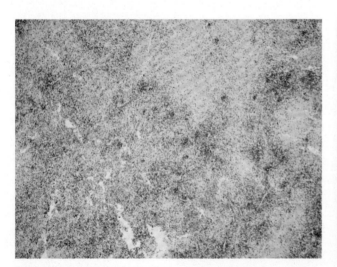

Figure 7.3. SLL: CD3 highlights the background T-cells.

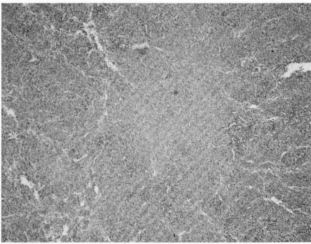

Figure 7.4. SLL: In comparison, you can see that there is dual expression of CD5 with the reactive T-cells being strong, while the neoplastic B-cells have weak expression.

composed of larger lymphoid cells with more abundant cytoplasm and occasional nucleoli. These areas can be highlighted by Ki-67 since there is increased proliferation in these areas, mimicking a germinal center and may have expression of cyclin D1 protein as well as MYC but lack these rearrangements.[1] At times, these proliferation centers can become more confluent and be concerning for large-cell transformation (Richter syndrome). Richter syndrome is commonly the diffuse large B-cell lymphoma (DLBCL) type with sheets of large atypical cells (Figures 7.8-7.10), and in some of these cases, there is no clonal relationship detected by IgVH mutational analysis between the low-grade component and transformed component.[2] The other form, which is less common, is the Hodgkin-like transformation of Richter syndrome and typically has discrete areas of Hodgkin lymphoma with a prominent inflammatory background consisting of T-cells, histiocytes, and eosinophils (Figures 7.11 and 7.12). The Hodgkin cells are positive for CD30 and may have variable expression of the B-cell program (Figures 7.13 and 7.14).

Figure 7.5. SLL: The tumor cells are positive for CD23.

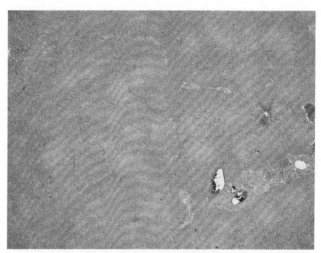

Figure 7.6. SLL: Low-power magnification; one can appreciate the pale areas consistent with proliferation centers that may mimic germinal centers.

Figure 7.7. SLL: Low-power magnification showing the proliferation centers that are pale.

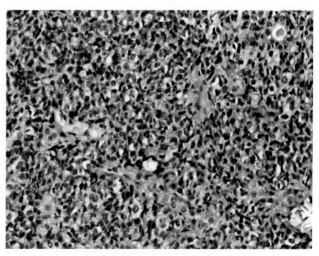

Figure 7.8. SLL with Richter syndrome: High-power magnification showing large neoplastic cells characteristic of DLBCL.

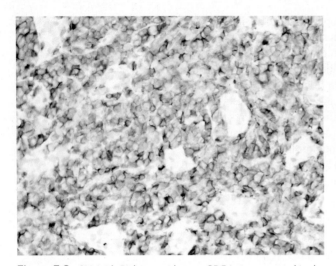

Figure 7.9. SLL with Richter syndrome: CD5 is coexpressed in the large tumor cells.

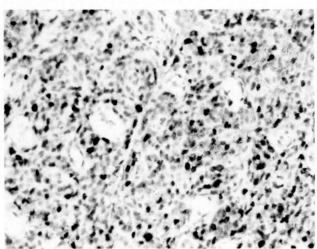

Figure 7.10. SLL with Richter syndrome: The proliferation index seen with Ki-67 is high.

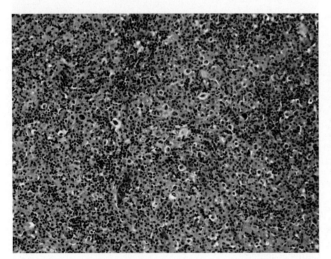

Figure 7.11. SLL with Richter syndrome: A type of Richter syndrome with cHL transformation. Medium magnification shows scattered Hodgkin cells.

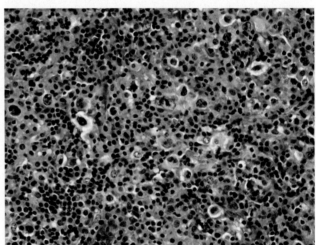

Figure 7.12. SLL with Richter syndrome: The Hodgkin cells are large with vesicular chromatin and prominent nucleoli.

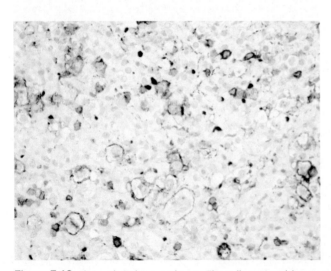

Figure 7.13. SLL with Richter syndrome: The cells are variably positive for CD20.

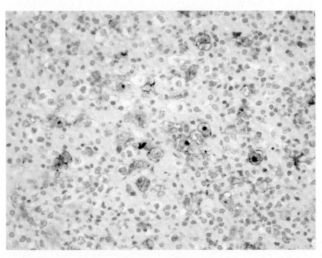

Figure 7.14. SLL with Richter syndrome: CD30 is positive in the Hodgkin cells with membrane and golgi staining.

MANTLE CELL LYMPHOMA

Mantle cell lymphoma typically is a monomorphic lymphoid proliferation that may have a mantle zone pattern or diffuse pattern. The morphology of the typical cases shows small- to medium-size cells with slight to markedly irregular nuclear contours, coarse chromatin, and indistinct nucleoli (Figure 7.15). Pink histiocytes can often be seen in the background (Figure 7.16). The immunophenotype of mantle cell lymphoma is positive for CD20, CD5, and cyclin D1 (Figures 7.17 and 7.18). SOX11 is also positive and is useful in identifying cyclin D1–negative mantle cell lymphomas.[3] Flow cytometry can be helpful since mantle cell lymphoma generally has moderate expression of CD20 and surface immunoglobulin and is negative for CD23 (Figure 7.19). This is in contrast to chronic lymphocytic leukemia (CLL) which has dim to negative CD20 and surface immunoglobulin and is positive for CD23. Cases with a blastoid and pleomorphic morphology have cells that are medium to large in size with irregular nuclear contours, fine chromatin, and occasional nucleoli. These cases usually have a diffuse pattern with notable mitotic figures, and the proliferation index is usually high seen with Ki-67. It is important to recognize blastoid/pleomorphic mantle cell lymphoma due to the prognostic implication as well as diagnostic consideration of DLBCL. In cases where the lymph node architecture is predominantly intact, a mantle zone growth pattern can be seen and an in situ mantle cell lymphoma needs to be considered.

PEARLS & PITFALLS

If you are reviewing a case that shows small- to medium-sized cells with clefted nuclei and scattered pink histiocytes and is positive for CD5 but is negative for cyclin D1 protein, performing a SOX11 immunostain might identify or rule out a cyclin D1–negative mantle cell lymphoma.

DIFFUSE FOLLICULAR LYMPHOMA

There are rare cases of follicular lymphoma that predominantly have a diffuse pattern (Figure 7.20). These cases usually have small follicles in the surrounding tissue (so-called microfollicles), and these cases are consistently lacking the *IGH/BCL2* translocation and have weak to absent BCL2 protein staining by immunohistochemistry. A common location of involvement is the inguinal lymph nodes. The tumor cells are positive for CD10, and most cases have CD23 expression in the cells (Figures 7.21 and 7.22). A common genetic aberration is deletion in 1p36 which contains the *TNFRSF14* gene as well as these cases showed *STAT6* mutations.[4,5] At times, interfollicular neoplastic centrocytes can be mistaken as diffuse areas. Also, determining a diffuse component on needle core biopsies may prove challenging.

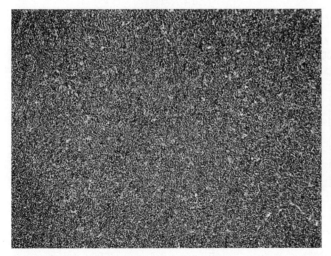

Figure 7.15. Mantle cell lymphoma: Low-power magnification of MCL with a diffuse pattern and scattered pink histiocytes.

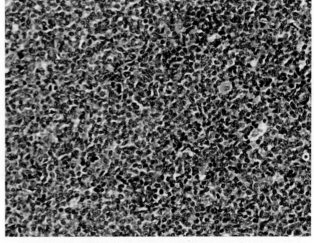

Figure 7.16. Mantle cell lymphoma: The cells are medium to small in size with irregular nuclear contours and course chromatin. Again the characteristic pink histiocytes are seen in the background.

PEARLS & PITFALLS

Diffuse follicular lymphoma should have predominantly centrocytes with only occasional centroblasts (<15/hpf). If you see areas with increased number or centroblasts (>15/hpf), a diagnosis of DLBCL may be warranted.

Figure 7.17. Mantle cell lymphoma: The tumor cells are positive for CD20.

Figure 7.18. Mantle cell lymphoma: They are positive for cyclin D1.

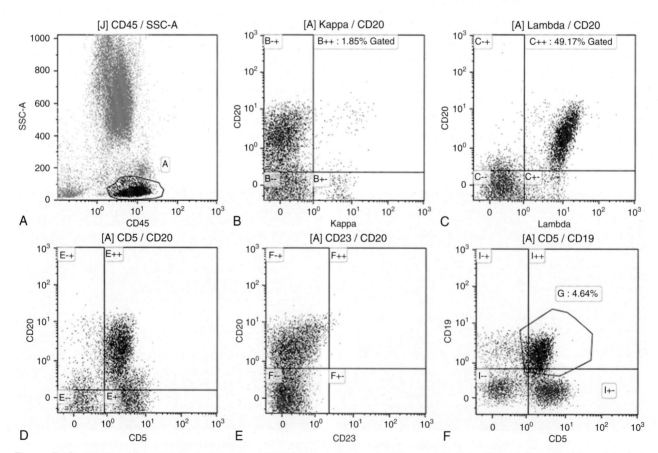

Figure 7.19. Mantle cell lymphoma: An example of the flow cytometry showing the tumor cells positive for CD20 (moderate), lambda restricted (moderate), and CD5- and CD23-positive.

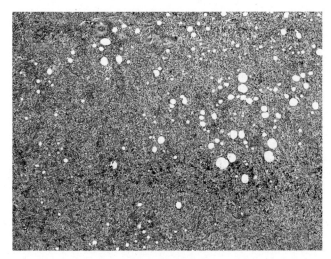

Figure 7.20. Diffuse follicular lymphoma: Low-power magnification showing the effaced nodal architecture of an inguinal node.

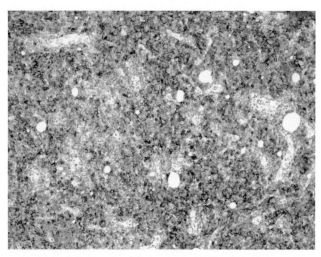

Figure 7.21. Diffuse follicular lymphoma: The tumor cells are positive for CD10.

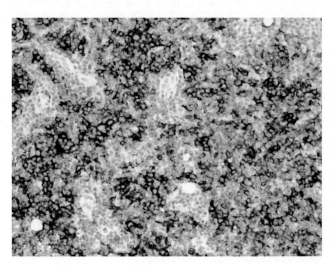

Figure 7.22. Diffuse follicular lymphoma: The tumor cells are positive for CD23.

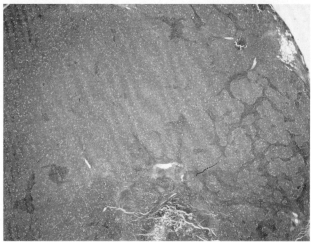

Figure 7.23. Follicular lymphoma with transformation to DLBCL: Low-power magnification showing areas of FL in the lower right area, while the top left showing a more diffuse pattern with sheets of neoplastic cells.

FOLLICULAR LYMPHOMA WITH TRANSFORMATION TO DLBCL

The most common type of histologic transformation of FL is to DLBCL, but high-grade B-cell lymphoma or B-lymphoblastic lymphoma has also been seen typically by acquiring a second "hit" such as the *MYC* translocation. The risk of transformation goes up 2% each year. The histology of the cells is typical of that seen in DLBCL or high-grade B-cell lymphoma (Figures 7.23-7.25). It is important to have good sampling of excisional lymph nodes, particularly cases with high fluorodeoxyglucose (FDG) uptake on PET, so a transformed component is not missed. Additionally, the follicular lymphoma component may be inconspicuous in cases of DLBCL and at the edge of the high-grade component or mimicking reactive follicle structures. Immunostaining for CD21, Ki-67, and BCL2 may be helpful, but some high-grade FLs may be negative for BCL2 protein[6] (Figure 7.26).

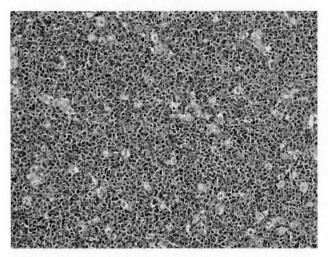

Figure 7.24. Follicular lymphoma with transformation to DLBCL: The diffuse areas show large atypical cells with numerous apoptotic bodies giving a starry-sky appearance.

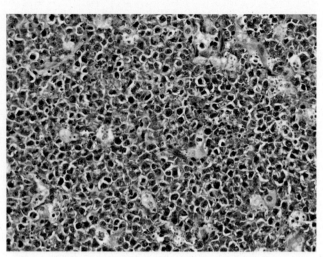

Figure 7.25. Follicular lymphoma with transformation to DLBCL: Higher magnification showing the large neoplastic cells of the DLBCL component.

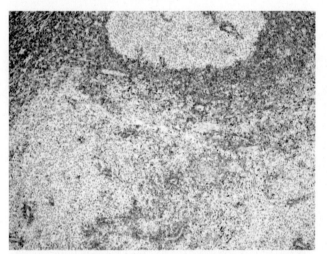

Figure 7.26. Follicular lymphoma with transformation to DLBCL: BCL2 immunostaining shows the follicular lymphoma component, as well as the DLBCL component, is negative for this protein.

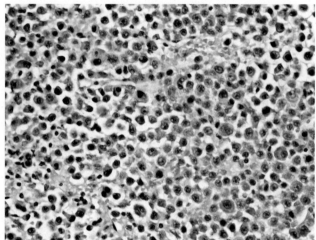

Figure 7.27. Plasma cell myeloma: High-power magnification showing sheets of mature plasma cells.

PEARLS & PITFALLS

In cases of DLBCL, it is important to examine the immunostains for BCL2 and Ki-67 at the edge of the lesion or in reactive-appearing follicles to ensure that a low-grade follicular lymphoma is not missed. The low-grade FL will have positivity in the germinal centers with BCL2, and the proliferation index is lower than that seen with reactive follicular hyperplasia.

PLASMACYTOMA/PLASMA CELL MYELOMA

Extraosseous plasmacytomas can occur in the upper respiratory tract, central nervous system, as well as lymph nodes. There may be complete effacement of the lymph node architecture by sheets of plasma cells, and the morphology can vary from typical benign plasma cells (Figure 7.27) to anaplastic or pleomorphic. The cells are positive for CD138 and are light chain restricted (Figures 7.28-7.30) but negative for Epstein-Barr encoding region (EBER). Consideration of other lymphomas, particularly marginal zone lymphoma, needs to be considered since these may be difficult to delineate as marginal zone lymphomas with marked plasmacytic differentiation can look identical to primary plasma cell neoplasm.

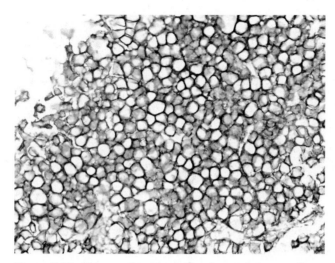

Figure 7.28. Plasma cell myeloma: The sheets of plasma cells are positive for CD138.

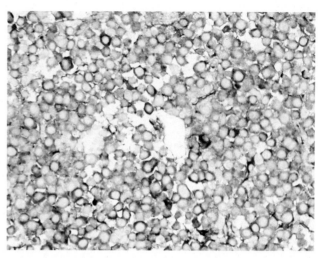

Figure 7.29. Plasma cell myeloma: The plasma cells are kappa restricted.

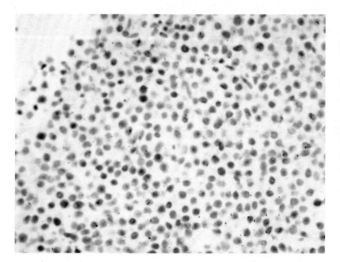

Figure 7.30. Plasma cell myeloma: The plasma cells are negative for lambda immunostaining.

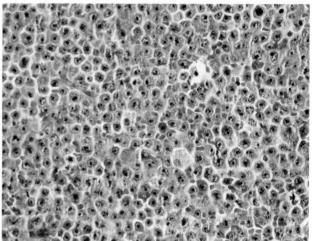

Figure 7.31. Diffuse large B-cell lymphoma: High magnification shows the immunoblastic variant with a prominent central nucleolus.

DIFFUSE LARGE B-CELL LYMPHOMA, NOT OTHERWISE SPECIFIED

The most common lymphoma that shows a diffuse infiltrate composed of large atypical cells forming sheets is DLBCL. The morphology of the cells can vary from immunoblastic (Figure 7.31), anaplastic (Figures 7.32 and 7.33), and centroblastic (Figure 7.34). The most common variant is the centroblastic variant and shows round nuclear contours, fine chromatin, and multiple small nucleoli. Immunoblastic variant shows a single centrally located nucleolus. The anaplastic variant shows bizarre pleomorphic nuclei that may resemble Hodgkin Reed-Sternberg cells as well as cells seen in anaplastic large-cell lymphoma. This variant is fairly rare. Typically, small T-lymphocytes can be seen but are mostly inconspicuous in the background. A starry-sky pattern with tingible-body macrophages creating a punched-out appearance can be seen. This finding can also be seen with lymphoblastic lymphomas as well as Burkitt lymphoma or processes with a high proliferation index. Focal necrosis as well as apoptotic cells can be seen due to the high turnover in some cases (Figure 7.35). Typically, DLBCL is categorized by germinal center phenotype (GCB) or activated B-cell (ABC)–like, which is determined by gene expression profiling (GEP).[7] Using the Hans algorithm as a surrogate to GEP, one can determine the cell of origin by performing a panel of immunostains (CD10, BCL6, and MUM1).[8] Generally, the centroblastic variant has a GCB versus immunoblastic morphology has a nongerminal center (eg, ABC) phenotype by GEP.

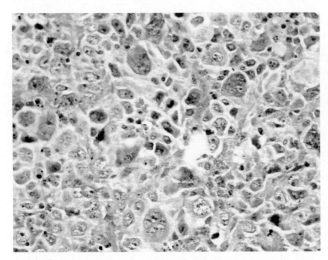

Figure 7.32. Diffuse large B-cell lymphoma: This is an example of the anaplastic/pleomorphic variant of DLBCL. Cells are large with multiple lobulations and multiple prominent nucleoli.

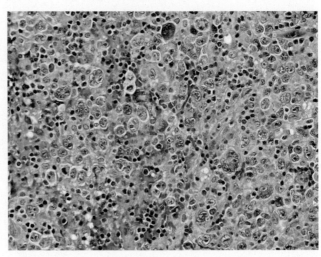

Figure 7.33. Diffuse large B-cell lymphoma: Another example of an anaplastic/pleomorphic variant of DLBCL.

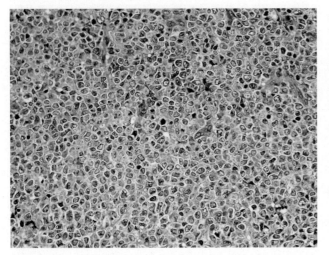

Figure 7.34. Diffuse large B-cell lymphoma: An example of centroblastic DLBCL. The cells have round nuclear contours, open chromatin, and multiple small nucleoli.

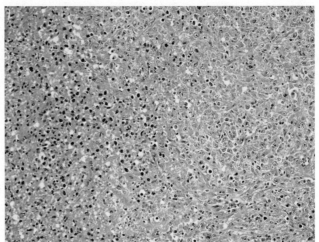

Figure 7.35. Diffuse large B-cell lymphoma: Some cases of DLBCL show tumor necrosis (left) as in the example.

T-CELL–/HISTIOCYTE-RICH LARGE B-CELL LYMPHOMA

T-cell–/histiocyte-rich large B-cell lymphoma (THRLBL) will also show an effaced nodal architecture with a diffuse pattern (Figures 7.36 and 7.37). However, the majority of the cells are histiocytes and/or T-cells with only occasional large B-cells seen (Figures 7.38-7.41). These large B-cells can be inconspicuous and are prominently seen with a CD20 stain or B-cell marker, highlighting the scattered large atypical cells, with the rich microenvironment in the background (Figures 7.42-7.47). The large atypical cells do not form sheets or large aggregates and are singly distributed. These large cells can mimic the neoplastic cells seen in nodular lymphocyte–predominant Hodgkin lymphoma (NLPHL) (LP cells) as well as those seen in classical Hodgkin lymphoma (cHL). Occasionally, a THRLBL can be seen concurrently arising from NLPHL. Therefore, careful evaluation of the areas surrounding the diffuse areas for residual NLPHL should be evaluated. The large atypical cells express B-cell markers as well as BCL6 and generally negative for CD30.

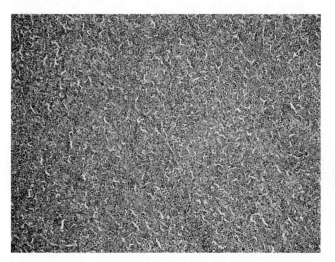

Figure 7.36. T-cell–/histiocyte-rich large B-cell lymphoma: Low-power magnification showing effaced nodal architecture with scattered, somewhat inconspicuous, large cells.

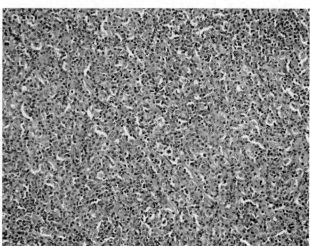

Figure 7.37. T-cell–/histiocyte-rich large B-cell lymphoma: The background shows mostly small lymphocytes which are T-cells and histiocytes.

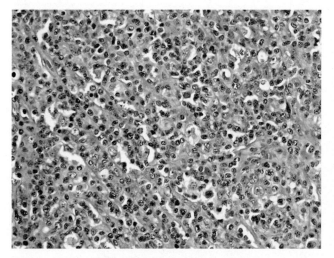

Figure 7.38. T-cell–/histiocyte-rich large B-cell lymphoma: Scattered large atypical cells are appreciated at high magnification.

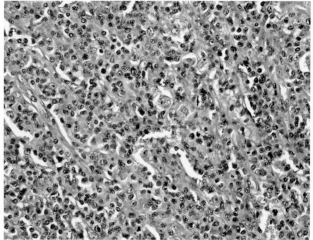

Figure 7.39. T-cell–/histiocyte-rich large B-cell lymphoma: Another example showing the large cells with vesicular chromatin and prominent nucleoli.

PLASMABLASTIC LYMPHOMA

This is a type of DLBCL which is most commonly seen in patients with immunodeficiency, most commonly HIV infection. Extranodal regions are more common such as the nasal cavity, but other sites can be seen and rarely lymph nodes. Posttransplant-associated plasmablastic lymphoma (PBL) can present with nodal involvement. This lymphoma shows sheets of large atypical cells with a predominant morphology of immunoblasts or plasmablasts (Figure 7.48). Areas of geographic necrosis are common, and some cases can have a "starry-sky" appearance. Tumor cells lack CD20, PAX5, and CD45. Plasma cell transcription factors are commonly expressed such as CD38, CD138, and MUM1. The proliferation index is typically high and above 90% when seen with Ki-67. EBER is expressed in 70% of

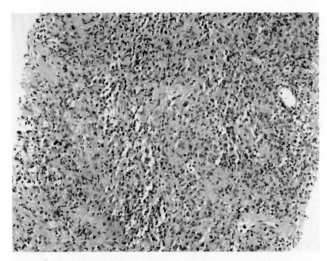

Figure 7.40. T-cell–/histiocyte-rich large B-cell lymphoma: Medium magnification of a needle core biopsy showing mostly histiocytes and scattered indistinct large cells.

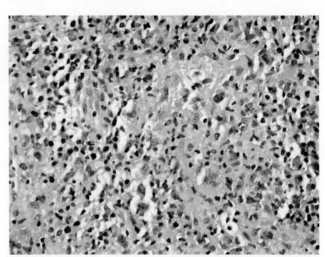

Figure 7.41. T-cell–/histiocyte-rich large B-cell lymphoma: Higher magnification showing large atypical cells which are the minority of the cellular population.

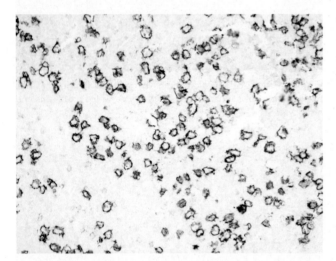

Figure 7.42. T-cell–/histiocyte-rich large B-cell lymphoma: CD20 highlights the large atypical B-cells. Notice how there are almost no small B-cells present.

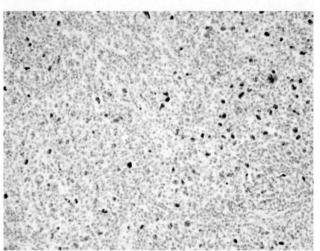

Figure 7.43. T-cell–/histiocyte-rich large B-cell lymphoma: Many of these cases show large cells are also positive for BCL6.

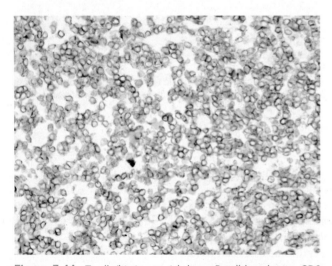

Figure 7.44. T-cell–/histiocyte-rich large B-cell lymphoma: CD3 highlights the prominent background T-cell population.

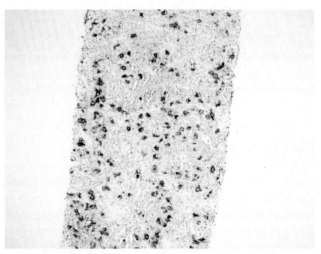

Figure 7.45. T-cell–/histiocyte-rich large B-cell lymphoma: A needle core biopsy with CD20 showing the scattered large atypical cells.

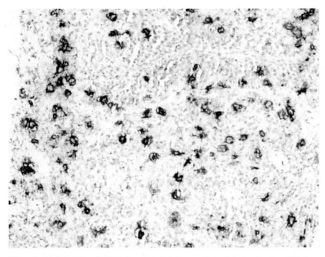

Figure 7.46. T-cell-/histiocyte-rich large B-cell lymphoma: Higher magnification showing the large atypical cells highlighted with CD20.

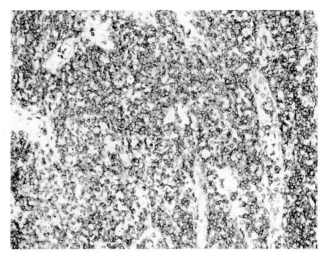

Figure 7.47. T-cell-/histiocyte-rich large B-cell lymphoma: On the needle core, the CD3 stains the numerous T-cells. Occasional rosettes can be seen.

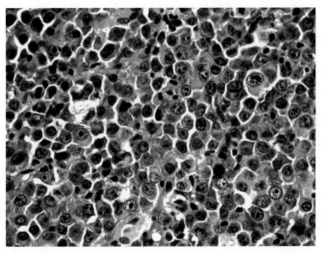

Figure 7.48. Plasmablastic lymphoma: High magnification of large atypical cells with eosinophilic cytoplasm, round nuclear contours, and prominent nucleolus.

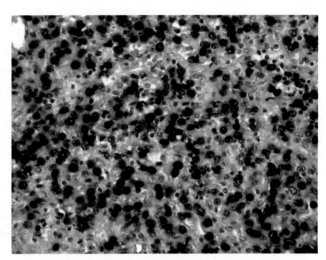

Figure 7.49. Plasmablastic lymphoma: EBER-ISH stain highlights the tumor cells associated with EBV.

cases, and this is the most helpful marker (Figure 7.49) since there is both morphologic and immunophenotypic overlap of PBL and plasma cell myeloma with plasmablastic features. *MYC* translocations are seen in about half of the cases.

PEARLS & PITFALLS

The distinction between PBL and plasma cell myeloma with plasmablastic features is often challenging. The majority of immunostains such as CD79a, CD138, MYC, and Ki-67 are not helpful in making this differentiation since there is considerable overlap. Additionally, FISH analysis for *MYC* translocations can be seen in both entities. EBER positivity would be diagnostic of a PBL, but if this is negative (30% of cases), reliance on the clinical history such as immunodeficiency (iatrogenic, viral) and myeloma workup is necessary (bone scan, SPEP/IFE, renal function).

PRIMARY MEDIASTINAL LARGE B-CELL LYMPHOMA

This tumor presents in the anterior mediastinum and has a female predominance compared to males. Patients will have symptoms of a large mediastinal mass such as superior vena cava syndrome. The cells are large to medium in size with variation in histology from immunoblastic, anaplastic, centroblastic, spindle, and Hodgkin-like cells can be present. There is usually abundant cytoplasm which is often clear. Sclerosis is common and can be delicate or dense collagen (Figures 7.50-7.52). Primary mediastinal large B-cell lymphoma (PMBL) expresses pan B-cell markers (Figures 7.53-7.55) and frequently expresses CD23 (70% of cases) (Figure 7.56). CD30 is commonly positive but does not show strong uniform staining as seen in Hodgkin lymphoma or gray zone lymphomas (B-cell lymphoma, unclassifiable, intermediate between DLBCL and cHL) (Figures 7.57 and 7.58). EBER is negative. One of the main differentials for PMBL is cHL, nodular sclerosis subtype, which can express pan B-cell markers, but the latter typically has a rich inflammatory background with eosinophils and may express CD15 but lacks CD45. Needle core biopsies also represent a challenge, and that distinction may not be made unless a larger biopsy or excision is performed. Transcriptions factors (OCT2 and BOB1) may be useful since these are positive in PMBL and usually negative or weakly positive in cHL.

KEY FEATURES
- PMBL typically shows a fine fibrotic background.
- PMBL should have intact B-cell markers such as CD20, PAX5, and CD79a.
- CD23 is helpful as most of the cases show some positivity in the tumor cells.
- CD30 may be positive but is usually weak and focal.

B-CELL LYMPHOMA, UNCLASSIFIABLE, WITH FEATURES INTERMEDIATE BETWEEN DIFFUSE LARGE B-CELL LYMPHOMA AND CLASSICAL HODGKIN LYMPHOMA (GRAY ZONE LYMPHOMA)

The cytologic appearance of these tumors varies with some areas resembling cHL and other more like PMBL.[9] Tumor density is usually high, and cells have a sheetlike growth pattern (Figures 7.59 and 7.60). Discordance of the immunophenotype is common (cases with morphology of cHL having the phenotype of PMBL and vice versa). Cases with a cytologic appearance of cHL are CD45-positive and have intact B-cell program such as CD20, CD79a, and CD30 and/or CD15 may be expressed (Figures 7.61-7.65). In cases with a histologic appearance of PMBL, there is loss of B-cell antigens but positivity with CD30 and CD15. Transcriptions factors are usually expressed such as PAX5, OCT2, and BOB1. The inflammatory background is typically sparse.

BURKITT LYMPHOMA

Burkitt lymphoma also shows a diffuse infiltrate typically with a starry-sky pattern (Figure 7.66). The cells are usually medium sized with round nuclear contours, finally clumped chromatin, and multiple small nucleoli (Figures 7.67 and 7.68). The cells are generally monomorphic, and nuclear irregularity would favor more of a typical DLBCL especially if there is variation in size. The starry-sky pattern is due to the presence of numerous tingible-body macrophages which can be explained by the high proliferation index seen in these tumors. Burkitt lymphoma has intact B-cell markers as well as germinal center markers (CD10 and BCL6) and lacks BCL-2 protein expression (Figures 7.69-7.72). The proliferation index is at or close to 100% seen with Ki-67. T-cells as well as other reactive cells are generally not seen in the background, and the former can best be seen with a concurrent CD3 stain (Figure 7.73). The Burkitt-like lymphoma with 11q aberration shows a similar morphologic finding as classic Burkitt lymphoma. However, these cases can have a high degree of cytologic pleomorphism (Figures 7.74 and 7.75).

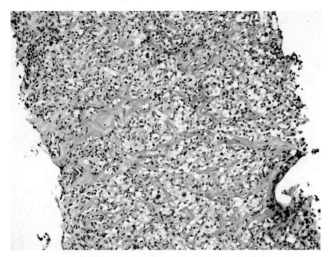

Figure 7.50. Primary mediastinal large B-cell lymphoma: Medium magnification of a needle core with compartmentalization of medium to large atypical cells by fine and coarse fibrosis.

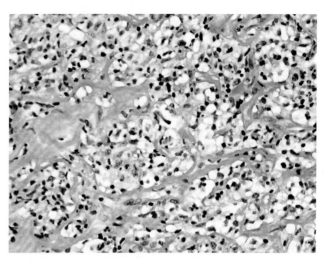

Figure 7.51. Primary mediastinal large B-cell lymphoma: Higher magnification showing medium to large atypical tumor cells with moderate clear cytoplasm.

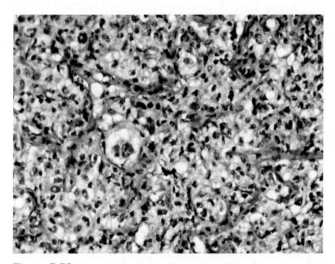

Figure 7.52. Primary mediastinal large B-cell lymphoma: Another high-power magnification showing compartmentalization by fibrosis with occasional lacunar-like Hodgkin cells.

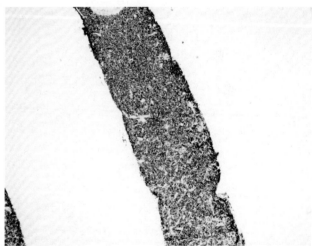

Figure 7.53. Primary mediastinal large B-cell lymphoma: The CD20 shows sheets of atypical B-cells.

FAQ: Can any 11q abnormality be considered in the Burkitt lymphomas lacking t(8;14) if the morphology fits?

Answer: No, the aberration should show a pattern with amplifications in 11q23.2-23.3 in conjunction with the telomeric loss in 11q24.1-qter.[10,11]

HIGH-GRADE B-CELL LYMPHOMA

High-grade B-cell lymphoma is a new category in the 2017 World Health Organization (WHO) classification,[12] with half showing morphologic features of DLBCL, not otherwise specified (NOS) and the other half of cases showing a blastoid morphology composed of medium-sized cells resembling centroblasts (Figures 7.76 and 7.77). Blastoid-variant mantle cell lymphoma may show similar morphologic features and therefore should be excluded. The majority of high-grade B-cell lymphoma are so-called double-hit lymphoma with rearrangements/translocations of *MYC* and *BCL2*. Of note, occasional cases of lymphoblastic

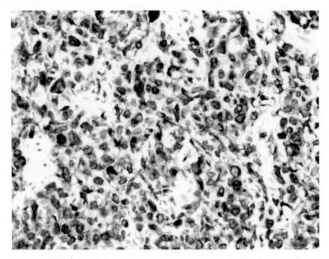

Figure 7.54. Primary mediastinal large B-cell lymphoma: These cells are also positive with CD79a.

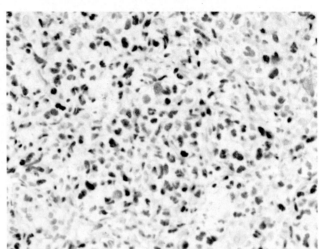

Figure 7.55. Primary mediastinal large B-cell lymphoma: These cells are also positive with PAX5.

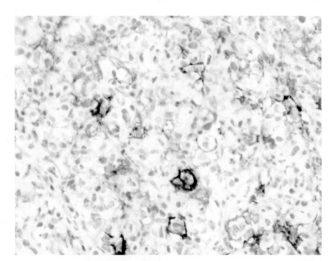

Figure 7.56. Primary mediastinal large B-cell lymphoma: The tumor cells have variable staining with CD30 in contrast to cHL.

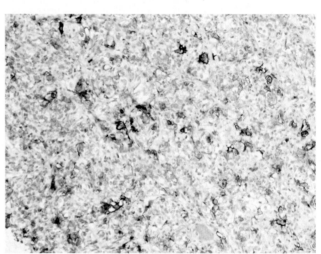

Figure 7.57. Primary mediastinal large B-cell lymphoma: CD30 staining shows scattered and variable staining.

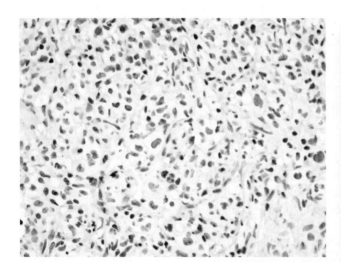

Figure 7.58. Primary mediastinal large B-cell lymphoma: CD15 is typically negative in these cases.

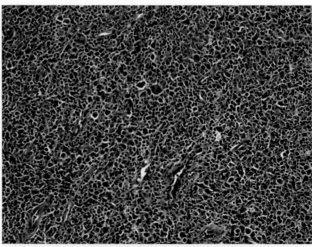

Figure 7.59. B-cell lymphoma, unclassifiable, intermediate between cHL and DLBCL: Medium magnification showing sheets of medium to large atypical cells.

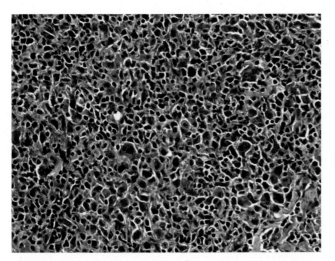

Figure 7.60. B-cell lymphoma, unclassifiable, intermediate between cHL and DLBCL: Higher magnification showing scattered Hodgkin cells and large atypical cells.

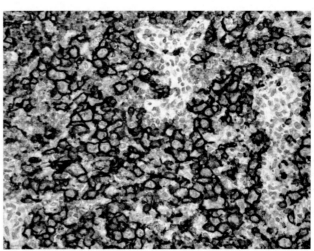

Figure 7.61. B-cell lymphoma, unclassifiable, intermediate between cHL and DLBCL: CD20 is diffuse and strong staining.

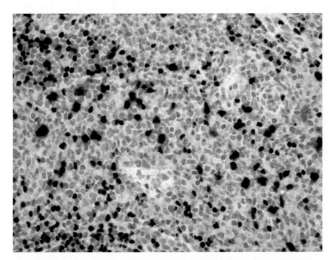

Figure 7.62. B-cell lymphoma, unclassifiable, intermediate between cHL and DLBCL: PAX5 is intact and strong.

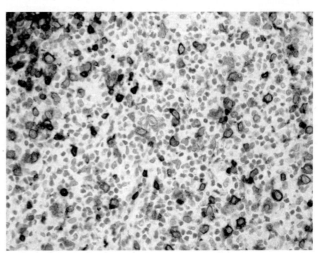

Figure 7.63. B-cell lymphoma, unclassifiable, intermediate between cHL and DLBCL: Another B-cell marker, CD79a is positive.

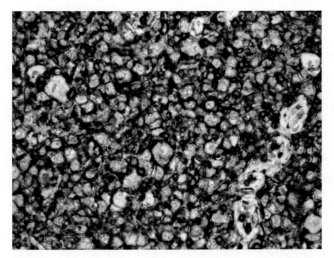

Figure 7.64. B-cell lymphoma, unclassifiable, intermediate between cHL and DLBCL: CD45 is also positive in the cells.

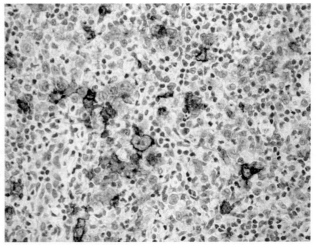

Figure 7.65. B-cell lymphoma, unclassifiable, intermediate between cHL and DLBCL: CD30 shows variable staining with some of the large cells being negative.

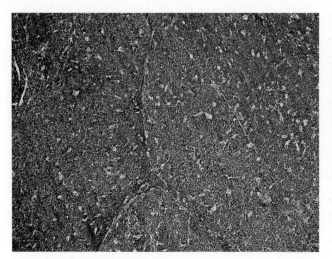

Figure 7.66. Burkitt lymphoma: Sheets of medium-sized atypical cells with a starry-sky appearance.

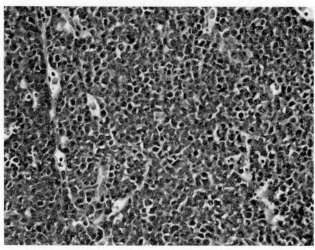

Figure 7.67. Burkitt lymphoma: The cells are medium in size with round nuclear contours and small nucleoli.

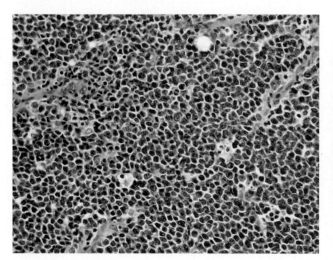

Figure 7.68. Burkitt lymphoma: The cells have a "jig-saw" appearance.

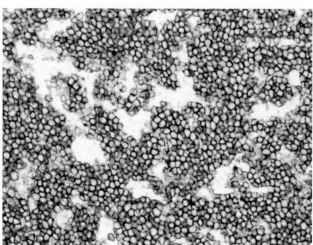

Figure 7.69. Burkitt lymphoma: Tumor cells are positive for CD20.

lymphoma can have overlapping morphology as well as cytogenetic abnormalities similar to these double-hit lymphomas. Generally, FISH analysis for *BCL6*, *BCL2*, and *MYC* should be performed in cases concerning for DLBCL and high-grade B-cell lymphoma to determine if the case is a double- or triple-hit lymphoma.

CHECKLIST: Testing in High-Grade B-Cell Lymphoma or DLBCL

☐ *Immunostaining panel:* CD20, CD19, CD3, CD5, CD10, BCL2, BCL6, MUM1, MYC, and Ki-67

☐ *FISH analysis: MYC* breakapart, *MYC/IGH*, *BCL2/IGH*, and *BCL6/IGH*

☐ Although most double-hit lymphomas are of GCB origin, there are some cases with a non-GCB phenotype that are double-hit lymphomas. In cases where the MYC IHC is >40%, it is important to also perform FISH for MYC probes.

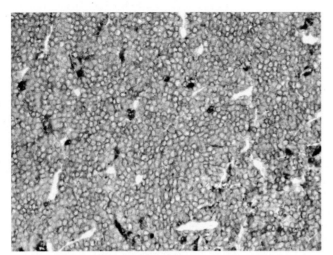

Figure 7.70. Burkitt lymphoma: Tumor cells are positive for CD10.

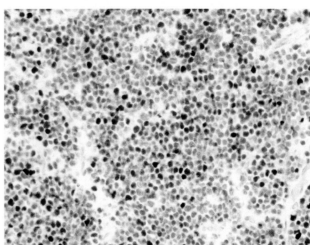

Figure 7.71. Burkitt lymphoma: Tumor cells are positive for BCL6.

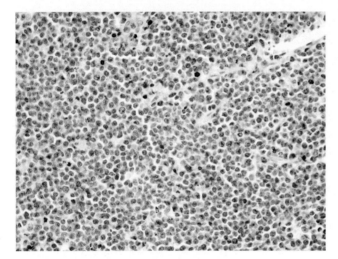

Figure 7.72. Burkitt lymphoma: Tumor cells are negative for BCL2.

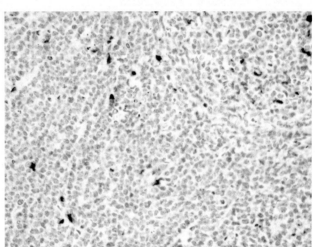

Figure 7.73. Burkitt lymphoma: CD3 highlights the low number of T-cells within the tumor.

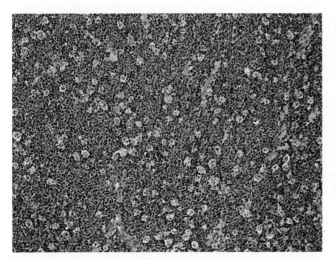

Figure 7.74. Burkitt lymphoma: Medium magnification of a Burkitt lymphoma with 11q abnormalities also showing a starry-sky appearance.

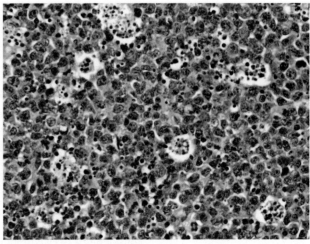

Figure 7.75. Burkitt lymphoma: These cases with 11q abnormalities show more nuclear pleomorphism compared to the classic Burkitt lymphomas.

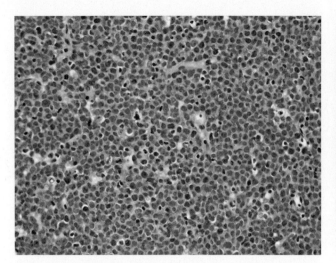

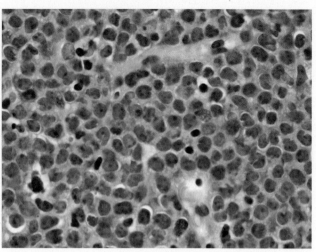

Figure 7.76. High-grade B-cell lymphoma with triple-hit: Sheets of medium-sized atypical cells with fine chromatin and small nucleoli. Numerous mitotic figures are appreciated.

Figure 7.77. High-grade B-cell lymphoma with triple-hit: Higher magnification shows the fine chromatin and multiple small nucleoli.

T-CELL LYMPHOMAS

ANAPLASTIC LARGE-CELL LYMPHOMA

Patients present with lymphadenopathy, and extranodal involvement is less common. Cases with cutaneous involvement need systemic workup, but if the skin is the only site, these cases are diagnosed as primary cutaneous anaplastic large cell lymphoma (ALCL). Systemic ALCL can be anaplastic lymphoma kinase (ALK)-positive or ALK-negative, and the latter usually has a poorer prognosis. The pattern of infiltration of typically sinusoidal but cases with diffuse effacement of the lymph node can be seen (Figures 7.78-7.87). Hallmark cells are characteristic of this disease and have horseshoe-shaped nuclei, but pleomorphic cells can also be observed (Figure 7.88). CD30 is strong and diffusely positive (Figure 7.89). T-cell markers are seen (CD3, CD2, CD4) but are frequently lost (Figures 7.90-7.94). Some cases may lack all T-cell markers and are noted as null-cell phenotype. Although PAX5 is a useful B-cell marker, it can be expressed in some cases of ALCL. ALK-negative ALCLs with *DUSP22-IRF4* rearrangements typically lack cytotoxic markers (TIA1, granzyme B, perforin) that are frequently seen in ALCL and have a good prognosis like ALK-positive ALCL.[13]

PEARLS & PITFALLS

PAX5 is a gene that encodes the B-cell lineage specific activator protein and is an excellent immunostain to determine B-cell lineage in such instances as B-lymphoblastic lymphoma in addition to cHL. However, there are instances of T-cell lymphomas, particularly ALCL that can have weak expression of PAX5.

PERIPHERAL T-CELL LYMPHOMA

The morphology of peripheral T-cell lymphoma (PTCL), NOS is very broad. The pattern of involvement can be interfollicular, paracortical, or diffuse. In this chapter, we will focus on the diffuse pattern of involvement. Many cases show medium to large atypical cells with irregular nuclear contours, some with clear cytoplasm (Figures 7.95-7.99). There is typically an admixture of reactive cells such as small lymphocytes, histiocytes, B-cells, plasma cells, and eosinophils. At times, it is challenging to see the atypical cells since the predominant population may be inflammatory cells. CD3 immunostaining can help with highlighting the T-cells and their cytologic atypia. We also find that eosinophils should clue the pathologist in considering a T-cell lymphoma. In some cases of PTCL, with Hodgkin-like cells are seen with angioimmunoblastic T-cell lymphoma or nodal T-cell lymphoma with follicular helper T-cell (TFH) phenotype (Figures 7.100-7.107), which can mimic cHL (Figures 7.98 and 7.99).

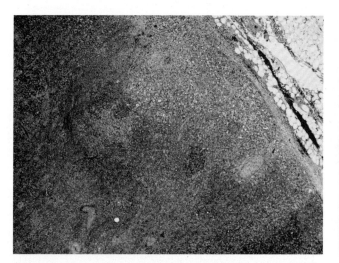

Figure 7.78. Anaplastic large-cell lymphoma, ALK-positive: Lymph node showing a sinusoidal infiltration by neoplastic cells.

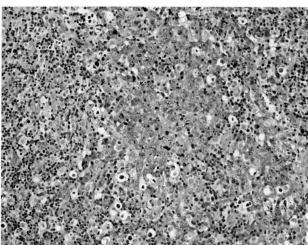

Figure 7.79. Anaplastic large-cell lymphoma, ALK-positive: The large cells have pleomorphic nuclei and moderate basophilic cytoplasm.

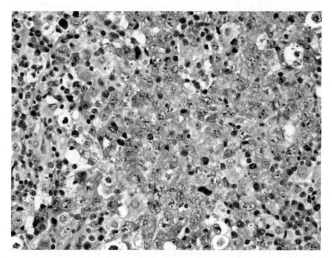

Figure 7.80. Anaplastic large-cell lymphoma, ALK-positive: Higher magnification showing the pleomorphic large cells.

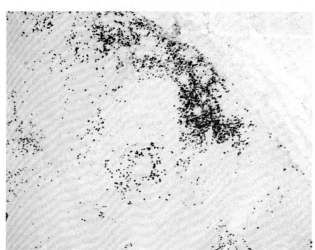

Figure 7.81. Anaplastic large-cell lymphoma, ALK-positive: Low-power magnification with ALK IHC showing the sinusoidal distribution.

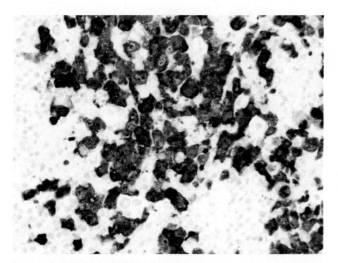

Figure 7.82. Anaplastic large-cell lymphoma, ALK-positive: High magnification with ALK IHC showing the tumor cells are positive.

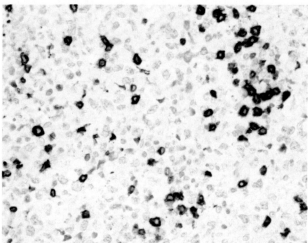

Figure 7.83. Anaplastic large-cell lymphoma, ALK-positive: High magnification shows the tumor cells are negative for CD3.

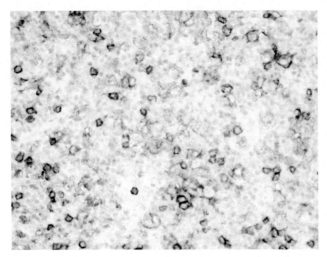

Figure 7.84. Anaplastic large-cell lymphoma, ALK-positive: The neoplastic cells are weakly positive for CD4.

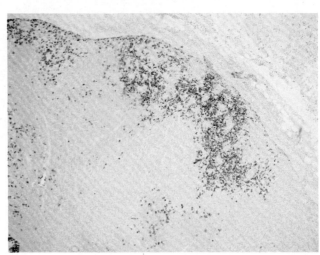

Figure 7.85. Anaplastic large-cell lymphoma, ALK-positive: CD30 at low magnification also highlights the sinusoidal distribution.

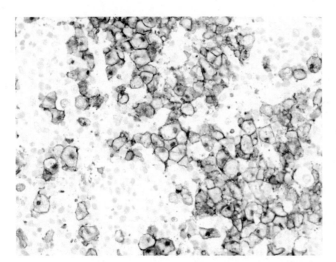

Figure 7.86. Anaplastic large-cell lymphoma, ALK-positive: High magnification shows the membranous and golgi staining with CD30.

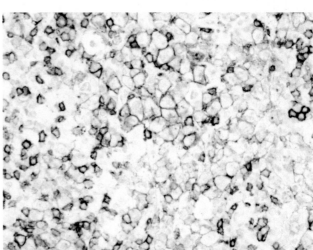

Figure 7.87. Anaplastic large-cell lymphoma, ALK-positive: Tumor cells are also positive with CD43.

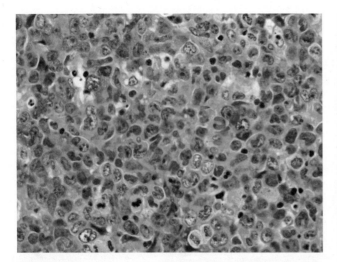

Figure 7.88. Anaplastic large-cell lymphoma, ALK-negative: This case shows at high magnification the characteristic hallmark cells seen in this disease.

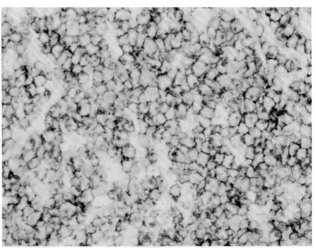

Figure 7.89. Anaplastic large-cell lymphoma, AlK-negative: CD30 is diffusely positive with membrane and golgi staining.

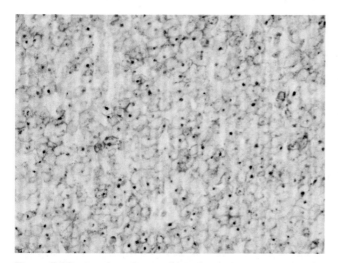

Figure 7.90. Anaplastic large-cell lymphoma, ALK-negative: In this case, the tumor cells are positive with CD2.

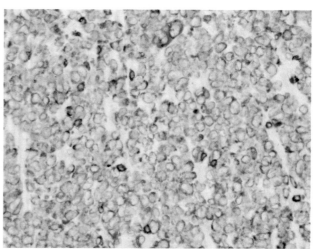

Figure 7.91. Anaplastic large-cell lymphoma, ALK-negative: Tumor cells are also positive with CD3.

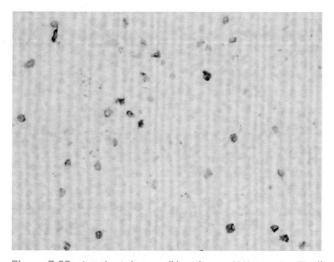

Figure 7.92. Anaplastic large-cell lymphoma, ALK-negative: T-cell markers are typically lost in ALCL such as CD5.

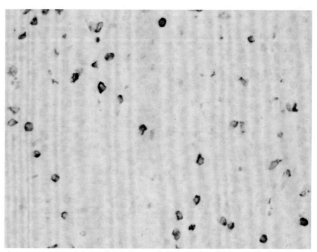

Figure 7.93. Anaplastic large-cell lymphoma, ALK-negative: Tumor cells are negative for CD7.

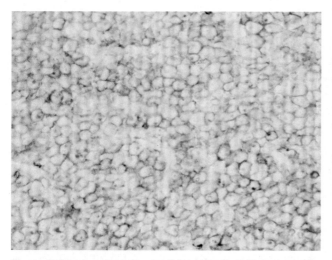

Figure 7.94. Anaplastic large-cell lymphoma, ALK-negative: This case showed expression with CD8.

Figure 7.95. Peripheral T-cell lymphoma with TFH phenotype: Low-power magnification shows effaced architecture with increased vascularity.

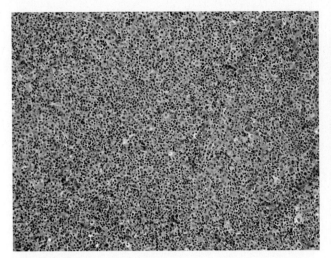

Figure 7.96. Peripheral T-cell lymphoma with TFH phenotype: Medium magnification shows clear cells.

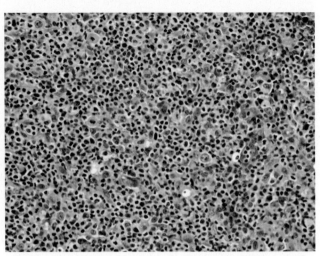

Figure 7.97. Peripheral T-cell lymphoma with TFH phenotype: Higher magnification shows clear cells and scattered immunoblasts.

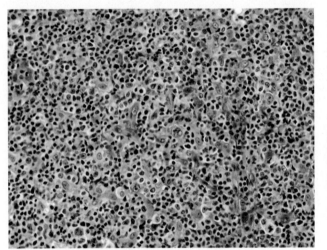

Figure 7.98. Peripheral T-cell lymphoma with TFH phenotype: Numerous clear cells admixed with large cells characteristic of immunoblasts.

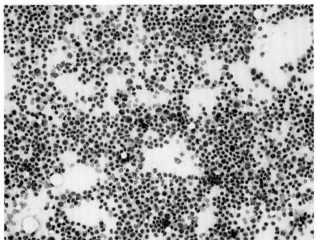

Figure 7.99. Peripheral T-cell lymphoma with TFH phenotype: Touch imprint of the same case shows monotony of cells that are medium-sized cells with moderate clear cytoplasm and scattered larger cells.

These Hodgkin-like cells can also be EBER-positive (Figures 7.108-7.110). If plasma cells are prominent, performing IHC for kappa and lambda is prudent to determine if there is a clonal plasma cell or B-cell process that is Epstein-Barr virus (EBV)–positive, which can be seen in conjunction with the PTCL. Molecular studies for T-cell–receptor gene rearrangement should always be performed to prove a clonal process and immunoglobulin gene rearrangement in the cases with prominent plasma cells or atypical B-cells.

LYMPHOEPITHELIOID VARIANT OF PTCL (LENNERT LYMPHOMA)

A variant of PTCL can have abundant histiocytes which can obscure the neoplastic cells which are typically small with only slight cytologic atypia (Figures 7.111-7.115). Background inflammatory cells include Hodgkin-like cells, plasma cells, as well as eosinophils. This variant tends to be confined to lymph nodes and extranodal involvement is uncommon. CD3 is helpful in highlighting the neoplastic cells, and T-cell lymphomas, in general, can lose bcl-2 expression which is helpful in determining a neoplastic process (Figures 7.116 and 7.117).

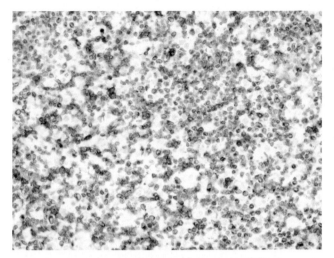

Figure 7.100. Peripheral T-cell lymphoma with TFH phenotype: Neoplastic cells are positive with CD3 and highlight atypia.

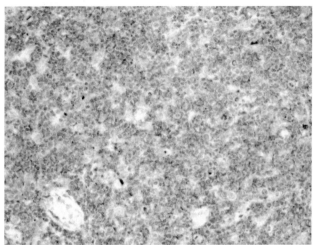

Figure 7.101. Peripheral T-cell lymphoma with TFH phenotype: Majority of tumor cells are positive with CD4.

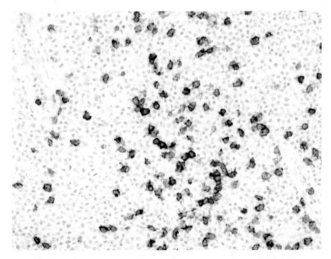

Figure 7.102. Peripheral T-cell lymphoma with TFH phenotype: Only scattered CD8-positive cells staining likely reactive T-cells.

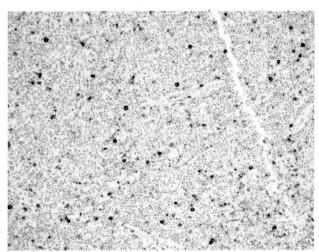

Figure 7.103. Peripheral T-cell lymphoma with TFH phenotype: The tumor cells are negative for CD7.

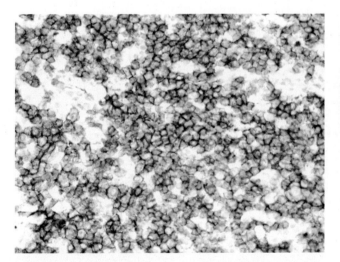

Figure 7.104. Peripheral T-cell lymphoma with TFH phenotype: PD1 shows strong expression.

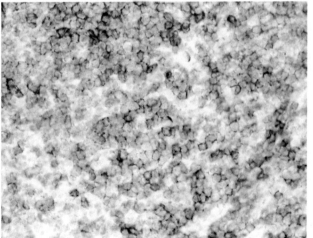

Figure 7.105. Peripheral T-cell lymphoma with TFH phenotype: ICOS (CD278) is also positive.

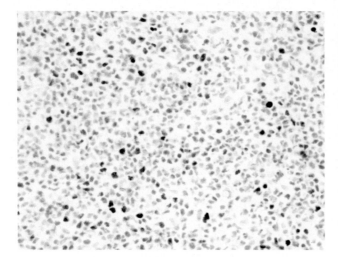

Figure 7.106. Peripheral T-cell lymphoma with TFH phenotype: BCL6 stains the abnormal T-cells.

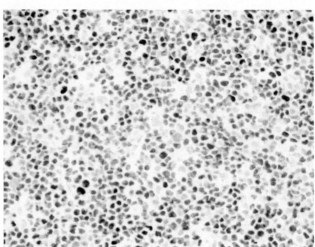

Figure 7.107. Peripheral T-cell lymphoma with TFH phenotype: GATA3 is also positive in the abnormal T-cells.

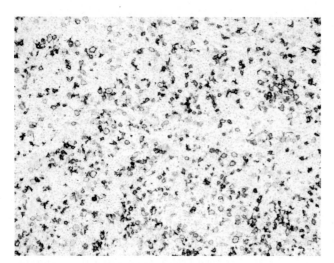

Figure 7.108. Peripheral T-cell lymphoma with TFH phenotype: CD20 highlights the increased immunoblasts.

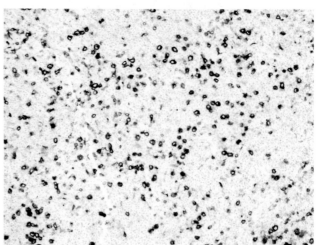

Figure 7.109. Peripheral T-cell lymphoma with TFH phenotype: CD30 highlights these immunoblasts.

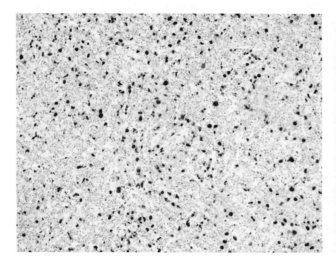

Figure 7.110. Peripheral T-cell lymphoma with TFH phenotype: EBER-ISH stains the immunoblasts.

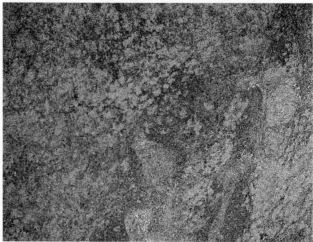

Figure 7.111. Peripheral T-cell lymphoma, Lennert type: Low-power magnification shows many collections of histiocytes with only focal areas of lymphoid cells.

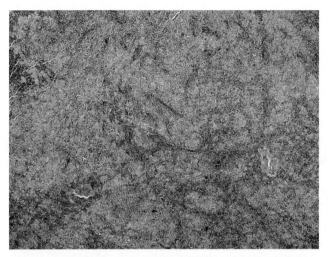

Figure 7.112. Peripheral T-cell lymphoma, Lennert type: Another low-power magnification showing predominately histiocyte clusters.

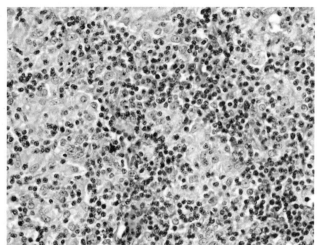

Figure 7.113. Peripheral T-cell lymphoma, Lennert type: High magnification shows mostly pink histiocyte collections and small lymphocytes with bland cytology.

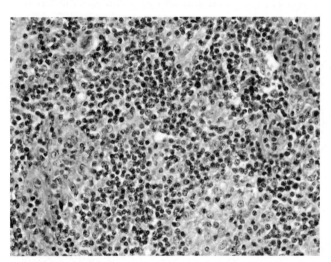

Figure 7.114. Peripheral T-cell lymphoma, Lennert type: High magnification showing bland cytology and inconspicuous nature of the tumor cells.

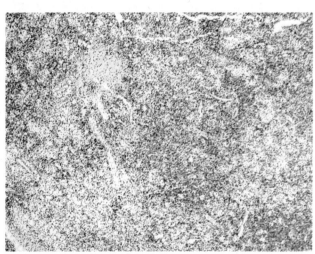

Figure 7.115. Peripheral T-cell lymphoma, Lennert type: CD3 shows numerous T-cells in the section.

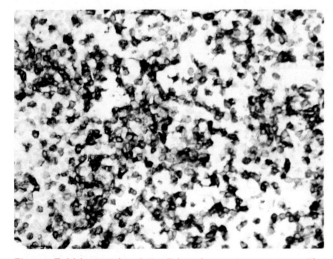

Figure 7.116. Peripheral T-cell lymphoma, Lennert type: The T-cells are highlighted by CD3 staining.

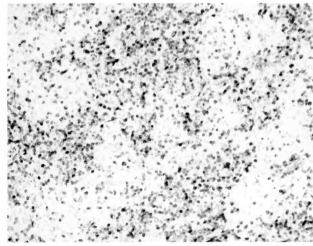

Figure 7.117. Peripheral T-cell lymphoma, Lennert type: Compared to the CD3, bcl-2 is decreased which is common in PTCL.

KEY FEATURES

- The epithelioid histiocytes may mask or be the predominant feature of the lesion.
- Neoplastic lymphocytes may not have prominent atypia.
- Eosinophils may be a clue to an underlying T-cell lymphoma.
- Performing T-cell gene rearrangements is necessary to prove clonality.

PRECURSOR LESION

MYELOID SARCOMA

A myeloid sarcoma can present in nearly any site in the body with the most common being skin and lymph nodes. Myeloid sarcomas can also be seen in isolation in patients that have undergone allogeneic stem cell transplantation and may be the initial manifestation of relapsed disease. A significant proportion of cases are of the myelomonocytic differentiation. There has to be architectural effacement in order to be considered a myeloid sarcoma. The infiltration is sheet-like and composed of large cells with round nuclear contours, open chromatin with occasional nucleoli (Figures 7.118 and 7.119). Carcinoma and melanoma should also be a consideration as well as other precursor lesions of B- or T-cell origin. Lesions are often positive for CD33, CD163, CD43, and CD68, but these stains are not specific (Figures 7.120 and 7.121). CD34, CD117, lysozyme, CD4, CD123, and MPO are helpful especially in the setting of blastic morphology but may not be sensitive (Figures 7.122-7.129). Many of the lesions may be of myelomonocytic differentiation, therefore stains such as CD68, lysozyme, CD163, CD4, CD123 are particularly helpful. Since blastic plasmacytoid dendritic cell neoplasms (BPDCNs) can also have the same morphology and similar phenotype (positive for CD4, CD56, CD123, TCL1 but negative for lysozyme), this needs to be ruled out and part of the differential. If fresh cells are available from the lesion, flow cytometry would be extremely helpful or diagnostic. Of note, the myeloid sarcoma phenotype may not match the phenotype seen in the bone marrow. For example, we have encountered acute myeloid leukemia that are positive for CD34 in the bone marrow but negative at the extramedullary site.

FAQ: Can a myeloid sarcoma occur without the presence of acute myeloid leukemia in the bone marrow?

Answer: Yes. In about a quarter of the cases, a myeloid sarcoma can occur without any disease in the bone marrow. Myeloid sarcomas can also be seen in patients with myelodysplastic/myeloproliferative neoplasms (MDSs or MPNs).

CHECKLIST: Workup for a Myeloid Sarcoma in Tissue

- ☐ Clinical history of MDS, MPN, or AML
- ☐ Laboratory values: CBC, peripheral blood smear
- ☐ IHC: Sensitive but not specific (CD33, CD68, lysozyme, CD4, CD43). More specific but not sensitive (CD34, CD117, CD123, MPO). Need to rule out BPDCN (include CD56 and TCL1), carcinoma (keratin), and melanoma

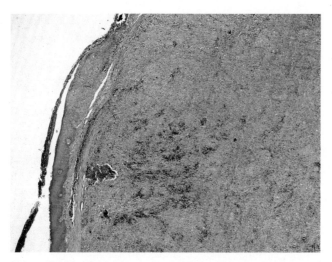

Figure 7.118. Myeloid sarcoma: Sections show sheets of atypical cells effacing the architecture (low magnification).

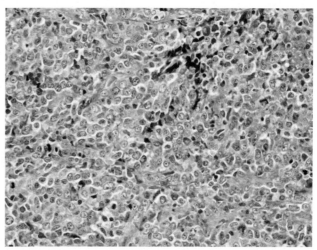

Figure 7.119. Myeloid sarcoma: High-power magnification shows sheets of blastic cells with fine chromatin and prominent nucleoli.

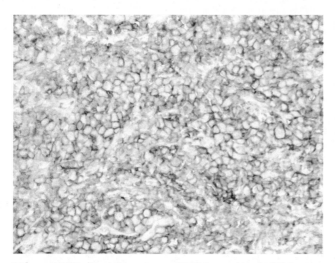

Figure 7.120. Myeloid sarcoma: CD33 is sensitive in MS but not specific. This tumor is positive.

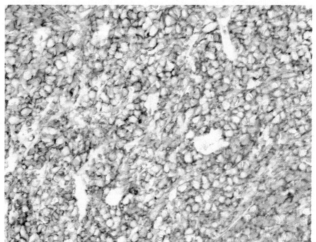

Figure 7.121. Myeloid sarcoma: CD43 is also sensitive for MS but not specific. This tumor is positive.

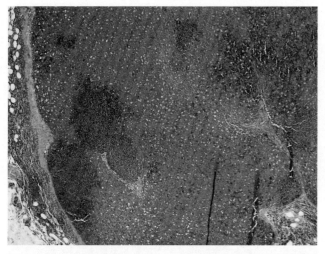

Figure 7.122. Myeloid sarcoma: Low-power magnification shows sheets of neoplastic cells with occasional residual lymphoid cells (dark areas).

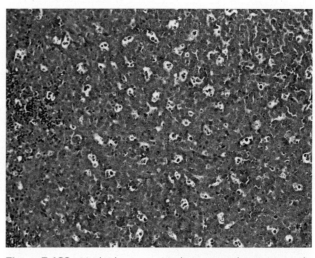

Figure 7.123. Myeloid sarcoma: Medium power shows a starry-sky appearance.

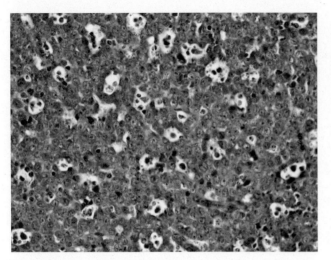

Figure 7.124. Myeloid sarcoma: High magnification shows the tin-gible-body macrophages with sheets of large atypical blastic cells with prominent nucleoli.

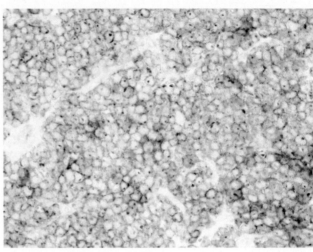

Figure 7.125. Myeloid sarcoma: Tumor cells are positive for CD4 consistent with a monocytic origin.

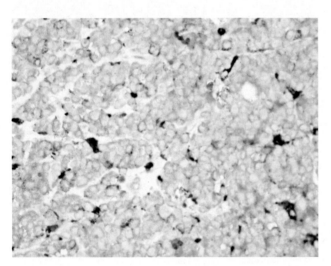

Figure 7.126. Myeloid sarcoma: Tumor cells are positive for CD68 which is a sensitive but not specific stain.

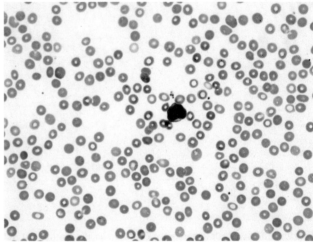

Figure 7.127. Myeloid sarcoma: In the same patient, there was blood and bone marrow disease. The peripheral blood shows cir-culating blasts.

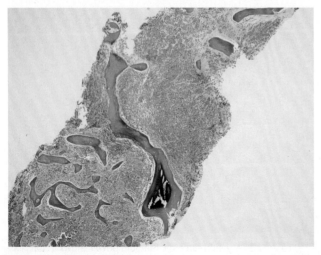

Figure 7.128. Myeloid sarcoma: The bone marrow is hypercellular and shows sheets of blasts.

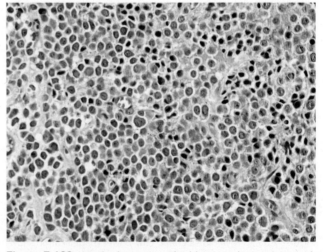

Figure 7.129. Myeloid sarcoma: The blasts are large in size with round nuclear contours, fine chromatin, and prominent nucleoli.

B-LYMPHOBLASTIC LYMPHOMA

B-lymphoblastic lymphoma (B-LBL) usually presents as skin or lymph node involvement. B-LBL rarely involves the mediastinum, in contrast to T-lymphoblastic lymphoma. The morphology is heterogeneous and can be small with condensed chromatin and indistinct nucleoli or larger cells with blue cytoplasm, dispersed chromatin, and nucleoli (Figures 7.130 and 7.131). Smears can also show cytoplasmic vacuoles which can also be seen in Burkitt lymphoma. The morphology and phenotype of B-LBL and B-lymphoblastic leukemia (B-ALL) are indistinguishable, and the distinction is based on the tissue distribution. The blasts are positive for CD19, PAX5, CD79a, TdT, and CD10 and can have variable staining with CD20 (Figures 7.132-7.135). Nearly all cases of B-LBL/B-ALL have rearrangement of the immunoglobulin heavy-chain gene. The current WHO classification defines B-LBL/B-ALL by recurrent genetic abnormalities such as *BCR-ABL1* or Ph-like.

T-LYMPHOBLASTIC LYMPHOMA

T-LBL is mostly found in the mediastinum and presents with high white blood cell counts, organomegaly, and lymphadenopathy. Unlike the B-cell lesions, the abnormal immature T-cells have a range in cytology from small and round to large cells with irregular nuclear contours and moderate amounts of cytoplasm. The chromatin varies as well from condensed to dispersed (Figures 7.136-7.139). Just as other high-grade lesions, a starry-sky appearance with scattered tingible-body macrophages can be seen. The blasts are positive for TdT and CD3 (cytoplasmic) with variable expression of CD1a, CD2, CD4, CD5, CD7, and CD8 (Figures 7.140-7.143).

PEARLS & PITFALLS

In T-LBL, CD7 is a sensitive marker but can also be expressed in acute myeloid leukemia or myeloid sarcomas. CD3 is lineage specific for T-LBL and is usually cytoplasmic.

NEAR MISSES

BLASTOID VARIANT OF MANTLE CELL LYMPHOMA

The blastoid variant of mantle cell lymphoma typically has sheets of medium-sized monomorphic cells resembling lymphoblasts with round nuclear contours, fine chromatin, and inconspicuous nucleoli (Figure 7.144). Mitotic figures are commonly seen and tingible-body macrophages are usually present, giving a starry-sky appearance. These cases can mimic lymphoblastic lymphoma, high-grade B-cell lymphoma, and DLBCL. In cases with blastoid morphology, performing CD5 and cyclin D1 should be considered and if positive (Figures 7.145-7.148), should be followed up with FISH analysis for *CCND1* since some cases of DLBCL can also express CD5 and cyclin D1 protein.[14,15]

SAMPLE NOTES

Lymph node, left axillary, excisional biopsy:

• Mantle cell lymphoma, blastoid variant, see comment.

Comment: The neoplastic cells have fine chromatin and distinct nucleoli consistent with a blastoid variant of mantle cell lymphoma. Consistent with this diagnosis is the high proliferation index of 80% seen with Ki-67.

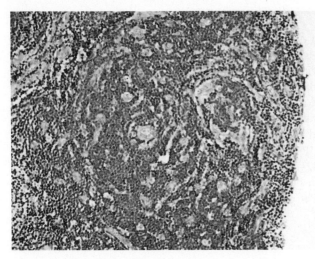

Figure 7.130. B-lymphoblastic lymphoma: Low-power magnification showing small- to medium-sized cells with fine and open chromatin.

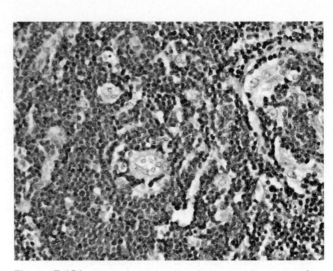

Figure 7.131. B-lymphoblastic lymphoma: Medium magnification showing these blastic cells with open chromatin and indistinct nucleoli.

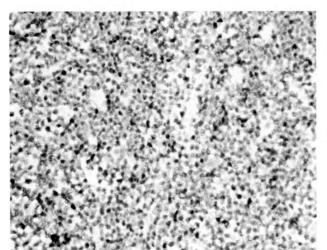

Figure 7.132. B-lymphoblastic lymphoma: Tumor cells are positive for PAX5.

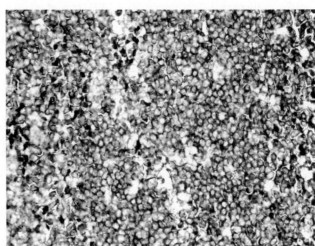

Figure 7.133. B-lymphoblastic lymphoma: Tumor cells are positive for CD34.

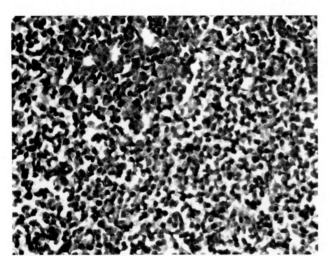

Figure 7.134. B-lymphoblastic lymphoma: Tumor cells are positive for TdT.

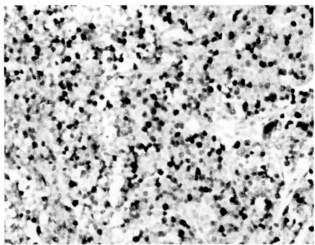

Figure 7.135. B-lymphoblastic lymphoma: Ki-67 shows a high proliferation index.

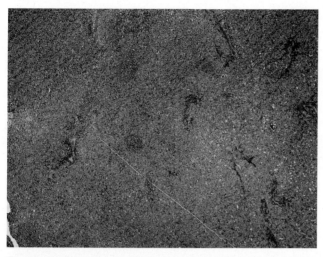

Figure 7.136. T-lymphoblastic lymphoma: Low magnification shows an effaced nodal architecture.

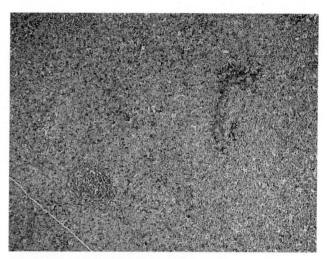

Figure 7.137. T-lymphoblastic lymphoma: Medium magnification shows a monotonous blastic population.

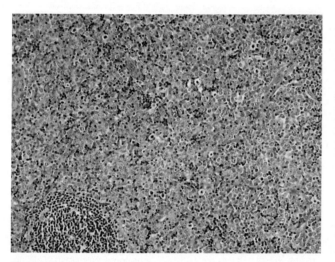

Figure 7.138. T-lymphoblastic lymphoma: Higher magnification shows rare residual follicles and adjacent sheets of blastic cells.

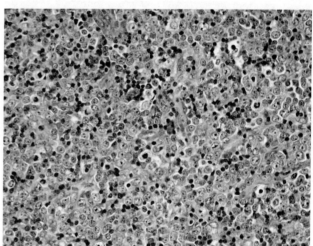

Figure 7.139. T-lymphoblastic lymphoma: High magnification showing large atypical cells with multiple small nucleoli.

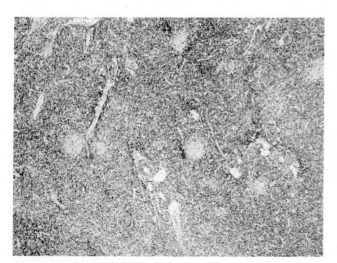

Figure 7.140. T-lymphoblastic lymphoma: Tumor cells are positive for CD2.

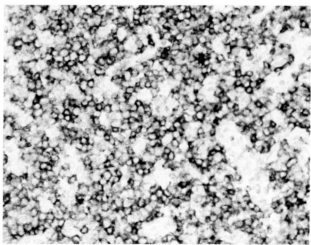

Figure 7.141. T-lymphoblastic lymphoma: High magnification. Tumor cells are positive for CD2.

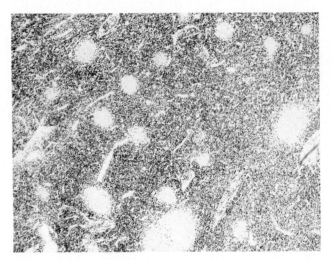

Figure 7.142. T-lymphoblastic lymphoma: Tumor cells are positive for CD1a.

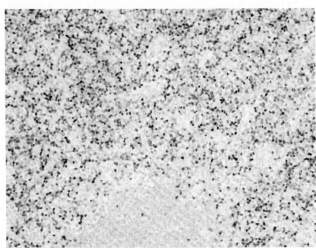

Figure 7.143. T-lymphoblastic lymphoma: The proliferation index is high seen with Ki-67.

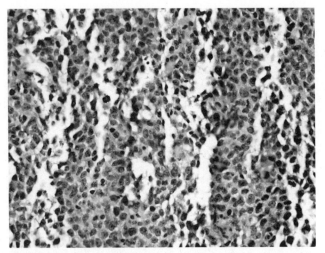

Figure 7.144. Blastoid mantle cell lymphoma: Sheets of medium-sized cells with fine chromatin and blastic appearance.

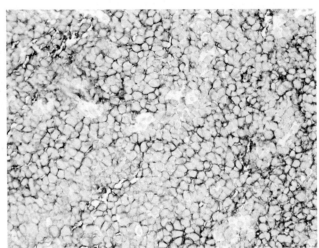

Figure 7.145. Blastoid mantle cell lymphoma: Neoplastic cells are positive for CD20.

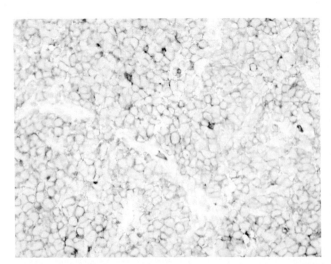

Figure 7.146. Blastoid mantle cell lymphoma: Tumor cells are weakly positive for CD5.

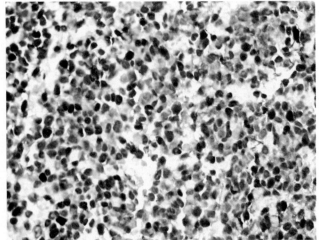

Figure 7.147. Blastoid mantle cell lymphoma: Cyclin D1 shows intense nuclear staining.

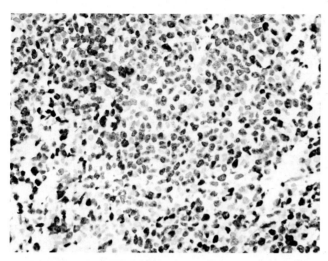

Figure 7.148. Blastoid mantle cell lymphoma: The proliferation index is high seen with Ki-67.

NODAL INVOLVEMENT BY CD30-POSITIVE T-CELL LYMPHOPROLIFERATIVE DISORDER

When reviewing lymph node biopsies from patients with a history of cutaneous T-cell lymphoma (mycosis fungoides, lymphomatoid papulosis, cutaneous ALCL), you may encounter morphologic findings similar to systemic ALCL or cHL.[16] It is important to make that distinction since the management varies depending on the diagnosis rendered. The tumor cells from the cutaneous lesions can drain into contiguous lymph nodes and show architectural disruption or effacement such as a sinusoidal pattern as seen in ALCL with the tumor cells being positive for CD30 and positive for T-cell markers. Some cases can show partial effacement of the nodal architecture with bands of fibrosis and scattered Hodgkin cells admixed with inflammatory cells (eosinophils, plasma cells, and histiocytes) consistent with cHL (Figures 7.149 and 7.150). These tumor cells are also positive for CD30 (Figures 7.151 and 7.152) and in some instances, for CD15; however, the tumor cells are negative for B-cell markers, and PAX5 negativity is especially helpful (Figures 7.153-7.155). There is usually loss of T-cell markers, but CD2 may be present in addition to cytotoxic markers (TIA1, granzyme B, or perforin) (Figures 7.156-7.160). Molecular studies for T-cell–receptor gene rearrangements are useful, but macrodissection may be necessary for enrichment, especially in focal involvement. An identical T-cell clone is typically seen in the lymph node tumor cells and cutaneous lesion. In this particular example, the patient had a long history of lymphomatoid papulosis with axillary lymphadenopathy.

SAMPLE NOTES

Lymph node, right inguinal, excisional biopsy:
• Nodal CD30-positive T-cell lymphoproliferative disorder; see comment.

Comment: In a patient with a history of cutaneous ALCL or LyP, this may represent nodal involvement by the cutaneous T-cell lymphoma rather than a PTCL. Nodal involvement by cutaneous T-cell lymphoma commonly occurs in contiguous nodes to the skin lesions. We recommend staging and clinical correlation.

PERIPHERAL T-CELL LYMPHOMA WITH HODGKIN-LIKE CELLS

PTCL with TFH phenotype such as angioimmunoblastic T-cell lymphoma may have Hodgkin-like cells (Figures 7.161-7.164) of B-cell lineage, and these are typically

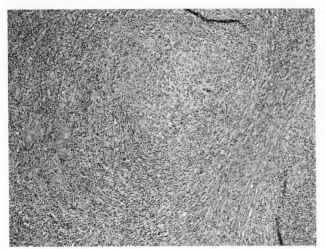

Figure 7.149. CD30-positive T-cell lymphoma: Low magnification shows a vaguely nodular effaced architecture.

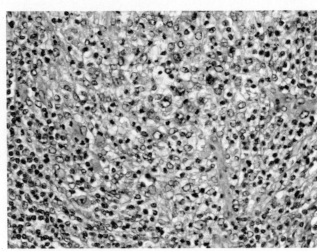

Figure 7.150. CD30-positive T-cell lymphoma: There are clusters or Hodgkin-like cells admixed with small- to medium-sized cells and eosinophils.

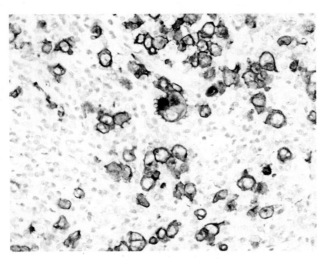

Figure 7.151. CD30-positive T-cell lymphoma: CD30 immunostain highlights the Hodgkin-like cells.

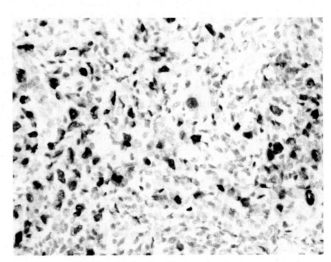

Figure 7.152. CD30-positive T-cell lymphoma: MUM1 stains the increased number of Hodgkin-like cells.

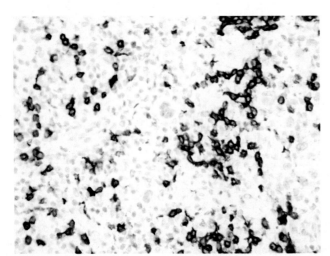

Figure 7.153. CD30-positive T-cell lymphoma: CD79a stains the background B-cells and is negative in the Hodgkin-like cells.

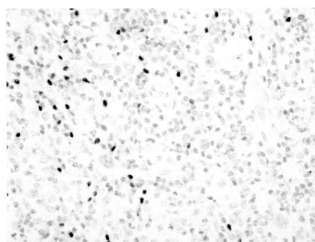

Figure 7.154. CD30-positive T-cell lymphoma: PAX5 is also negative in the Hodgkin-like cells.

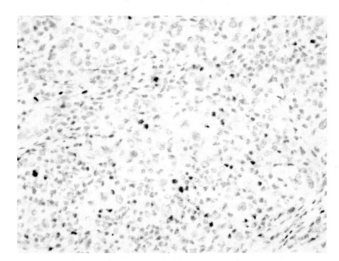

Figure 7.155. CD30-positive T-cell lymphoma: Oct2 which is a B-cell transcription factor is also negative in the large atypical cells.

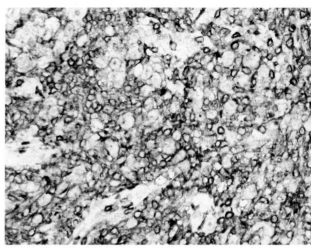

Figure 7.156. CD30-positive T-cell lymphoma: CD4 is weakly positive in the large atypical Hodgkin-like cells.

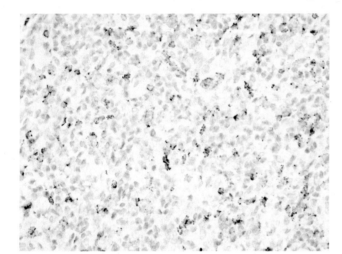

Figure 7.157. CD30-positive T-cell lymphoma: The large atypical cells have expression with TIA1.

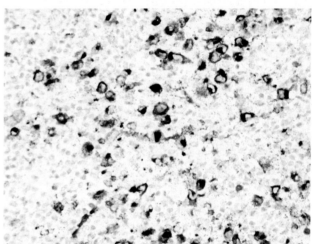

Figure 7.158. CD30-positive T-cell lymphoma: The Hodgkin-like cells also show high expression of granzyme B.

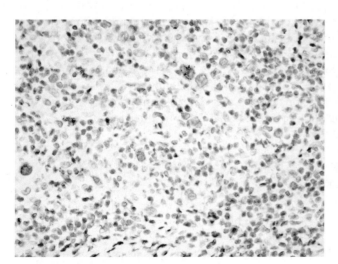

Figure 7.159. CD30-positive T-cell lymphoma: A subset of the Hodgkin-like cells express perforin.

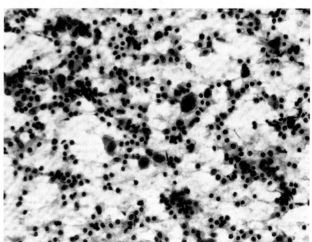

Figure 7.160. CD30-positive T-cell lymphoma: Touch imprint of the same node shows scattered Hodgkin-like cells, which could be a diagnostic pitfall.

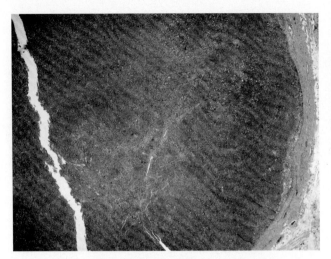

Figure 7.161. PTCL with Hodgkin-like cells: Low-power magnification shows an effaced architecture with a vaguely nodular pattern.

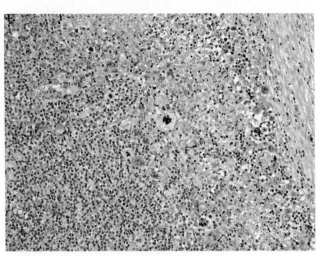

Figure 7.162. PTCL with Hodgkin-like cells: Sinuses show increased large atypical Hodgkin-like cells.

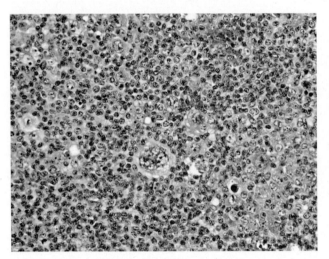

Figure 7.163. PTCL with Hodgkin-like cells: Some of these cells have bizarre morphology.

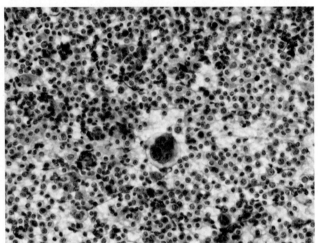

Figure 7.164. PTCL with Hodgkin-like cells: The touch imprint shows scattered large Hodgkin-like cells.

EBER-positive. This can be a diagnostic pitfall and misdiagnosed as cHL. The neoplastic cells are positive for PAX5, CD30, and CD15 and may express CD20 (Figures 7.165-7.168). The background T-cells may show minimal atypia or be overlooked. In many cases, the Hodgkin-like cells are cohesive or form clusters resembling ALCL. Performing immunostains to determine the density of TFH cells such as PD1, ICOS, CXCL13, CD10 (Figures 7.169-7.171), and BCL6 is helpful as well as T-cell–receptor gene rearrangement studies for clonality. For this particular case, flow cytometry also detected the abnormal population of T-cells which were negative for surface CD3 and positive for CD4 and CD10.

ANAPLASTIC LARGE-CELL LYMPHOMA WITH ABERRANT EXPRESSION OF PAX5

Anaplastic large-cell lymphoma commonly can lose most of the T-cell–specific antigens such as CD2, CD3, CD5, and CD7 by immunohistochemistry (Figures 7.173-7.178). Occasional cases of ALCL can aberrantly express PAX5 (Figure 7.179), which is a sensitive and fairly specific marker for B-cell origin. ALCL has also shown expression of cyclin D1 as in this case (Figure 7.180). The combination of the loss of pan T-cell antigens with expression of PAX5 can compound the problem of determining the lineage. Other markers such as CD4, CD8, or cytotoxic markers (TIA1, granzyme B, and perforin) can aid in the diagnosis of ALCL.

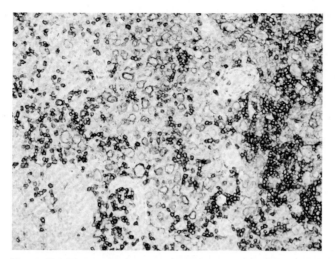

Figure 7.165. PTCL with Hodgkin-like cells: The Hodgkin-like cells are positive for CD20.

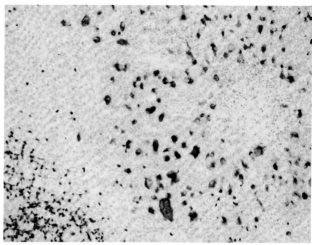

Figure 7.166. PTCL with Hodgkin-like cells: The Hodgkin-like cells are positive for PAX5, which is strong.

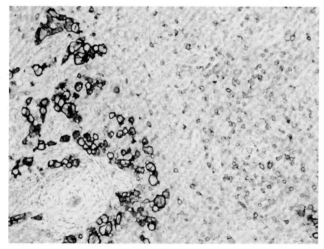

Figure 7.167. PTCL with Hodgkin-like cells: The Hodgkin-like cells are positive for CD30, which is strong.

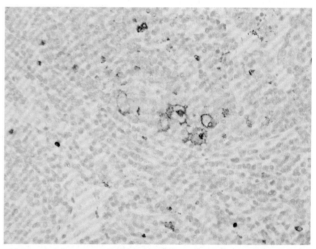

Figure 7.168. PTCL with Hodgkin-like cells: A subset of the Hodgkin-like cells are positive for CD15.

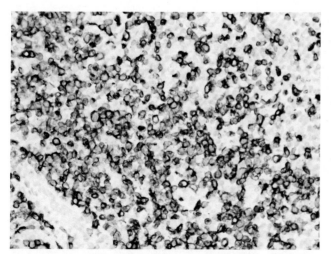

Figure 7.169. PTCL with Hodgkin-like cells: In other areas, there are increased number of T-cells, and CD3 highlights the atypia in these cells.

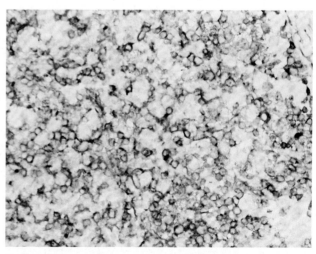

Figure 7.170. PTCL with Hodgkin-like cells: CD4 is positive in these neoplastic T-cells.

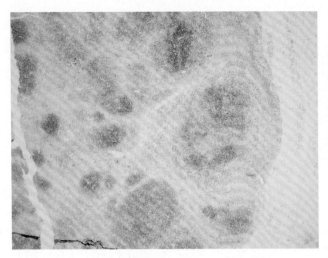

Figure 7.171. PTCL with Hodgkin-like cells: Low-power magnification shows the nodular areas with T-cells and coexpression with CD10.

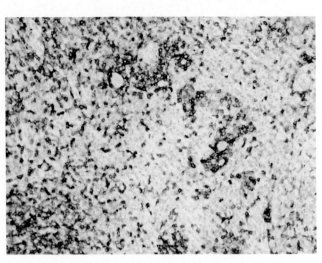

Figure 7.172. PTCL with Hodgkin-like cells: A subset of the neoplastic T-cells are positive for ICOS.

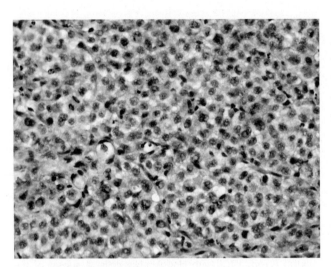

Figure 7.173. ALCL with PAX5 expression: High-power magnification showing sheets of pleomorphic cells.

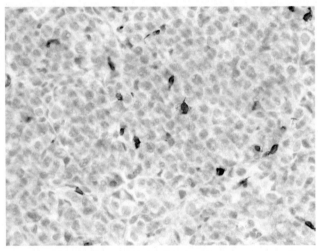

Figure 7.174. ALCL with PAX5 expression: These tumor cells are mostly negative for CD3.

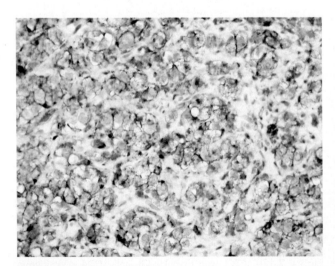

Figure 7.175. ALCL with PAX5 expression: The neoplastic cells are positive for CD4.

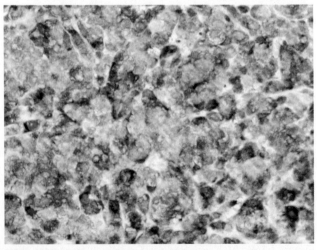

Figure 7.176. ALCL with PAX5 expression: The neoplastic cells are positive with ALK1 staining.

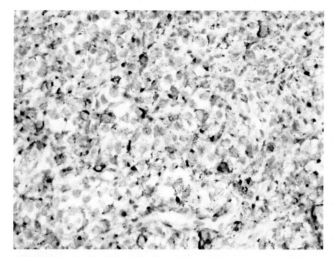

Figure 7.177. ALCL with PAX5 expression: The neoplastic cells are positive for granzyme B.

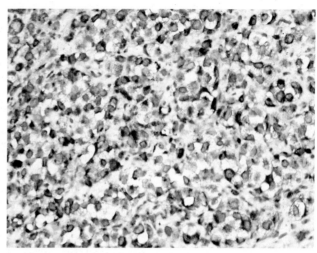

Figure 7.178. ALCL with PAX5 expression: The neoplastic cells are positive for perforin.

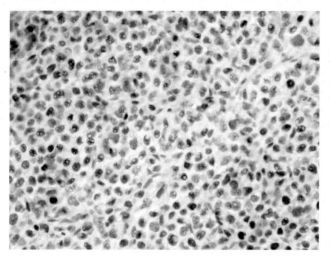

Figure 7.179. ALCL with PAX5 expression: The neoplastic cells also express PAX5 which is a typical B-cell marker.

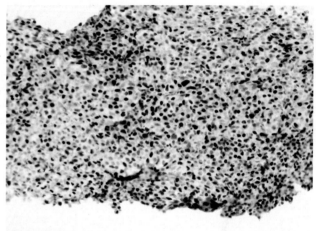

Figure 7.180. ALCL with PAX5 expression: In addition, the tumor cells express cyclin D1 protein but lack the translocation by FISH analysis (not shown).

References

1. Gradowski JF, Sargent RL, Craig FE, et al. Chronic lymphocytic leukemia/small lymphocytic lymphoma with cyclin D1 positive proliferation centers do not have CCND1 translocations or gains and lack SOX11 expression. *Am J Clin Pathol*. 2012;138(1):132-139.

2. Mao Z, Quintanilla-Martinez L, Raffeld M, et al. IgVH mutational status and clonality analysis of Richter's transformation: diffuse large B-cell lymphoma and Hodgkin lymphoma in association with B-cell chronic lymphocytic leukemia (B-CLL) represent 2 different pathways of disease evolution. *Am J Surg Pathol*. 2007;31(10):1605-1614.

3. Mozos A, Royo C, Hartmann E, et al. SOX11 expression is highly specific for mantle cell lymphoma and identifies the cyclin D1-negative subtype. *Haematologica*. 2009;94(11):1555-1562.

4. Siddiqi IN, Friedman J, Barry-Holson KQ, et al. Characterization of a variant of t(14;18) negative nodal diffuse follicular lymphoma with CD23 expression, 1p36/TNFRSF14 abnormalities, and STAT6 mutations. *Mod Pathol*. 2016;29:570.

5. Launay E, Pangault C, Bertrand P, et al. High rate of TNFRSF14 gene alterations related to 1p36 region in de novo follicular lymphoma and impact on prognosis. *Leukemia*. 2012;26(3):559-562.

6. Schraders M, de Jong D, Kluin P, Groenen P, van Krieken H. Lack of Bcl-2 expression in follicular lymphoma may be caused by mutations in the BCL2 gene or by absence of the t(14;18) translocation. *J Pathol.* 2005;205(3):329-335.

7. Alizadeh AA, Eisen MB, Davis RE, et al. Distinct types of diffuse large B-cell lymphoma identified by gene expression profiling. *Nature.* 2000;403(6769):503-511.

8. Hans CP, Weisenburger DD, Greiner TC, et al. Confirmation of the molecular classification of diffuse large B-cell lymphoma by immunohistochemistry using a tissue microarray. *Blood.* 2004;103(1):275-282.

9. Traverse-Glehen A, Pittaluga S, Gaulard P, et al. Mediastinal gray zone lymphoma: the missing link between classic Hodgkin's lymphoma and mediastinal large B-cell lymphoma. *Am J Surg Pathol.* 2005;29(11):1411-1421.

10. Salaverria I, Martin-Guerrero I, Wagener R, et al. A recurrent 11q aberration pattern characterizes a subset of MYC-negative high-grade B-cell lymphomas resembling Burkitt lymphoma. *Blood.* 2014;123(8):1187-1198.

11. Feldman AL, Law ME, Inwards DJ, Dogan A, McClure RF, Macon WR. PAX5-positive T-cell anaplastic large cell lymphomas associated with extra copies of the PAX5 gene locus. *Mod Pathol.* 2010;23(4):593-602.

12. Swerdlow S, Campo E, Harris NL, et al. *WHO Classification of Tumours of Haematopoietic and Lymphoid Tissues.* Lyon: International Agency for Research on Cancer; 2017.

13. Luchtel RA, Dasari S, Oishi N, et al. Molecular profiling reveals immunogenic cues in anaplastic large cell lymphomas with DUSP22 rearrangements. *Blood.* 2018;132(13):1386-1398.

14. Yamaguchi M, Seto M, Okamoto M, et al. De novo CD5+ diffuse large B-cell lymphoma: a clinicopathologic study of 109 patients. *Blood.* 2002;99(3):815-821.

15. Ehinger M, Linderoth J, Christensson B, Sander B, Cavallin-Stahl E. A subset of CD5− diffuse large B-cell lymphomas expresses nuclear cyclin D1 with aberrations at the CCND1 locus. *Am J Clin Pathol.* 2008;129(4):630-638.

16. Eberle FC, Song JY, Xi L, et al. Nodal involvement by cutaneous CD30-positive T-cell lymphoma mimicking classical Hodgkin lymphoma. *Am J Surg Pathol.* 2012;36(5):716-725.

CHAPTER OUTLINE

INTRODUCTION

Necrosis is a common finding in both reactive and neoplastic conditions involving the lymph node. This chapter focuses on the presence of necrosis in the lymph nodes and diseases associated with it. The characteristics of necrosis include the extent, what type of necrosis, what cell type is necrotic, and clinical history (eg, prior lymphoma or treatment history), which can provide useful clues to the disease process.

LYMPHOMA/AGGRESSIVE LYMPHOPROLIFERATIVE NEOPLASMS

Tumor necrosis (necrosis/infarction with ghost cells) is commonly seen with aggressive lymphomas particularly due to the proliferation beyond blood supply, high turnover, or destruction of the underlying cell population or architecture. Although nearly all aggressive lymphomas can cause some degree of necrosis, we will highlight common and interesting examples in this chapter.

PEARLS & PITFALLS

Many causes of necrosis in the lymph node are incited by Epstein-Barr virus (EBV) either in reactive conditions or neoplastic. I usually order an EBER-ISH stain when necrosis is present to determine if EBV is the cause and what types of cells are infected (B- or T-cell). This in conjunction with the clinical history will help to determine the diagnosis. If ample tissue is available, stains for microorganisms are also helpful (acid-fast bacilli [AFB] and Grocott Methenamine Silver [GMS]).

B-CELL LYMPHOMA

B LYMPHOBLASTIC LYMPHOMA

B lymphoblastic lymphoma (B-LBL) can occasionally involve the lymph node and may only show paracortical involvement with preservation of the follicles. Other extranodal sites may be involved such as the skin, tonsil, and gastrointestinal tract. Unlike T lymphoblastic lymphoma, mediastinal involvement is not typical in B-LBL. The cells are medium-sized and have a uniform morphology and usually show "starry sky" appearance but may be focal as compared to Burkitt lymphoma. Necrosis can be present as well. Immunostains show the neoplastic cells are positive for CD19, PAX5, CD10, CD79a, and TdT (Figures 8.1-8.3). TdT is extremely helpful in distinguishing it from mature high-grade B-cell lymphomas such as double-hit or Burkitt lymphoma. The proliferation index is generally high and greater than 80% seen with Ki-67.

PEARLS & PITFALLS

There are instances where it is exceedingly challenging to determine if the lymph node or extranodal site that is involved by a high-grade B-cell process is immature (B-ALL) or mature (high-grade B-cell lymphoma and Burkitt lymphoma). If TdT is positive in the tumor cells, then it is more consistent with B-ALL. Flow cytometry is also helpful to see if there is any surface light chain expressed and restricted as this would favor a mature B-cell lymphoma.

DIFFUSE LARGE B-CELL LYMPHOMA, NOT OTHERWISE SPECIFIED

Diffuse large B-cell lymphoma (DLBCL) forms sheets of neoplastic cells and usually has a high proliferation index. Apoptotic bodies are frequently seen. On occasion, necrosis (Figures 8.4-8.6) can be seen in DLBCL and is predominately composed of necrotic tumor cells, "ghost cells." You can usually still see the monotony of the tumor cells in these necrotic areas. These "ghost cells" are frequently positive with CD20 but usually negative for other immunostains due to the loss of antigens by the dead cells, and usually a two-tone staining pattern can be seen with the viable cells being strongly positive for CD20 and diminished or weak CD20 in the nonviable cells. Nuclear stains usually are negative in the necrotic cells as well as EBER-ISH since the RNA is degraded. Therefore, EBV status should never be determined just in the necrotic areas and the focus should be on the more viable cells. Biopsies of patients on treatment may only show necrosis and performing a CD20 immunostain may at least give a clue that the necrotic cells were part of the disease process.

SAMPLE NOTE

Lymph node, axillary, left, needle core biopsy:

- Necrotic tissue with no viable cells present, see comment.

Comment: The patient has a history of DLBCL and post chemotherapy. The biopsy is entirely necrotic, and no viable cells are present. CD20 stains the necrotic areas, consistent with cell death of the tumor cells in this disease. These findings are consistent with treatment effect.

PEARLS & PITFALLS

CD20 is a helpful stain in determining if the necrosis is from a B-cell process such as a DLBCL.
EBER-ISH will not stain in nonviable or necrotic areas.

EBV-POSITIVE DIFFUSE LARGE B-CELL LYMPHOMA, NOT OTHERWISE SPECIFIED

EBV-positive DLBCL, not otherwise specified (NOS) is a new entity in the 2017 WHO classification.[1] These lesions are usually seen in patients older than 50 years but can be seen in younger adults as well. Sites of involvement are usually extranodal, but lymph node involvement is not unusual.[2] Geographic necrosis is characteristic but not always present in these lesions (Figure 8.7). There are two histologic variants seen, polymorphic and monomorphic. The monomorphic has a pattern consistent with typical de novo DLBCL with sheets of transformed cells, while the polymorphic shows a range of B-cell maturation with small lymphocytes, immunoblasts, plasma cells, and occasional Hodgkin-like cells (Figures 8.8-8.11). The latter also shows a prominent inflammatory background with histiocytes and may have a low density of large tumor cells mimicking a T-cell/histiocyte-rich large B-cell lymphoma (Figures 8.9 and 8.10).

PEARLS & PITFALLS

EBV-positive DLBCL, NOS was previously called "EBV-positive DLBCL of the elderly." These lesions have been increasingly found in younger patients; therefore, the WHO classification has been updated in the 2017 version. These lesions need to be distinguished from EBV+ mucocutaneous ulcer (MCU) (provisional entity in the 2017 WHO classification) since MCU has a limited growth potential and responds to conservative measures such as reduction of immunosuppressive therapy. MCU is usually localized and limited to mucosal sites.

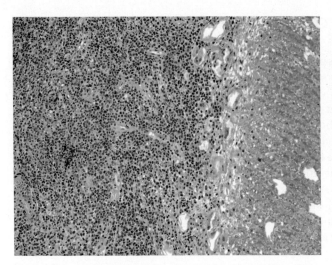

Figure 8.1. **B lymphoblastic lymphoma:** Low magnification shows sheets or monomorphic atypical cells with adjacent necrosis (right).

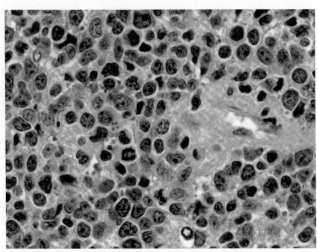

Figure 8.2. **B lymphoblastic lymphoma:** Higher magnification shows these cells have round nuclear contours, fine chromatin, and occasional nucleoli with apoptotic bodies and mitoses seen.

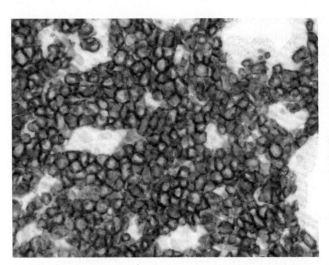

Figure 8.3. **B lymphoblastic lymphoma:** The tumor cells are diffusely positive for CD19 immunostain.

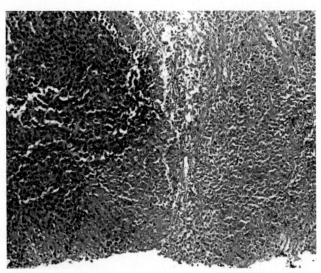

Figure 8.4. **Diffuse large B-cell lymphoma:** Low-power magnification shows sheets of large atypical cells. Adjacent to these tumor cells is a large area of necrosis (right).

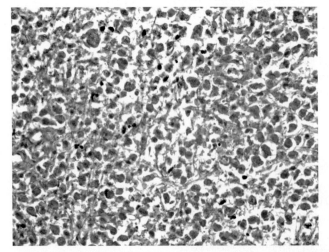

Figure 8.5. **Diffuse large B-cell lymphoma:** The necrotic area shows "ghost cells" and one can appreciate the monomorphic appearance of the nonviable tumor cells.

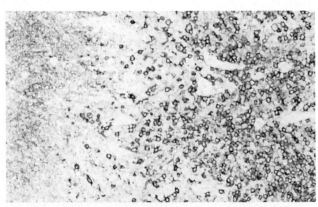

Figure 8.6. **Diffuse large B-cell lymphoma:** CD20 immunostaining shows stronger staining in the viable tumor cells (right) as compared with the weaker staining in the coagulative necrotic area (left).

POST-TRANSPLANT LYMPHOPROLIFERATIVE DISORDER

Although post-transplant lymphoproliferative disorder (PTLD) can have overlapping features with EBV-positive DLBCL, NOS, the history is critical as these patients have a history of transplantation. Most of these lesions occur in the setting of solid organ transplantation, but some cases arise from allogeneic stem cell transplantation. These lesions can be categorized as nondestructive versus destructive (**Checklist**). Necrosis is usually present in the infectious mononucleosis (IM) PTLD as well as in the destructive PTLDs (polymorphic, monomorphic, classical Hodgkin lymphoma [CHL]). In this example of polymorphous PTLD, there is geographic necrosis (Figures 8.12 and 8.13) and a spectrum of B-cell maturation from small lymphocytes, plasma cells, and Hodgkin-like cells (Figure 8.14). CD20 usually is variable since there is downregulation of the B-cell program in EBV-positive lesions (Figures 8.15 and 8.16). Light chain restriction with kappa and lambda can be detected in clonal lesions (Figures 8.17 and 8.18).

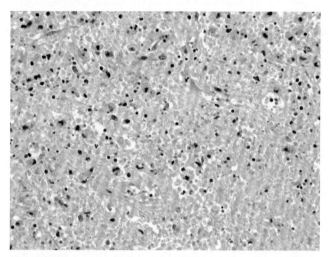

Figure 8.7. **Epstein-Barr virus–positive diffuse large B-cell lymphoma:** Areas of necrosis are present.

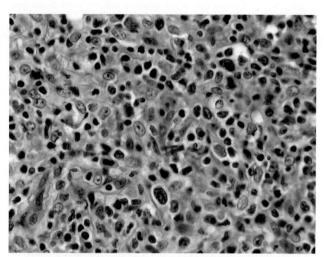

Figure 8.8. **Epstein-Barr virus–positive diffuse large B-cell lymphoma:** High-power magnification shows a polymorphous infiltrate of small to large atypical cells.

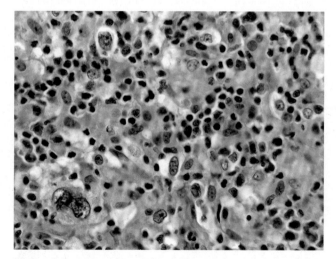

Figure 8.9. **Epstein-Barr virus–positive diffuse large B-cell lymphoma:** Scattered large atypical cells are present, some reminiscent of Hodgkin cells.

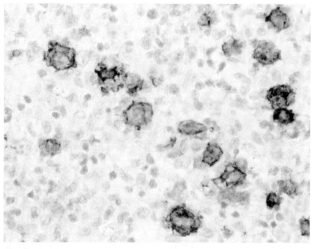

Figure 8.10. **Epstein-Barr virus-positive diffuse large B-cell lymphoma:** Immunostaining shows the large atypical cells are positive for CD20 and has a T-cell/histiocyte-rich-like large B-cell lymphoma pattern.

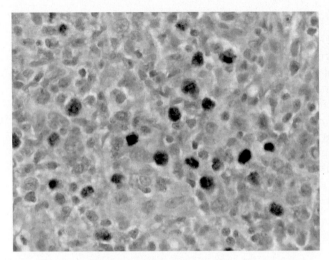

Figure 8.11. Epstein-Barr virus–positive diffuse large B-cell lymphoma: These large cells are positive for EBER-ISH.

Figure 8.12. Polymorphous post-transplant lymphoproliferative disorder: An effaced nodal architecture is seen with areas of necrosis.

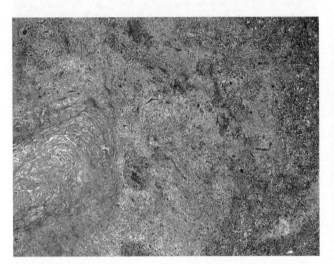

Figure 8.13. Polymorphous post-transplant lymphoproliferative disorder: In some areas, the necrosis is large.

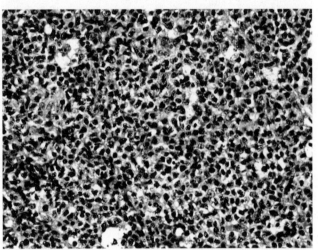

Figure 8.14. Polymorphous post-transplant lymphoproliferative disorder: High-power magnification shows a spectrum with small to large atypical cells. Some cells are reminiscent of Hodgkin cells and lacunar cells.

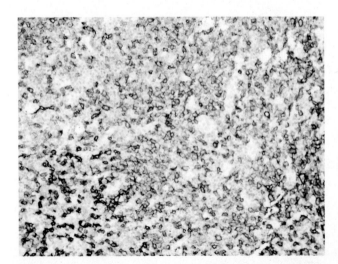

Figure 8.15. Polymorphous post-transplant lymphoproliferative disorder: CD20 immunostain shows variability with staining.

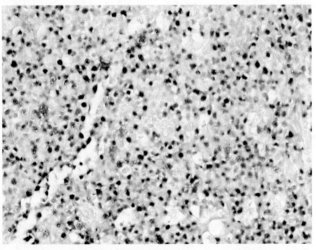

Figure 8.16. Polymorphous post-transplant lymphoproliferative disorder: EBER-ISH shows numerous B-cells are positive.

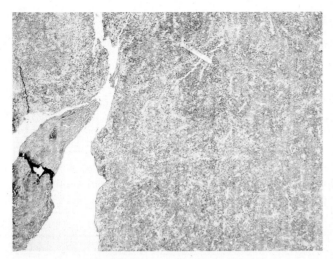

Figure 8.17. **Polymorphous post-transplant lymphoproliferative disorder:** Kappa is restricted in the neoplastic cells.

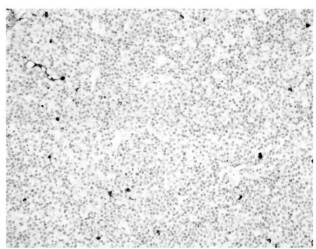

Figure 8.18. **Polymorphous post-transplant lymphoproliferative disorder:** Lambda is negative.

Checklist

Post-transplant Lymphoproliferative Disorder	Histology	Other Findings
Nondestructive	May have architectural distortion but no loss of architecture	May spontaneously regress
Plasmacytic hyperplasia	Increased sinusoidal plasma cells forming sheets	EBV+ PC
Infectious mononucleosis (IM)	Similar to typical IM with mixture of immunoblasts, PC, and FH	EBV+ immunoblasts
Florid follicular hyperplasia[a]	Follicular hyperplasia	Germinal centers EBV+, polytypic B, IGH–
Destructive	Loss of architecture	
Polymorphic	Full range of B-cell maturation with HRS-like cells	Many EBV+ cells (range), IGH+, TCR +/–
Monomorphic	Fits lymphoma definition in WHO. B-cell most common type (eg, DLBCL)	EBV+/–, IGH+ (B-cell type)
Classical Hodgkin lymphoma	Commonly mixed cellularity	EBV+ (latency II)

FH, follicular hyperplasia; HRS, Hodgkin/Reed-Sternberg; IGH, immunoglobulin gene rearrangements; PC, plasma cells; TCR, T-cell receptor gene rearrangements.
[a]New entity in 2017 WHO classification.

PLASMABLASTIC LYMPHOMA

This is an entity mostly seen in immunodeficiency such as HIV/AIDS patients. These lesions are usually extranodal such as in the head/neck, oral cavity, nasal cavity, and less commonly lymph nodes. The architecture is effaced and shows sheets of neoplastic cells that are predominately immunoblasts and plasmablasts. Geographic necrosis is frequently seen (Figure 8.19). The phenotype is that of plasma cells and usually lacks expression of CD20, CD45, and PAX5 (Figure 8.20). The cells are frequently positive for CD38, CD138, MUM1, and CD30 (Figure 8.21). Cytoplasmic light chain restriction can be seen, and it is recommended to perform in situ hybridization for kappa and lambda rather than immunohistochemistry (IHC), which may present nonspecific staining (Figures 8.22 and 8.23). The lymphoma cells are positive for EBV by EBER-ISH in about 70% of cases but HHV8 is negative (Figure 8.24).

PEARLS & PITFALLS

Since plasmablastic lymphoma (PBL) may lack many of the normal B-cell markers or lymphoid markers (eg, PAX5 or CD45) as well as have aberrant expression of other nonspecific markers (eg, CD30), it is crucial to confirm that one is dealing with a PBL rather than other overlaps such as melanoma or a poorly differentiated carcinoma.

SAMPLE NOTE

Lymph node, neck, right, needle core biopsy:

- PBL, EBV-positive, HIV-associated, see comment.

Comment: The patient has a history of HIV/AIDS with a diminished CD4 T-cell count. Although the tumor cells lack expression of pan B-cell markers (PAX5 and CD20), there is expression of plasma cells markers such as CD138 and CD79a (partial) as well as cytoplasmic light chain restriction by ISH. EBER-ISH is also positive supporting a diagnosis of PBL.

CLASSICAL HODGKIN LYMPHOMA

Classical Hodgkin lymphoma frequently shows necrosis particularly in the nodular sclerosis subtype. The necrosis is usually focal, forming microabscesses. The lymph node architecture is effaced and has a nodular pattern with intervening fibrotic bands and within the nodules is a polymorphous population of cells composed of eosinophils, histiocytes, small lymphocytes, neutrophils, and varying numbers of Hodgkin/Reed-Sternberg (HRS) cells (Figures 8.25 and 8.26). The neoplastic cells usually have diminished B-cell program with CD20, Oct2, Bob1, and CD79a, but PAX5 is usually weakly positive. CD30 is always positive and a subset of cases have expression with CD15. EBER-ISH is only positive in a minority of nodular sclerosis CHL, but other variants have a higher incidence of EBV-positive Hodgkin cells. Variants such as mixed cellularity and lymphocyte-rich typically do not show necrosis.

T-CELL AND NK CELL LYMPHOMA

PERIPHERAL T-CELL LYMPHOMA, NOT OTHERWISE SPECIFIED

Peripheral T-cell lymphomas are a heterogeneous group of lymphomas that can show necrosis which is usually focal rather than large or geographic (Figure 8.27). Additional morphologic findings and phenotype can be seen in other chapters of this book (see Chapter 6).

NK/T-CELL LYMPHOMA

Nodal NK/T-cell lymphoma comprises of 10% of peripheral T-cell lymphomas, NOS. These cases are positive for EBV in most of the cells and have a cytotoxic phenotype, express CD8, and are usually of T-cell origin with a small minority of cases being NK cell origin. These lesions are also negative for CD4 and CD56. The cells usually show a centroblastoid morphology with Reed-Sternberg-like cells or multinucleated giant cells.

Extranodal NK/T-cell lymphoma can show nodal involvement in 30% of cases. The nasal cavity should always be investigated when the extranasal biopsy shows NK or T-cells that are EBV-positive. Extranodal NK/T-cell lymphomas are usually negative for CD4 and CD8 but positive for CD56 and cytotoxic markers. Surface CD3 is negative indicating an NK cell origin, but cytoplasmic CD3 is seen by immunohistochemistry. Necrosis is frequently seen (Figures 8.28-8.31).

Checklist

Lymphoma	Features	Phenotype/Genetics
Nodal NK/T-cell lymphoma	No nasal lesion. Centroblastic with occasional HRS-like cells.	Mostly T-cell. +CD8, −CD4, −CD56, +cytotoxic. EBV+ +TRG.
Extranodal NK/T-cell lymphoma	May have nasal lesions. Variable cytomorphology but usually no HRS-like cells.	Mostly NK cell. −CD4, −CD8, +CD56, +cytotoxic. EBV+ −TRG.

HRS, Hodgkin/Reed-Sternberg; TRG, T-cell receptor gene rearrangement.

FAQ: Why is the IHC for CD3 positive in extranodal NK/T-cell lymphoma when it is negative by flow cytometry?

Answer: In extranodal NK/T-cell lymphoma, there is no surface expression of CD3 but there will be cytoplasmic staining by IHC since the antibody has cross-reactivity with the CD3-epsilon which is expressed by NK-cells. Therefore, by flow cytometry, you will not detect surface CD3 in these cases but will see CD3 cytoplasmic staining by IHC.

ANAPLASTIC LARGE CELL LYMPHOMA

Anaplastic large cell lymphoma (ALCL) usually shows an effaced nodal architecture but can also show focal involvement mainly within the sinuses and subcapsular spaces (Figure 8.32). There are sheets of pleomorphic neoplastic cells that are predominately large in size with irregular nuclear contours and are often present with characteristic "hallmark" cells. These large cells have a horseshoe- or kidney-shaped nuclei with prominent paranuclear eosinophilic golgi (Figure 8.33). These cells are strongly positive for CD30 and express ALK1 by IHC if they have the translocation (Figure 8.34). Cases with the *ALK* translocation have a favorable prognosis compared to the ALK-negative cases. However, there is a subset of ALK-negative ALCL that have a *DUSP22* rearrangement, and these patients have a more favorable prognosis.[3]

KEY FEATURES of Anaplastic Large Cell Lymphoma

- Two entities: (1) ALK-positive and (2) ALK-negative ALCL.
- ALK-negative ALCL has a poorer prognosis compared with ALK-positive.
- There is a group of ALK-negative ALCL that have the *DUSP22* rearrangement that has a similar prognosis as ALK-positive cases.
- CD30 must be diffuse with strong positivity in the tumor cells because PTCL, NOS can have variable positivity with CD30.

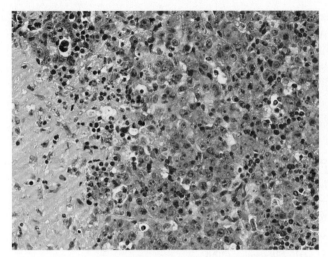

Figure 8.19. **Plasmablastic lymphoma:** High-power magnification with sheets of large atypical cells with prominent nucleoli (immunoblastic) and areas of necrosis (left).

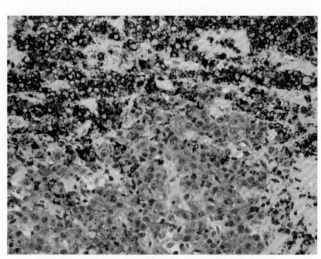

Figure 8.20. **Plasmablastic lymphoma (PBL):** CD45 immunostain shows the neoplastic cells are negative which is typical in PBL.

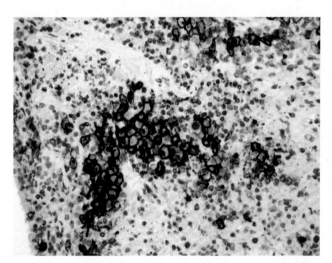

Figure 8.21. **Plasmablastic lymphoma (PBL):** Some cases of PBL can express CD30 by immunostaining.

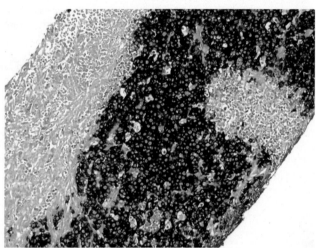

Figure 8.22. **Plasmablastic lymphoma:** In situ hybridization for kappa shows the neoplastic cells are restricted for light chains.

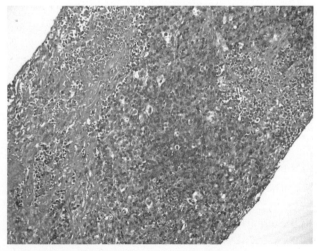

Figure 8.23. **Plasmablastic lymphoma:** In situ hybridization for lambda is negative.

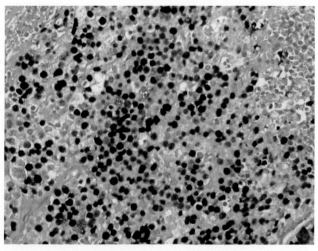

Figure 8.24. **Plasmablastic lymphoma:** EBER-ISH shows the neoplastic cells are positive.

Figure 8.25. **Classical Hodgkin lymphoma, NS:** Low-power magnification shows clusters of Hodgkin cells surrounding an area of necrosis (top) and bands of fibrosis surrounding the nodule.

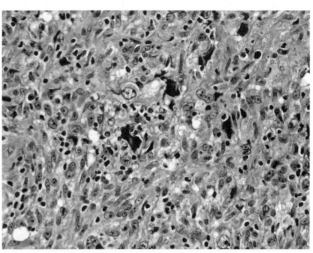

Figure 8.26. **Classical Hodgkin lymphoma, NS:** High-power magnification shows the Hodgkin cells as well as mummified cells admixed with histiocytes and small lymphocytes.

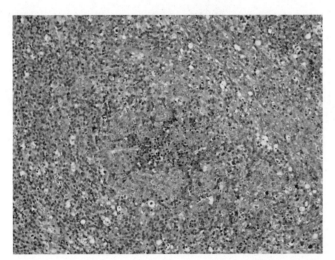

Figure 8.27. **Peripheral T-cell lymphoma, follicular helper type:** Clusters of large atypical cells with a microabscess seen in the center.

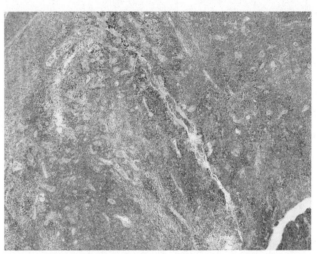

Figure 8.28. **NK/T-cell lymphoma:** Low-power magnification shows sheets of monomorphic cells with areas of necrosis (top left).

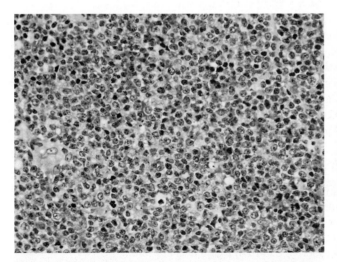

Figure 8.29. **NK/T-cell lymphoma:** High-power magnification shows numerous mitotic figures with a polymorphous population of atypical medium to large cells.

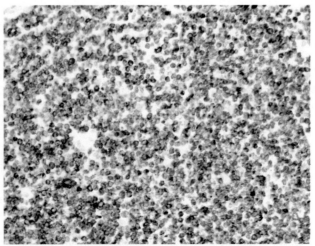

Figure 8.30. **NK/T-cell lymphoma:** Immunostain for CD3 shows the tumor cells are positive (mostly cytoplasmic).

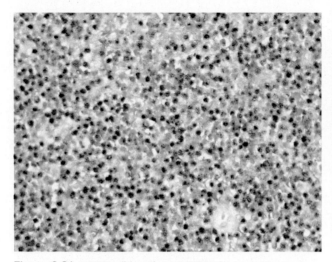

Figure 8.31. **NK/T-cell lymphoma:** EBER-ISH is positive in these cells.

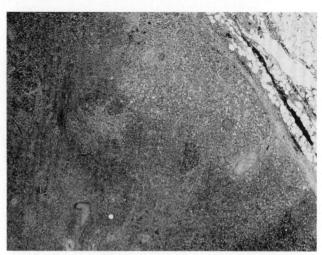

Figure 8.32. **Anaplastic large cell lymphoma, ALK+:** Sheets of neoplastic cells in the subcapsular sinus with focal necrosis.

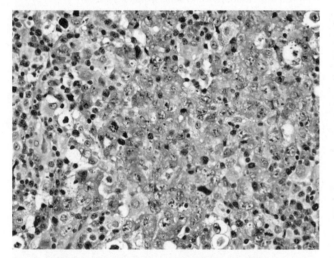

Figure 8.33. **Anaplastic large cell lymphoma, ALK+:** Large pleomorphic atypical cells are seen, some with horseshoe nuclei.

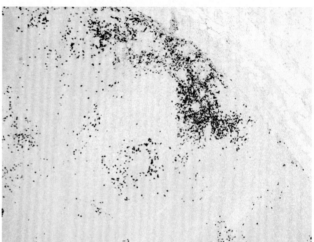

Figure 8.34. **Anaplastic large cell lymphoma, ALK+:** ALK1 immunostain highlights the sinusoidal pattern of the neoplastic cells.

INFECTIOUS ETIOLOGIES

MYCOBACTERIAL LYMPHADENITIS

Mycobacterial lymphadenitis can be caused by *Mycobacterium tuberculosis* or by nontuberculous mycobacteria such as *M. avium intracellulare, M. scrofulaceum, M. malmoense, M. celatum, M. fortuitum,* and *M. chelonei,* just to name a few. These typically cause lymphadenitis in children and usually involves the head and neck. Histologic features of mycobacterial lymphadenitis are similar showing a granulomatous inflammation with caseating necrosis, multinucleated giant cells, and capsular fibrosis (Figure 8.35). A Ziel-Neelsen stain can highlight the AFB, but this can be inconspicuous. It is also important to have these lymph nodes cultured if there is a high suspicion of infection to ensure speciation and proper management.

PEARLS & PITFALLS

The Ziel-Neelsen stain is important for identifying AFB. I find it helpful to start with the control to give yourself a reference with the color and size of the AFB. I then move to the tissue of interest in the granulomatous areas at high magnification and spend most of the time moving from area to area using the fine focus since the organism may only be seen in a certain plane and are rare.

Note: If AFB are identified but in unusual locations away from the inflammation or out of place, you will need to determine whether there is any contamination in the reagents used for staining.

CYTOMEGALOVIRUS INFECTION

In cytomegalovirus (CMV) lymphadenitis, there is a follicular and paracortical hyperplasia with scattered immunoblasts and HRS-like cells. There is usually a prominent monocytoid B-cell proliferation and these are the areas that the CMV-infected cells will be found. They have large acidophilic and intranuclear inclusions (Figures 8.36 and 8.37). Focal necrosis can be seen.

FAQ: How does one distinguish CMV infection from infectious mononucleosis (IM)?

Answer: CMV infection has a similar clinical picture as IM. However, the heterophile antibody test will be negative. Infection can be seen in both immunocompromised and immunocompetent patients. The morphology will be similar in both conditions, but immunocompetent patients may have fewer inclusions, which may be challenging to find, and they are usually in the T-cells rather than the B-cells.

HERPES SIMPLEX LYMPHADENITIS

Herpes simplex virus (HSV) (either type I or II) usually produces lymphadenitis localized to the inguinal nodes and is seen predominately in immunocompromised patients such as chronic lymphocytic leukemia. The histology of HSV can vary and be similar to the other viral infections (monocytoid B-cell hyperplasia, follicular hyperplasia with paracortical expansion), but there are usually areas of necrosis with neutrophils and occasional large cells with prominent nuclear "ground glass" inclusions (Figures 8.38-8.41).

CAT SCRATCH DISEASE

PEARLS & PITFALLS

The diagnosis of cat scratch disease (CSD) requires any three of the following four criteria:

1. Contact with a cat and presence of scratch
2. Positive skin or serologic test for CSD
3. Regional lymphadenopathy
4. Tissue biopsy showing histopathologic features of CSD

Individual assays (Steiner, polymerase chain reaction, IHC) have varying sensitivities; therefore, using them in combination may improve the identification of the organism.

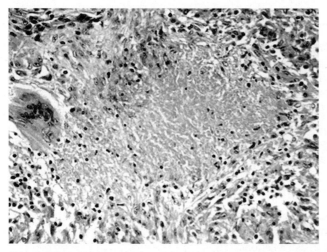

Figure 8.35. *Mycobacterium tuberculosis*: High-power magnification shows central necrosis with palisading histiocytes and a multinucleated giant cell.

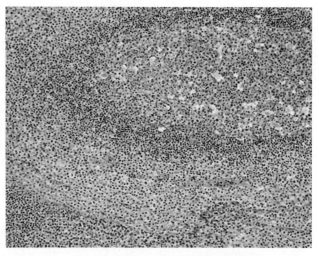

Figure 8.36. **Cytomegalovirus lymphadenitis:** Follicular hyperplasia is present as well as monocytoid B-cell hyperplasia.

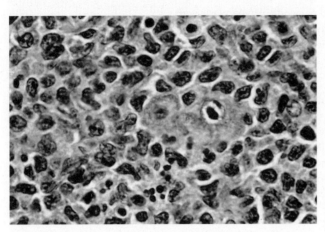

Figure 8.37. **Cytomegalovirus lymphadenitis:** In the areas of monocytoid B-cell hyperplasia, occasional large intranuclear inclusions are seen.

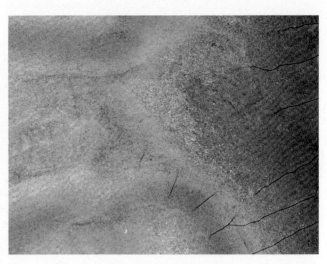

Figure 8.38. **Herpes simplex virus (HSV) and chronic lymphocytic leukemia (CLL):** Low-power magnification of a case with CLL and HSV. Note the large areas of geographic necrosis.

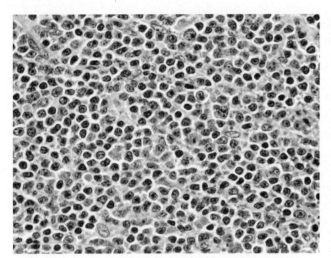

Figure 8.39. **Herpes simplex virus and chronic lymphocytic leukemia (CLL):** High-power magnification of an area with CLL showing a monotonous population of small lymphoid cells with coarse chromatin.

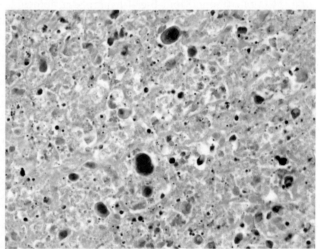

Figure 8.40. **Herpes simplex virus and chronic lymphocytic leukemia:** Within the necrotic areas are cells with "ground glass" nuclei with a background of cellular debris.

This disease is caused by *Bartonella henselae* (gram-negative coccobacilli) which is harbored in kittens and young cats. Most cases are seen in children and are transmitted by the infected cat claws. Usually the disease is localized and resolved spontaneously, but antibiotics may be necessary. The lymph node architecture is intact usually with follicular hyperplasia and some distortion caused by the necrosis that is often stellate with neutrophils and surround palisading histiocytes. A Steiner/Warthin-Starry stain can be used to identify the bacteria (Figures 8.42-8.44). Immunohistochemical stain is available for *B. henselae* but may be less sensitive.[4]

FUNGAL INFECTION/LYMPHADENITIS

Fungal infections of the lymph node show similar morphologic features with identification based on cultures and the morphology of the fungal element using a special stain such as GMS. Necrosis can be seen with calcifications.

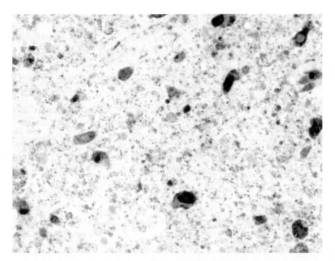

Figure 8.41. Herpes simplex virus (HSV) and chronic lymphocytic leukemia: Immunostain for HSV highlights these "ground glass" nuclei.

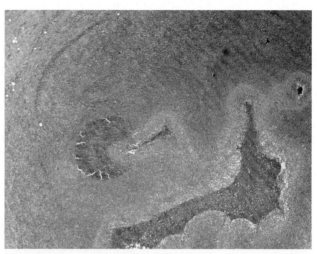

Figure 8.42. Cat scratch lymphadenitis: Low-power magnification shows lymphoid hyperplasia with areas of geographic necrosis with palisading histiocytes.

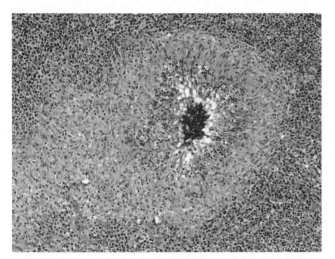

Figure 8.43. Cat scratch lymphadenitis: Higher magnification shows the focus of necrosis with the palisading histiocytes.

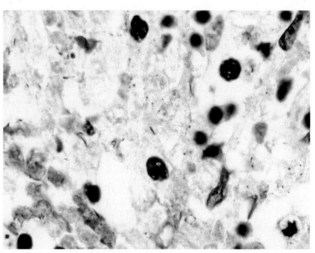

Figure 8.44. Cat scratch lymphadenitis: Steiner stain highlights the bacteria, *Bartonella henselae*, which are rod shaped.

Checklist

Fungus	Morphology	Vector/Etiology
Histoplasma capsulatum	Granulomas with necrosis. Small intracellular budding yeast.	Pigeon or bat dropping
Coccidioides immitis	Granulomatous with necrosis. Giant cells. Thick walled. Spherules containing endospores.	San Joaquin valley
Cryptococcus neoformans	Round to oval shape. Mucicarmine stain positive.	Immunosuppressed patient
Blastomyces dermatitidis	Neutrophilic infiltrate to necrotizing granulomatous inflammation with giant cells. Yeast lakes. Negative for mucicarmine.	Mississippi, Missouri, and Ohio rivers. Immunosuppressed patient.

BENIGN REACTIVE LYMPHOPROLIFERATIVE DISORDERS

SYSTEMIC LUPUS ERYTHEMATOSUS

Lymphadenopathy is present in approximately 60% of patients with systemic lupus erythematosus (SLE). The morphology can be nonspecific and includes follicular hyperplasia with expanded interfollicular areas and increased plasma cells. Necrosis is characteristic and generally large with abundant karyorrhectic debris and histiocytes (Figure 8.45). Like Kikuchi-Fujimoto lymphadenitis (KFL), there is a lack of neutrophils in the necrosis. Hematoxylin bodies (LE body) may be present (homogeneous basophilic particle consisting of degraded nuclear material) (Figure 8.46). Hematoxylin bodies are not seen in Kikuchi disease.

PEARLS & PITFALLS

SLE lymphadenopathy in some cases is histologically and immunophenotypically impossible to distinguish from Kikuchi disease. Therefore, it is always important to consider SLE in the differential diagnosis of Kikuchi disease and correlate with clinical history and presentation. Hematoxylin bodies are usually not seen in Kikuchi disease, which may be helpful in making that distinction.

NEAR MISSES

EPSTEIN-BARR VIRUS: INFECTIOUS MONONUCLEOSIS

IM shows lymphadenopathy and enlargement of the tonsils in adolescent and young adults with symptoms of sore throat and fever. The heterophile antibody test is positive. Early in the disease, the lymph node may show follicular hyperplasia with monocytoid B-cell aggregates. Later in the course, the architecture is distorted and there is a polymorphous infiltrate in the expanded paracortical regions composed of large immunoblasts admixed with plasma cells and small lymphocytes. Occasional HRS-like cells may be seen, and some areas may be more diffuse resembling DLBCL (Figure 8.47). There are increased CD8-positive T-cells with focal necrosis (Figure 8.48). Hodgkin disease is in the differential since the immunoblasts express CD30, but these large cells lack CD15 and express CD45.

CHECKLIST

Differential diagnosis of IM.

DLBCL: DLBCL will have architectural effacement with sheets of large atypical cells. IM will have intact architecture with presence of patent sinuses and high endothelial venules associated with immunoblasts.

CHL: Unlike CHL, IM large cells will have expression of CD45 and lack CD15. Also, EBV will be expressed in a spectrum of small to large cells as compared with CHL, which only has EBV-positive large cells.

KIKUCHI-FUJIMOTO LYMPHADENITIS

Histiocytic necrotizing lymphadenitis, also known as KFL, was originally described in Japan in 1972. It usually affects young women of Asian descent and most cases spontaneously resolve in a few months. Patients have cervical lymphadenopathy with fever or leukopenia. KFL typically has three stages: proliferative, necrotizing, and xanthomatous. The necrotic stage is seen in most cases and there is patchy necrosis in the interfollicular areas with abundant karyorrhectic nuclear debris (Figures 8.49 and 8.50). There are no neutrophils seen. Surrounding these areas are crescentic histiocytes and immunoblasts with aggregates of plasmacytoid dendritic cells which can be highlighted with CD123 immunostain (Figure 8.51). Immunoblasts at the edge of the necrosis are predominately CD8-positive T-cells

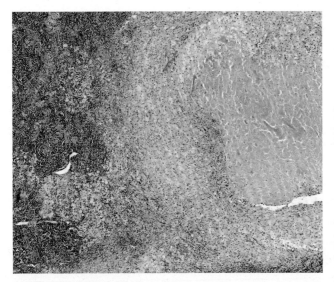

Figure 8.45. **Systemic lupus erythematosus:** Low-power magnification shows areas of necrosis surrounded by histiocytes and lymphoid hyperplasia.

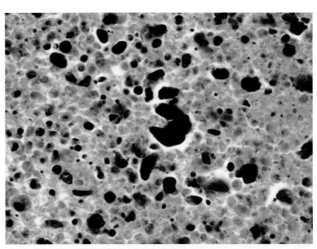

Figure 8.46. **Systemic lupus erythematosus:** High-power magnification shows the hematoxylin bodies that are composed of degraded nuclear material.

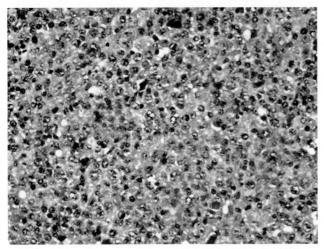

Figure 8.47. **Infectious mononucleosis:** High-power magnification shows sheets of large atypical cells concerning for diffuse large B-cell lymphoma. However, other areas of the lymph node show intact architecture.

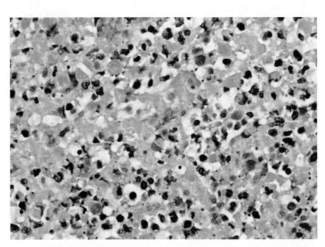

Figure 8.48. **Infectious mononucleosis:** Area of necrosis with apoptotic debris.

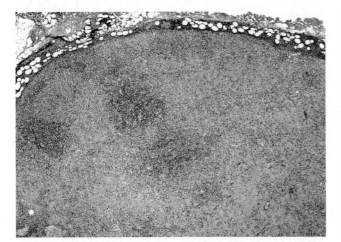

Figure 8.49. **Kikuchi disease:** Low-power magnification shows intact follicles but extensive necrosis in the interfollicular regions.

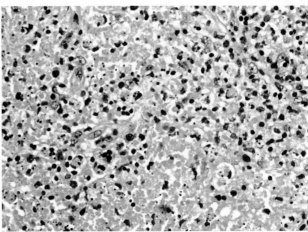

Figure 8.50. **Kikuchi disease:** Higher magnifications in the necrotic regions show numerous apoptotic debris, absence of neutrophils, and crescentic histiocytes.

which have variable CD30 expression (Figures 8.52 and 8.53). Histiocytes are positive for CD68 and myeloperoxidase (Figures 8.54 and 8.55). KFL can be confused with and misdiagnosed as a T-cell lymphoma since the necrosis can be alarming as well as the cytologic atypia seen in the CD8-positive T-cells. T-cell gene rearrangement studies are helpful as KFL is usually negative, while T-cell lymphomas will be positive.[5]

KEY FEATURES of Kikuchi-Fujimoto lymphadenitis

- Affects young Asian women.
- Cervical lymphadenopathy is common.
- Crescentic histiocytes surround the necrosis which lacks neutrophils. CD68 and MPO are positive in these histiocytes.
- Plasmacytoid dendritic cell clusters can be seen and highlighted with CD123.
- T-cell receptor gene rearrangements are usually negative.
- Differential diagnosis includes a peripheral T-cell lymphoma.

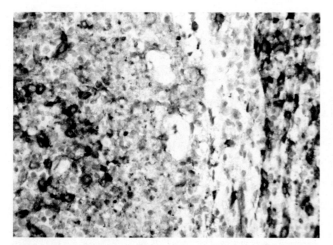

Figure 8.51. **Kikuchi disease:** Immunostain for CD123 highlights the plasmacytoid dendritic cells which are usually prominent.

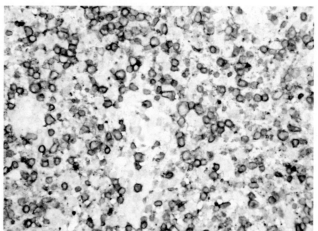

Figure 8.52. **Kikuchi disease:** CD3 immunostain highlights the large immunoblasts with cytologic atypia.

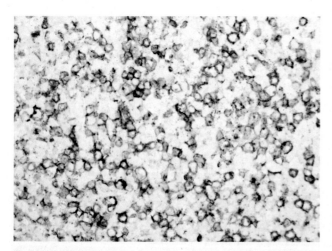

Figure 8.53. **Kikuchi disease:** These CD3-positive immunoblasts are also positive for CD8.

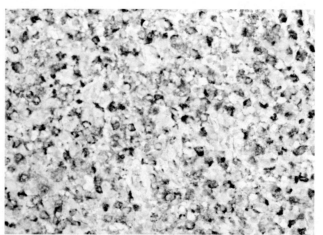

Figure 8.54. **Kikuchi disease:** There are increased histiocytes highlighted by CD68 immunostain.

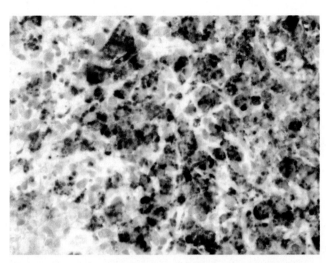

Figure 8.55. **Kikuchi disease:** There are no neutrophils usually seen in the necrosis, but the histiocytes are positive for myeloperoxidase.

References

1. Swerdlow S, Campo E, Harris NL, et al. *WHO Classification of Tumours of Haematopoietic and Lymphoid Tissues.* Lyon, France: International Agency for Research on Cancer; 2017.

2. Gibson SE, Hsi ED. Epstein-Barr virus-positive B-cell lymphoma of the elderly at a United States tertiary medical center: an uncommon aggressive lymphoma with a nongerminal center B-cell phenotype. *Hum Pathol.* 2009;40(5):653-661.

3. Luchtel RA, Dasari S, Oishi N, et al. Molecular profiling reveals immunogenic cues in anaplastic large cell lymphomas with DUSP22 rearrangements. *Blood.* 2018;132(13):1386-1398.

4. Caponetti GC, Pantanowitz L, Marconi S, Havens JM, Lamps LW, Otis CN. Evaluation of immunohistochemistry in identifying Bartonella henselae in cat-scratch disease. *Am J Clin Pathol.* 2009;131(2):250-256.

5. Bosch X, Guilabert A, Miquel R, Campo E. Enigmatic Kikuchi-Fujimoto disease: a comprehensive review. *Am J Clin Pathol.* 2004;122(1):141-152.

IMMUNOHISTOCHEMISTRY

9

CHAPTER OUTLINE

INTRODUCTION

Immunohistochemistry (IHC) is one of the most important ancillary tool for lymphoma diagnosis, more so than flow cytometry in some cases. All clinical IHC is performed on autostainers these days. From a technical perspective, most nuclear immunostains worked better with high pH retrieval. Also, nuclear immunostains are fairly sensitive to tissue fixation quality, and false negative staining is frequent in necrotic and autopsy tissues. This must be kept in mind as one orders stains. A full discussion of the most common and reliable close is not possible in this chapter, but the reader is referred to NordiQC website which has extensive data on most of the common antibodies with details on the most reliable clones of any specific antibody across several laboratories.[1,2]

Basic knowledge of the expected positive and negative markers in various lymphomas is necessary and further discussion of this will not be made in this chapter and the reader is referred to the WHO book 2016 for this. However, this chapter will discuss critical information related to all common antibodies with useful points related to clones, internal control cells, staining pattern, or finer aspects of interpretation, besides quick recognition of suboptimal stains. In addition, best practices for ordering immunostains, interpretation, and write-up of immunostain data in reports will also be discussed and illustrated.

KEY FEATURES RELATED TO TECHNICAL POINTS IN IMMUNOHISTOCHEMISTRY

1. Leica Bond instruments are generally better with nuclear immunostains compared with other IHC instruments.
2. For stains requiring additional serum blocking (like CD5, for example), Ventana instrument perform better, especially with bone marrow biopsies.
3. NordiQC lists the most common reliable clones for many of the antibodies and is a useful resource before picking antibodies.
4. Nuclear stains may sometimes just not work in the bone marrow–decalcified specimens and in B5-fixed specimens (Figures 9.1 and 9.2).

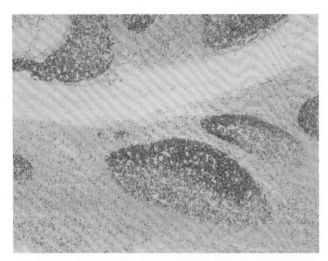

Figure 9.1. Ki-67 stain in with formalin-fixed tonsil demonstrating multiple proliferative secondary lymphoid follicles with polarization. Even dark and light zone distinction is apparent in this stain.

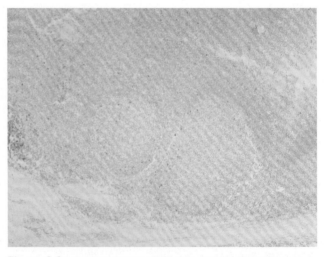

Figure 9.2. Ki-67 stain with B5 fixation in the same tissue as in figure 10.1, however, shows markedly decreased, nearly absent proliferative cells. Nuclear stains including proliferative markers are sensitive to the fixative and decalcification process. Hence, immunohistochemistry protocols must be optimized for alternate fixatives in such cases and proliferation should never be assessed in B5-fixed and/or decalcified tissues.

LIST OF COMMON ANTIBODIES IN LYMPHOMA IMMUNOHISTOCHEMISTRY

CD20 and PAX5: This is the staple stain in nearly every case of lymphoma. Typical staining pattern is membranous in B-cells of tonsillar germinal centers, mantle, and marginal zones that serve as controls. Interfollicular immunoblasts exhibit weaker expression of CD20 consistent with the shift to plasmacytic differentiation (Figure 9.3).

> **FAQ: Should I order both CD20 and PAX5 for confirming B-cell origin for a new diagnosis of lymphoma, or is either one of these sufficient?**
>
> For a new diagnosis, CD20 is usually sufficient for confirming B-cell lineage. Cases of chronic lymphocytic leukemia (CLL) with weak CD20 and blastoid processes that may turn out to be B-lymphoblastic lymphoma are often negative for CD20 and in these cases, PAX5 is more useful.

> **FAQ: What is the difference between "L-26" and CD20?**
>
> L-26 is the most common clone of CD20 antibody used. Sometimes, many labs will label the stains based on the common clone names or cluster designation names viz. MIB-1, CD279, and Ki-1 rather than antibody names KI-67, PD-1, or CD30, respectively.

PEARLS & PITFALLS

PAX8 immunostain cross-reacts with PAX5 and stains B-cells. Hence, undifferentiated PAX8+ neoplasms must be worked up for possible B-cell lymphoma (Figures 9.4-9.7).

CD3: Staining pattern for CD3 shows a corona of follicular helper T-cells inside germinal centers besides interfollicular T-cells. The common clone of this antibody recognizes both T-cells and NK cells in contrast to the flow cytometry clone, which is specific for CD3-epsilon and recognizes only T-cells and not NK cells (Figures 9.8-9.10).

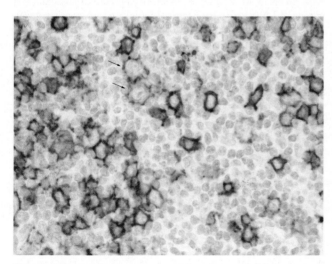

Figure 9.3. CD20 immunostain within the interfollicular regions demonstrate larger CD20 lymphoid cells with prominent nucleoli and weak membranous staining, consistent with immunoblasts (arrow). This patient is a 7-year-old, 5 years post orthotopic liver transplant at 2 years of age with evidence of EBV coinfection in the cells, consistent with infectious mononucleosis–like post-transplant lymphoproliferative disorder.

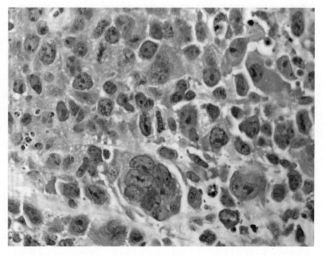

Figure 9.4. A 67-year-old female with a breast mass shows sheets of pleomorphic large cells thought to be anaplastic breast carcinoma. There was strong expression of PAX8 as seen here while all other markers including keratin were negative.

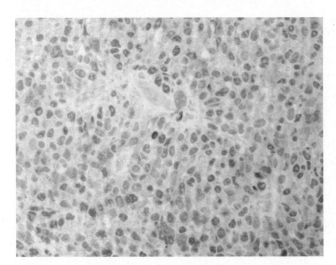

Figure 9.5. GATA3 immunostain to determine primary breast origin was also negative prompting further work-up. Scattered small GATA-3+ lymphoid cells consistent with T-cells are seen (internal control).

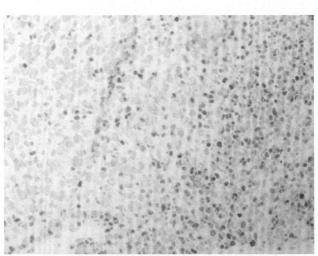

Figure 9.6. Additional CD45 stain in the neoplastic cells of the case above confirming hematopoietic origin. Background reactive lymphoid cells are positive for CD45 (right side of field).

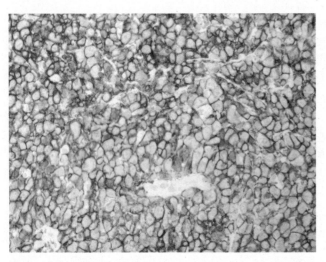

Figure 9.7. CD20 is positive supporting the diagnosis of diffuse large B-cell lymphoma which was positive for *MYC* and *BCL6* rearrangements corroborating double-hit lymphoma.

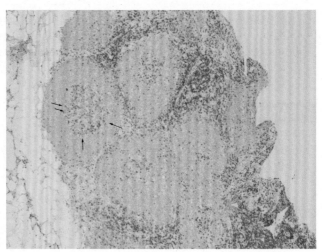

Figure 9.8. CD3 stain showing that T-cells are located in the paracortical regions. However, reactive lymphoid follicles contain a corona of T-cells within the germinal center (arrows), consistent with follicular helper T-cells which usually stain with CD4 and PD1.

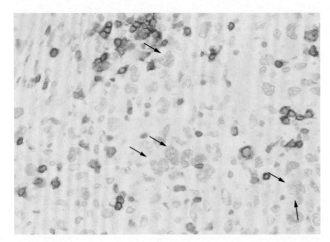

Figure 9.9. CD3 stain in a case of ALK-negative anaplastic large cell lymphoma demonstrating that the lymphoma cells are negative for CD3 (arrows) while background small T-cells are positive for CD3. Loss of CD3 is rather frequent in this T-cell lymphoma which often demonstrates null phenotype.

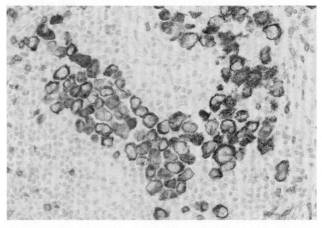

Figure 9.10. CD3 stain with strong aberrant cytoplasmic CD3 expression within plasmablastic cells of extracavitary primary effusion lymphoma. This can often be a pitfall unless the context of HIV is considered and additional EBV and HHV8 stains are performed.

NEAR MISS

CASE: CD20-NEGATIVE FOLLICULAR LYMPHOMA

Most cases of follicular lymphoma (FL) express CD20 at diagnosis, but this one was notable for negative CD20 at diagnosis and additional stains were performed only because the nodular architecture and lack of CD20 was not congruent. Although follicular T-cell lymphoma may show similar morphology, most cells within the nodular component were also CD3 negative (Figures 9.11-9.16).

PEARLS & PITFALLS

For identifying NK cells by IHC, a combination of CD3 and CD5 is useful since NK cells are positive for CD3 but negative for CD5 by IHC, whereas T-cells express both.

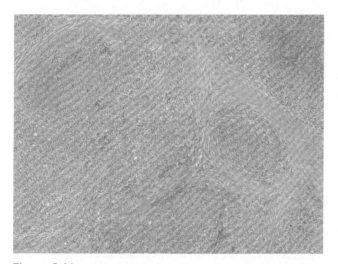

Figure 9.11. H&E image at low power demonstrating multiple nodular follicular structures.

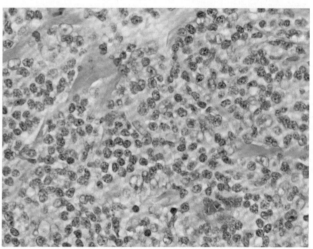

Figure 9.12. H&E image at high power demonstrates diffuse proliferation of centrocytes within the nodular structures.

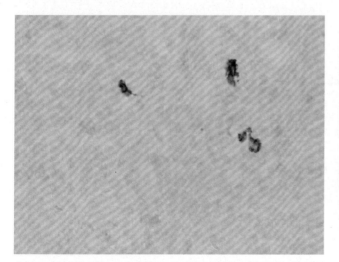

Figure 9.13. CD20 immunostain demonstrates only rare scattered small B-cells. No treatment with rituximab was given in this patient at diagnosis. PAX5 immunostain was strongly positive in this case supporting B-cell derivation.

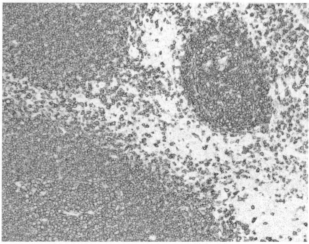

Figure 9.14. CD20 control tissue of the same case demonstrating strong staining within the follicular structures of the reactive tonsil.

CD5: CD5 stains with similar pattern as CD3 on the tonsils with T-cells serving as internal controls. Loss of CD5 is useful in T-cell malignancies, whereas dual-dim expression of CD5 is useful in small lymphocytic lymphoma (SLL) and mantle cell lymphoma (MCL; Figures 9.17-9.20).

CD10: CD10 stains not only germinal center B-cells (GCB) but also neutrophils since CD10 is a neutrophil endopeptidase. All malignancies of GCB origin express CD10 (FL, GCB diffuse large B-cell lymphomas [DLBCLs]) as well as a subset of T-cell malignancies of follicular helper T-cell (T$_{FH}$) origin[3] (Figures 9.21-9.25).

PEARLS & PITFALLS

Whenever incidental CD10 is performed on reactive lymph nodes, look for the intensity of CD10 within these follicles. In cases with abnormal bright CD10, BCL2 immunostain might be performed to assess for possible in situ follicular neoplasia (Figure 9.26).

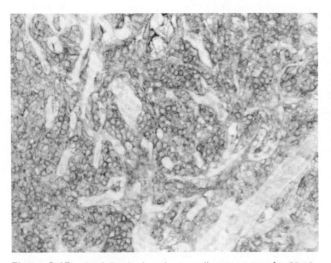

Figure 9.15. The follicular lymphoma cells are positive for CD10.

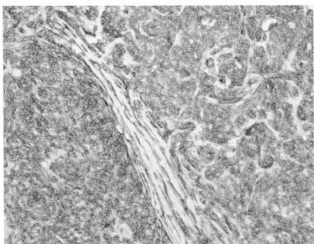

Figure 9.16. The follicular lymphoma (FL) cells are positive for BCL2. The combination of PAX5, CD10, and BCL2 supports designation as FL. Lack of CD20 is very unusual otherwise in FL.

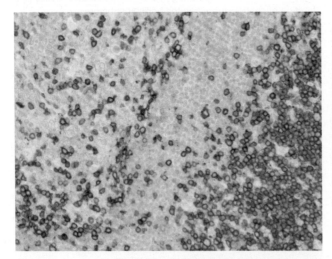

Figure 9.17. High-power view of the germinal center mantle and paracortex interface with germinal center to the left. Paracortical T-cells to the right expressed strong CD5 while germinal center follicular helper T-cells are also positive for CD5 (present at the interface of germinal center and mantle zones).

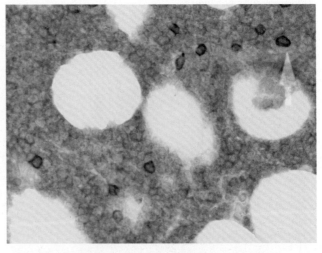

Figure 9.18. CD5 expression with bright scattered CD5+ T-cells (yellow arrow) with uniform dim CD5 expression in background mantle cell lymphoma cells. Similar biphasic pattern is useful in CLL. Internal controls (T-cells) are very useful in B-cell lymphomas with aberrant weak CD5 expression. Rarely there can be discordance between CD5 expression by flow cytometry and immunostains and hence, it is worthwhile performing immunostain for CD5 even though flow cytometry may be negative.

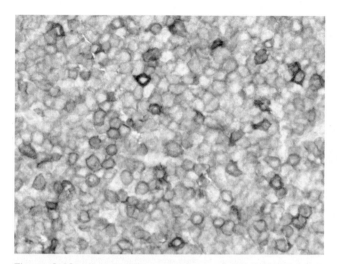

Figure 9.19. Biphasic CD5 expression in small lymphocytic lymphoma (SLL) with dim CD5 expression in SLL cells.

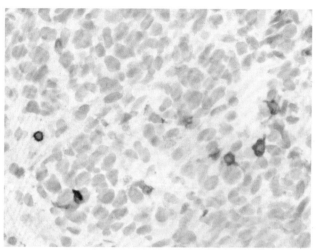

Figure 9.20. Loss of CD5 in anaplastic large cell lymphoma cells with scattered background CD5+ small T-cells.

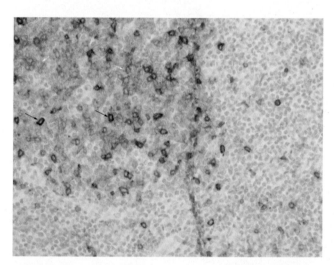

Figure 9.21. CD10 stain in reactive follicular hyperplasia. Reactive secondary lymphoid follicle usually demonstrates two populations of CD10+ cells: one of these populations demonstrates distinct bright staining (black arrow) corresponding to follicular helper T-cells while the (dim), background CD10 corresponds to germinal center B-cells (white arrows). Knowledge of this pattern is important in recognizing lymphomas.

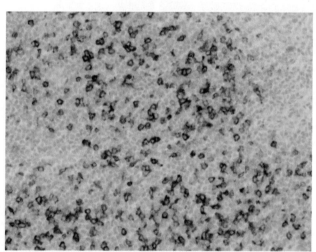

Figure 9.22. CD10 immunostain in a case of angioimmunoblastic T-cell lymphoma with so-called "pattern 2" morphology described by Attygalle et al. with multiple scattered nodular collections of neoplastic follicular helper T-cells.[10] Note that the nodules while resembling primary follicles do not demonstrate any of the weak CD10+ population corresponding to germinal center B-cells. Almost all CD10+ cells within the nodules correspond to bright lymphoid cells, which were positive for PD-1 consistent with the T-cell lymphoma diagnosis.

BCL6: BCL6 is a nuclear stain that marks GCB cells like CD10. However, on poorly fixed material, BCL6 works only in the peripheral areas of the tissue section which are better fixed compared to central areas. Usual control tissue is GC B-cells in tonsillar reactive second lymphoid follicles. T_{FH} cells also stain with BCL6 (Figure 9.27).

MUM1: A nuclear stain that stains plasma cells and a small subset of GCB and mostly post GCB. A subset of T-cells also stain with MUM1. It is useful in distinction of GCB vs non-GCB cell of origin in DLBCLs and to highlight cells with plasmacytic differentiation (Figure 9.28).

FAQ: Are both CD138 and MUM1 equally good for picking up plasmacytic differentiation?

MUM1 captures a broader range of plasmacytic differentiation compared to CD138. Many plasmablastic processes are positive for MUM1 as well as CD38 and BLIMP1 (two other markers of plasmacytic differentiation), whereas CD138 is useful only for terminally differentiated mature plasmacytic cells (Figure 9.29). Likewise, CD79a stains B-cells, plasma cells, and cells with intermediate differentiation especially after rituximab therapy (Figure 9.30).

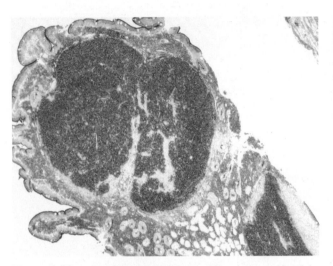

Figure 9.23. Unusual bright CD10 expression within the nodular structures of duodenal-type follicular lymphoma.

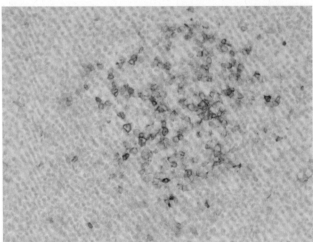

Figure 9.24. CD10 immunostain in reactive lymphoid follicle colonized by marginal zone lymphoma. Note the moth-eaten pattern demonstrating scattered clusters of germinal center B-cells weakly positive for CD10 with rare follicular helper T-cells noted at the bottom of the field. Majority of the cells within the follicle are negative corresponding to infiltrating CD10-negative extra-follicular marginal zone B-cells.

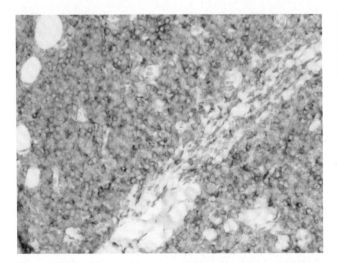

Figure 9.25. T-lymphoblastic lymphoma: Everything expressing weak CD10 does not correspond to B-cells. Weak CD10 expression is noted in this mediastinal mass with a cortical phenotype positive for CD10, CD1a, as well as CD4 and CD8. Lymphoblastic processes (B and T) as well as Burkitt lymphoma express CD10.

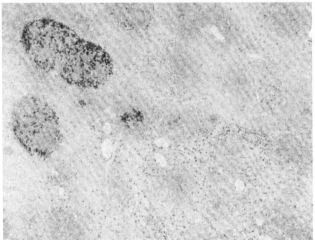

Figure 9.26. CD10 expression in in situ follicular neoplasia (ISFN). Note the three follicles on the top left with patchy unusual bright CD10 expression along with the rest of the follicles demonstrating weak CD10 expression, the latter consistent with reactive follicles. The bright CD10+ cells were positive for BCL2 consistent with ISFN. Morphologically, ISFN follicles appear reactive on H&E section with preserved mantle cuffs.

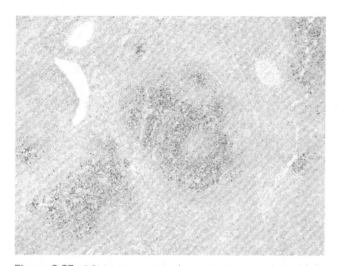

Figure 9.27. BCL6 immunostain demonstrating an enlarged folli-cle with multiple patchy areas of negative staining consistent with clusters of mantle zone cells within the germinal center supporting the diagnosis of progressive transformation of germinal center.

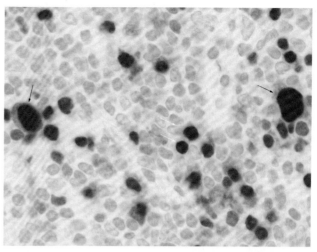

Figure 9.28. MUM1 immunostain in a case of classical Hodgkin lymphoma, interfollicular mixed cellularity subtype demonstrating strong staining in the nuclei of Hodgkin cells (black arrows). In addi-tion, background plasma cells express nuclear MUM1 (white arrows) and serve as internal controls. All plasmacytic and plasmablastic processes as well as post germinal center B-cells expressed MUM1. MUM1 is a particularly useful marker for identifying rare Hodgkin cells in a sclerotic piece of tissue, especially in mediastinal biopsies.

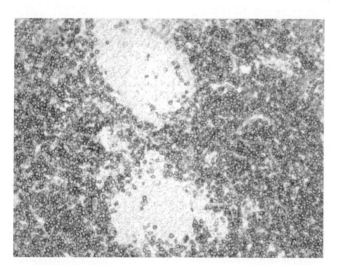

Figure 9.29. CD138 immunostain in a case of nodal marginal zone lymphoma with extensive plasmacytic differentiation. The interfol-licular plasmacytic component is diffusely positive for CD138 with light chain restriction. CD138, kappa, and lambda immunostains are especially useful in proving clonality on tissues where flow cytometry data are not available.

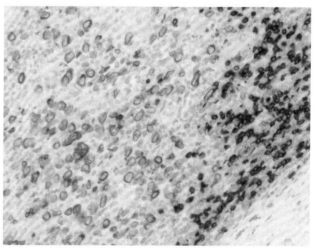

Figure 9.30. CD79a immunostain in a case of EBV + diffuse large B-cell lymphoma demonstrating moderate cytoplasmic staining in the neoplastic cells to the left of the field while scattered normal B-cells within primary follicles to the right express strong CD79a. Functionally, CD79a acts to tether the chains of the immunoglobulin molecule on the surface of the B-cell.

IgD: It is used mainly to highlight mantle zone lymphoid cells which are naïve B-cells. It is useful in several settings including progressive transformation of germinal center (PTGC), attenuated mantle zones in FL, and disrupted mantle zones in marginal zone lymphoma (MZL) with colonization of follicles by extrafollicular MZL cells (Figures 9.31-9.34). A small subset of nodular lymphocyte predominant Hodgkin lymphoma (NLPHL) may express IgD.[4]

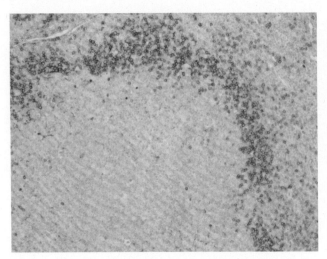

Figure 9.31. Reactive secondary lymphoid follicle at medium power demonstrating mantle zone cells expressing IgD.

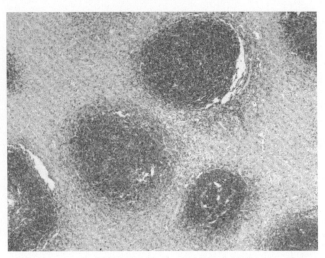

Figure 9.32. Primary lymphoid follicles in a patient with hyaline vascular Castleman disease demonstrating strong expression of IgD in keeping with the same phenotype as normal mantle zones of secondary lymphoid follicles.

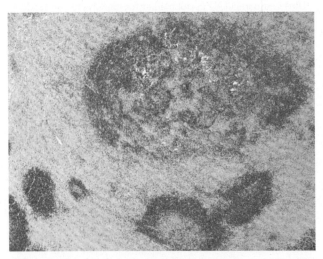

Figure 9.33. Progressive transformation of germinal centers. Markedly enlarged progressively transformed follicle is noted on the top with several primary and secondary reactive lymphoid follicles at the bottom of the field. Note the total loss of the germinal center–mantle zone distinction in the progressively transformed follicle containing numerous IgD + lymphoid cells within the germinal center disrupting the architecture.

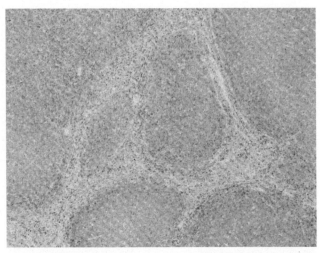

Figure 9.34. Splenic marginal zone lymphoma demonstrating expression of IgD on the lymphoma cells. Compared to nodal marginal zone lymphoma, splenic marginal zone lymphoma often expressed IgD. In addition, a subset of nodular lymphocyte predominant Hodgkin lymphoma in younger patients may express IgD on the lymphocyte predominant cells.

Kappa/lambda IHC and ISH: These are useful to assess clonality of plasmacytic cells in myeloma, plasmablastic processes, and lymphomas with plasmacytic component. The ISH is generally more useful for assessing clonality in plasma cells although it is more expensive to run. The IHC is typically more useful for assessing low levels of surface light expression as in lymphoid cells although the stain needs to be titrated appropriately to assess clonality on B-cells (Figures 9.35-9.39).

Ki-67: MIB-1 is the clone most labs use for this proliferation marker. This is useful in DLBCLs and correlates with high-grade biology as in most cancers. It is also useful in other low-grade processes to assess progression to more aggressive lymphoma/transformed lymphoma. Tonsillar germinal center dark zones serve as the best controls. Ki-67 should not, however, be interpreted in decalcified sections (Figure 9.40).

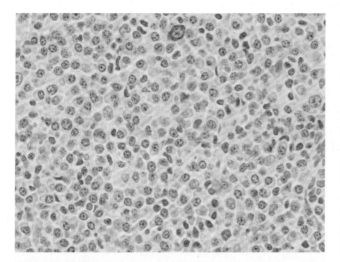

Figure 9.35. Lambda immunostain highlights rare immunoblast positive for lambda while all the plasmacytic cells in a marginal zone lymphoma with plasmacytic differentiation are negative.

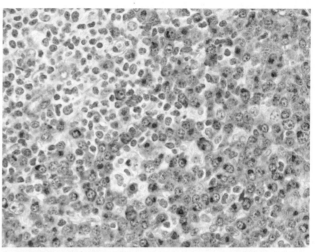

Figure 9.36. Kappa immunostain highlights strong cytoplasmic kappa light chain restriction while the lymphoid component in the top left is negative. High background stain is an issue with most kappa and lambda IHCs since these are used at high dilutions and bind nonspecifically to tissues.

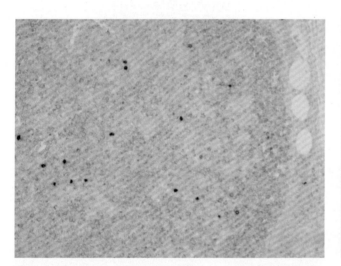

Figure 9.37. Kappa in situ hybridization stain in a case of immunosuppression-associated diffuse large B-cell lymphoma. Note dual population of plasmacytic cells including bright plasma cells while the majority of background lymphoma cells with partial plasmacytic differentiation show dim kappa expression.

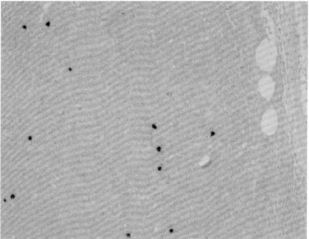

Figure 9.38. Lambda ISH in case above (IA-DLBCL) demonstrating scattered lambda + plasma cells without any staining in the lymphoma cells. This allows inference of polytypic plasma cells with kappa-restricted lymphoma cells. Both component should be carefully examined in such cases on kappa and lambda light chain stains.

MYC: The Y69 clone is the most commonly used clone and scattered intrafollicular MYC+ cells serve controls in reactive tonsillar germinal centers. With the recognition of double-hit and double-expressor lymphomas, this stain is more routinely used in most DLBCLs as part of the routine work-up (Figure 9.41).

BCL2: Clone 124 is the most common clone used in most labs. Normal mantle zone B-cells and normal T-cells are positive for BCL2 in the tonsils. The two major uses are in FL diagnosis and DLBCL prognostication (for identifying double-expressor/double-hit cases). Once CD3+/BCL2+ cells are excluded, BCL2 expression on neoplastic B-cells in FL supports the diagnosis (Figures 9.42-9.44).

PEARLS & PITFALLS

- BCL2 can also serve as a surrogate of IgD and can identify PTGC mantle zone B-cells.
- Rare cases of BCL2 clone 124 negative FL carry underlying mutations in the site recognized by the clone 124 antibody can be detected by the E17 or SP66 antibody[5] (Figures 9.45-9.47).
- All low-grade B-cell lymphomas are positive for BCL2 by IHC (Figure 9.48), but only in FL, BCL2 expression is secondary to an underlying translocation and hence the positivity has diagnostic utility. BCL2 expression should therefore not be misconstrued as being synonymous with FL in all instances.

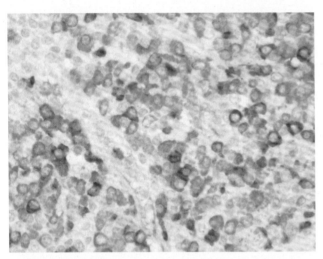

Figure 9.39. Dual kappa (brown)/lambda (red) double stain showing polytypic plasma cells in a case of angioimmunoblastic T-cell lymphoma. By convention, labeling for the first stain in brown while second is in red. However, red color tends to be brighter and give the impression of greater numbers relative to brown positive cells. One needs to avoid this fallacy in interpretation.

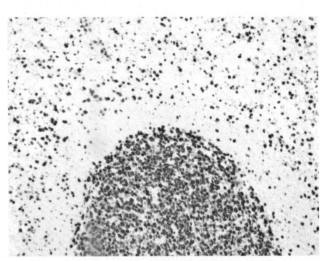

Figure 9.40. Ki-67 in a reactive follicle showing numerous proliferative cells with scattered interfollicular immunoblasts and occasional T-cells also showing proliferative staining.

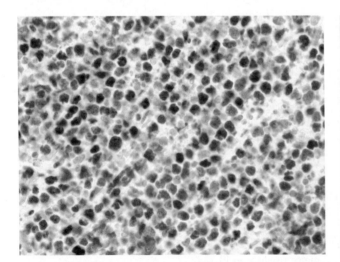

Figure 9.41. MYC immunostain in a patient with Burkitt lymphoma showing over 80% proliferative cells (>50% positive cells is considered as MYC IHC + while >80% staining usually correlates with underlying translocation).

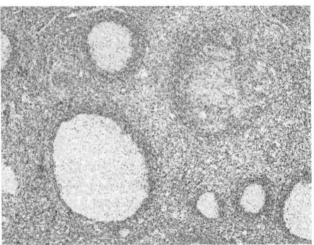

Figure 9.42. BCL2 immunostain in a patient with IgG4-related lymphadenopathy demonstrating reactive secondary lymphoid follicles demonstrating strong staining for BCL2 within the mantle zones and paracortical T-cells. Note the progressively transformed germinal centers at the top right demonstrating increased numbers of BCL2+ cells within the germinal center.

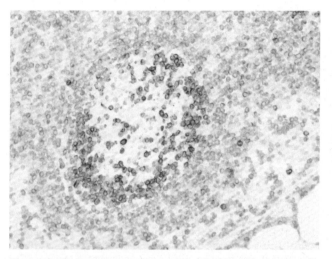

Figure 9.43. BCL2 immunostain demonstrating abnormal bright staining with reactive secondary lymphoid follicles consistent with in situ follicular neoplasia. The surrounding mantle zones demonstrate normal BCL2 expression. These latter cells serve as reference for intensity in internal control cells.

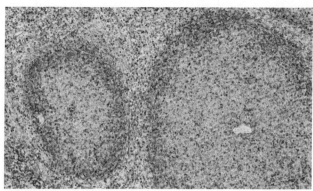

Figure 9.44. BCL2 immunostain is weakly positive in splenic marginal zone lymphoma cells. The lymphoma nodules are surrounded by residual mantle zones of the white pulp while the red pulp T-cells are also positive for BCL2.

Cyclin D1: Positivity in lymphoid cells indicates MCL. Internal control cells are histiocytes and endothelial cells (Figure 9.49). Therefore, an external positive control is unnecessary for this marker.

KEY FEATURES of Some Useful Prognostic Stains and Their Utility in Diagnosis in Various Settings

Stains	Utility	Comment
CD20	B-cell lineage	Cannot be used frequently in relapse after rituximab therapy
CD30	B- and T-cell lymphoma	Useful in T-cell lymphomas for selecting for upfront B-CHP regimen and in relapsed CD30+ lymphomas for anti-CD30 therapy
Ki-67	Proliferative marker	Useful in confirming high proliferation in Burkitt and high-grade B-cell lymphoma
PD-L1	Marks histiocytes and neoplastic cells	Useful in relapsed lymphomas selected for checkpoint inhibitor therapy
CD5	Confirming CLL/SLL or MCL and CD5+ diffuse large B-cell lymphoma	CD5 is sometimes negative by flow and should be tested by immunohistochemistry in such cases
CD19	B-cell lineage	Useful in relapsed lymphoma prior to CAR-T-cell therapy
MYC	>40% useful in BL and double-hit lymphomas	Patients with DHL are selected for EPOCH-R regimen upfront sometimes
BCL2	>50% useful in BL and DHL	Same as above; cases negative with clone 124 should be tested with clone SP66 or E17

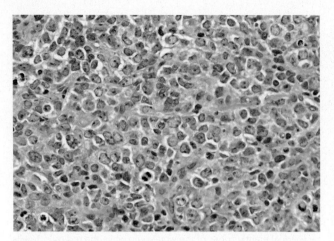

Figure 9.45. H&E image of blastoid double-hit lymphoma in a 47-year-old male with immunostains showing B-cell phenotype.

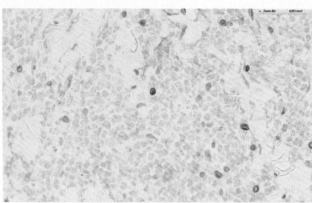

Figure 9.46. BCL2 immunostain in case above using the standard clone 124 is negative and the lymphoma cells while background normal T-cells serve as internal controls. However, due to cytogenetic studies documenting a BCL2 rearrangement, additional BCL2 immunostain was performed using clone SP66.

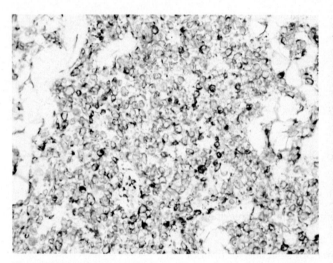

Figure 9.47. BCL2 immunostain in the above case is strongly positive using the SP66 antibody consistent with the underlying BCL2 rearrangement. Mutations in the BCL2 gene may occur in follicular lymphoma and high-grade lymphoma in rare instances and appropriate testing using an alternate antibody such as SP66 or E17 is recommended in such cases.[5]

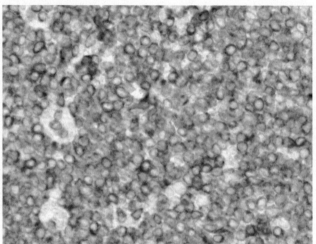

Figure 9.48. BCL2 immunostain in small lymphocytic lymphoma (SLL) demonstrating strong staining in the lymphoma cells. All low-grade lymphomas including mantle cell lymphoma, SLL, and many nodal marginal zone lymphoma are positive for BCL2-like follicular lymphoma, although none of those entities carry an underlying *IGH-BCL2* translocation driving BCL2 overexpression. However, such overexpression is useful from a therapeutic perspective inasmuch as anti-BCL2 therapies such as venetoclax and navitoclax remain potential options.

NEAR MISS

CASE: INCIDENTALLY MCL IN REACTIVE LOOKING NODE

The case is from a 65-year-old female with mediastinal adenopathy with mediastinal lymph nodes removed during a right lung lower lobe excision procedure which demonstrated adenocarcinoma (Figures 9.50-9.55). Incidentally, routine flow cytometry was performed on the lymph nodes accidently, which led to the identification of B-cell clone negative for CD5 and CD10. Additional immunostains were performed on the lymph node, and cyclin D1 was added only in the last round of immunostains. The overtly reactive lymph node and negative CD5 by flow cytometry and immunostains depicted below made it difficult to arrive at the diagnosis. There was evidence of underlying t(11; 14) translocation by FISH.

PEARLS & PITFALLS

Cyclin D1 can be positive in CLL proliferation centers and one must be cautious in such cases not to call it MCL. Tonsillar crypt epithelial cells are also positive for cyclin D1 and hence invaginated crypts within tonsillar lymphoid tissue can be misconstrued as MCL cells.

SOX11: There are no internal control tissues for this nuclear marker useful in documenting MCL. Also, positive in lymphoblastic processes and cyclin D1-negative MCL, this marker is usually positive in most nodal MCL (Figure 9.56).[6]

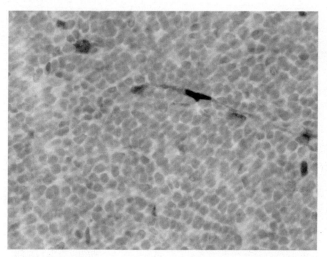

Figure 9.49. Cyclin D1 immunostain in a case of CLL showing scattered endothelial cells and histiocytes with nuclear staining for cyclin D1 while the lymphoma cells are negative for cyclin D1.

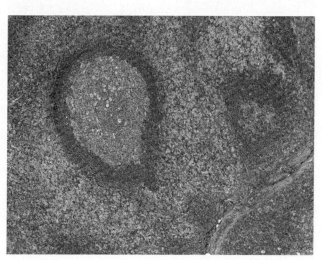

Figure 9.50. Low-power H&E image demonstrating multiple scattered reactive secondary lymphoid follicles with moderate paracortical hyperplasia. There was no lymph node architecture effacement.

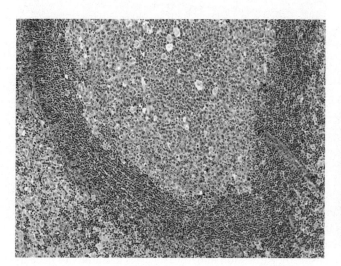

Figure 9.51. High-power H&E image demonstrating normal mantle zones with a mixed population of cells within the germinal center with some distortion of the light zone–dark zone interface.

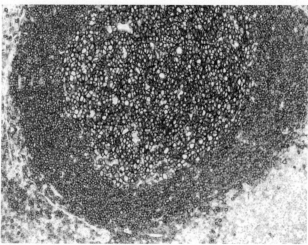

Figure 9.52. CD20 immunostain uniformly highlights germinal center B-cells and mantle zones consistent with the pattern expected for a reactive follicle.

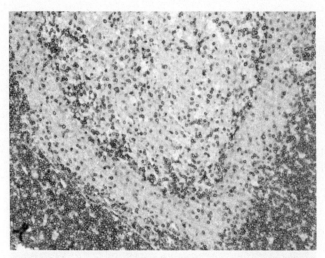

Figure 9.53. CD5 immunostain highlights follicular helper T-cells (white arrows) at the germinal center–mantle zone interface and additionally stains numerous paracortical T-cells. There is some suggestion of weak CD5 in a small subset of mantle zone cells. But most mantle zone cells are negative for CD5 by immunohistochemistry.

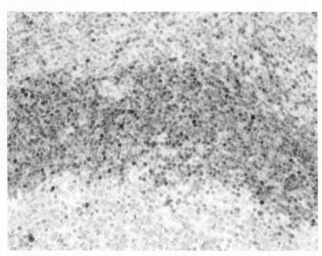

Figure 9.54. Cyclin D1 immunostain is uniformly positive in the mantle zones. The nucleus of tingible body macrophage within the germinal center is seen at the bottom left inside the germinal center.

Figure 9.55. SOX11 immunostain is uniformly negative. Although most nodal mantle cell lymphomas express both cyclin D1 and SOX11, this case is negative.

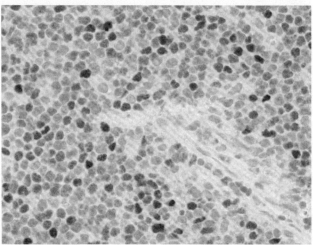

Figure 9.56. SOX11 immunostain demonstrating nuclear staining of lymphoma cells in a case of blastoid mantle cell lymphoma (MCL) with other areas demonstrating more typical classic MCL. This case was unusually negative for cyclin D1 with up regulation of CD10, BCL6 and MUM1 in the blastoid areas.

CD30: An activation marker with diagnostic and prognostic utility. The typical antibody clone which most labs use is either BerH2 or Ki-1. Utility is in diagnosis of classical Hodgkin lymphoma, anaplastic large cell lymphoma (ALCL), and all CD30+ LPDs including EBV + DLBCL, NOS. Prognostically, expression in neoplastic cells has utility in patients selected for treatment with anti-CD30 antibody conjugate, brentuximab. Internal control includes scattered perifollicular immunoblasts around reactive tonsillar secondary lymphoid follicles (Figure 9.57).

Checklist of Entities Expressing CD30

Entity	CD30 Numbers/ Intensity	Additional Diagnostic Points
B-cell entities		
Classical Hodgkin lymphoma (Figure 9.58)	Variable/strong	Weak PAX5/negative CD20
Mediastinal gray zone lymphoma (Figures 9.59-9.60)	Variable/strong	Variable strong CD20 and other B-cell markers
Primary mediastinal (thymic) large B-cell lymphoma (Figure 9.61)	Numerous/ weak-moderate	Compartmentalizing sclerosis; CD23+
EBV + large B-cell lymphoma (Figure 9.62)	Variable/strong	Strong CD20 and EBV
Post-transplant lymphoproliferative disorder (polymorphic and monomorphic) (Figure 9.63)	Variable/variable	Clinical context; otherwise indistinguishable from cHL or EBV + DLBCL
Plasmablastic processes	Variable	Cellular cytomorphology
EBV + mucocutaneous ulcer (Figure 9.64)	Variable/strong band-like mucosal	GI location and context
EBV reactivation	Variable/strong	Older patient; preserved architecture
Infectious mononucleosis	Variable/strong, variable size of cells	Young patient; tonsillar location
CMV lymphadenitis and other reactive proliferations (Figure 9.65)	Strong scattered cells	High degree of suspicion
T-cell entities		
Anaplastic large cell lymphoma (Figure 9.66)	Numerous/strong	CD3-/cytotoxic markers+
Angioimmunoblastic T-cell lymphoma (Figure 9.67)	Variable/variable	Hypervascular with EBV/T-cell clone
Peripheral T-cell lymphoma with Hodgkin-like cells (Near miss case below)	Scattered/variable	High degree of suspicion/T_{FH} markers and polymerase chain reaction for T-cell clonality
CD30+ cutaneous lymphoproliferative disorders	Variable (LyP A and B scattered) Numerous (LyP C, D, E)	Clinical context

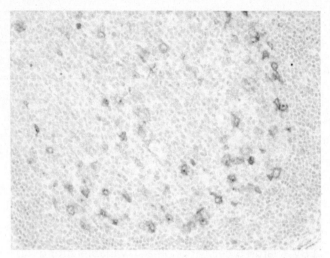

Figure 9.57. CD30 immunostain in reactive follicular hyperplasia showing immunoblasts expressing CD30 at the periphery of the germinal center abutting the mantle zones. At times, these immunoblasts are also seen in the immediate perifollicular location. This is the typical reactive pattern of immunoblasts, and this should not be confused with Classical Hodgkin lymphoma cells.

NEAR MISS

CASE: PERIPHERAL T-CELL LYMPHOMA WITH HODGKIN-LIKE CELLS OF B-CELL DERIVATION

This is a 63-year-old man who had extensive lymphadenopathy extending from the supraclavicular regions extending into the mediastinum. Several discrete bone lesions were also noted besides splenomegaly and hypercalcemia (Figures 9.68-9.75). Several scattered Hodgkin-like cells are present with identical immunophenotype as classical Hodgkin lymphoma but present within a hypervascular background with several scattered background immunoblasts. However, scattered extra-follicular CD21+ dendritic cell meshworks were identified. Despite the lack of EBV and a clonal T-cell gene rearrangement, the clinical picture and morphology supported designation as peripheral T-cell lymphoma with Hodgkin-like B-cells.[7] These entities are often treated with an etoposide-based regimen and hence distinction from classical Hodgkin lymphoma is critical in these instances.

CD15: LeuM1 is the most common clone and the main use for this marker is in diagnosis of cHL. Neutrophils express high CD15, whereas monocytes express weak CD15. These two cells serve as internal controls in all tissues and hence a positive external control is not necessary for this marker. One must take time when screening for CD15 in cHL since expression can be very focal and weak (Figure 9.76).

T-cell receptor (TCR) IHC: Most benign T-cells as well as T-cell neoplasms express surface TCR-beta with very few expressing TCR-delta. Good antibodies are available for TCR-beta and TCR-delta to identify these markers. T-cell malignancies sometimes are silent for both TCRs and this is especially useful and there is no obvious antigenic abnormalities such as abnormal CD4:CD8 ratio or loss of T-cell antigens. In such cases, total absence of both TCRs by IHC can be especially useful in identifying an abnormal phenotype on sections (Figures 9.77-9.79).

Programmed cell death receptor-1 (PD-1) is a marker specific for follicular helper T-cells, a special class of CD4 T-cells present at the interface of germinal center and mantle zones of reactive follicles. Neoplasms arising from these cells are positive for PD1 and include angioimmunoblastic T-cell lymphoma as well as follicular T-cell lymphoma (Figures 9.80 and 9.81).

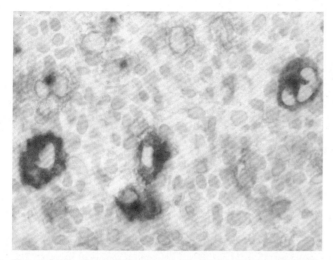

Figure 9.58. Classical Hodgkin lymphoma with scattered Hodgkin/Reed-Sternberg cells demonstrating strong membranous, cytoplasmic staining for CD30 with Golgi accentuation.

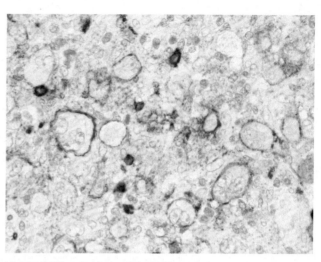

Figure 9.59. Mediastinal gray zone lymphoma showing one focus with Hodgkin-like cells with variable weak CD20.

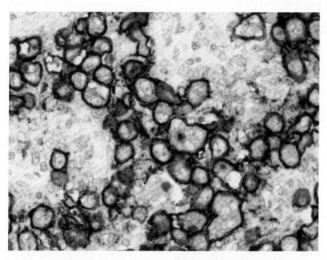

Figure 9.60. Mediastinal gray zone lymphoma showing other areas with sheets of large B-cells strongly expressing CD20. This case expressed strong CD79a with weak PAX5 and variable CD30. Morphologically and immunophenotypically, there were distinct components allowing a diagnosis of composite GZL.

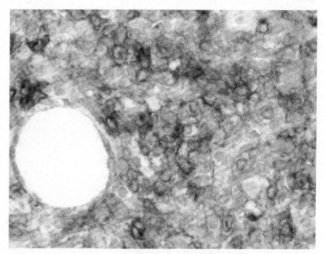

Figure 9.61. Primary mediastinal (thymic) large B-cell lymphoma with variable weak to moderate staining for CD30. Frequently, there is coexpression of CD23 with characteristic cytomorphology. Patients are typically young females.

Programmed cell death protein ligand-1 (PD-L1) is the ligand for PD-1. Neoplastic cells such as large B-cell lymphoma cells and Hodgkin lymphoma cells express PD-L1, which interacts with PD1+ microenvironment lymphoid cells and results in energy and evasion of tumor-specific immune response. Both of these markers are relevant in lymphoma due to significant benefit in frontline and relapse setting with checkpoint blockade therapy. Background macrophages demonstrate strong expression of PD-L1 and serve as internal controls and most lymphoma tissues (Figures 9.82 and 9.83).

PEARLS & PITFALLS

Mere positivity for PD-1 in diffuse processes does not connote lymphoma such as angioimmunoblastic T-cell lymphoma automatically. Increased numbers of PD-1+ lymphoid cells are often observed in the background microenvironment nodes in patients with autoimmune conditions and lymphoma (HL as well as NLPHL). Correlation with other stains and molecular studies is important before arriving at the appropriate diagnosis.

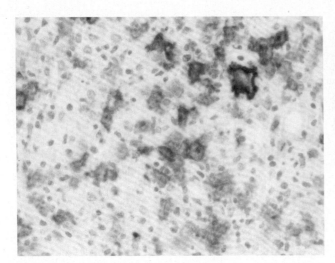

Figure 9.62. EBV-positive large B-cell lymphoma demonstrating variable numbers of CD30- Hodgkin-like cells that range in size from medium to large with variability in expression. Most cases usually demonstrate strong CD20 compared to classical Hodgkin lymphoma. However, it must be remembered that EBV can lead to downregulation of B-cell, germinal center program, and surface light chain expression.

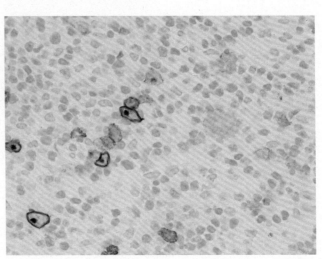

Figure 9.63. EBV-positive polymorphic post-transplant lymphoproliferative disorder with scattered variably sized CD30 positive lymphoid cells. The right side of the field contains large Hodgkin-like cells with weak staining with several scattered smaller brightly staining immunoblasts on the left side of the field. The distinction between classical Hodgkin lymphoma, EBV + large B-cell lymphoma, and polymorphic PTLD can often be very difficult and requires correlation with clinical context to a large extent. Such cases often may be best classified as EBV + gray zone lymphoma. These latter entities require aggressive treatment with regimens used for diffuse large B-cell lymphoma, whereas the regimens used for PTLD and classical Hodgkin lymphoma are very different and hence the distinction is critical from a therapeutic standpoint.

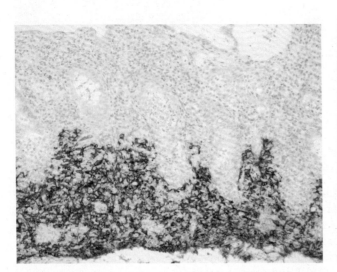

Figure 9.64. EBV-positive mucocutaneous ulcer demonstrating strong CD30+ cells present as sheets with a bandlike pattern subjacent to ulcerated epithelium. These are self-limited lesions described more recently in the context of immunosuppression from a variety of sources and may also occur in the post-transplant setting. Presence of serum EBV DNA indicates a more systemic process such as PTLD in cases with similar morphology.[11]

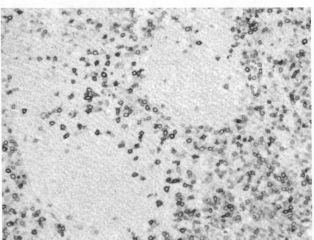

Figure 9.65. Florid reactive immunoblastic proliferation mistaken for anaplastic large cell lymphoma. This patient had extensive lymphadenopathy with florid immunoblastic proliferation in the paracortex with numerous T-cells. However, it was difficult to identify if the CD30+ cells were B-cells or T-cells. These cells were hard to identify on CD20 but better picked up on MUM1 highlighting large nuclei consistent with immunoblastic differentiation. EBV was, however, negative and the exact cause of this immunoblastic proliferation was uncertain.

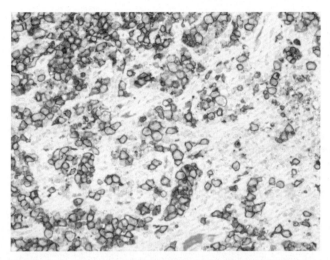

Figure 9.66. Angioimmunoblastic T-cell lymphoma with numerous varying sized CD30+ lymphoid cells. Scattered Hodgkin-like cells in addition to several smaller immunoblast-like cells are noted. Varying numbers of EBV-positive cells are also seen in these cases similar in size and distribution to the CD30+ B lymphoid cells. Frequently, this entity is also confused with other EBV-positive processes including classical Hodgkin lymphoma, EBV + DLBCL, and EBV + polymorphic PTLD. On occasions, clonal proliferations can arise from these EBV-infected cells with coexistent EBV + DLBCL arising within angioimmunoblastic T-cell lymphoma.

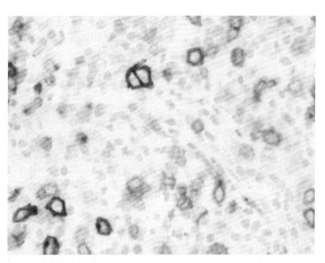

Figure 9.67. Anaplastic large cell lymphoma (ALCL), ALK-demonstrating diffuse strong CD30 expression in all lymphoma cells. The expression of CD30 is universal in this T-cell lymphoma. Rare peripheral T-cell lymphoma may express diffuse CD30 and CD15 without the characteristic morphology of ALCL and care should be taken not to classify these as ALCL or classical Hodgkin lymphoma.[12].

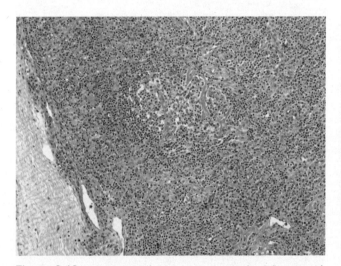

Figure 9.68. Low power demonstrating capsular sclerosis with obliteration of the subcapsular sinus. Regressed peripheral cortical lymphoid follicle with some increase in vascularization is noted in H&E.

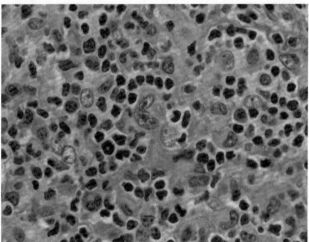

Figure 9.69. At higher power, scattered multinucleated and mononuclear cells compatible with Hodgkin/Reed-Sternberg cells are noted.

CD68: Tumors of myeloid, monocytic, and histiocytic origin are positive for CD68. Hence, the distinction of myeloid sarcoma from histiocytic sarcoma may sometimes be difficult based just on CD68 and multiple markers may be required. The two common clones used are PGM1 and KP-1.

S100: Tumors of dendritic origin such as Langerhans cells, interdigitating dendritic cells, and histiocytes of Rosai-Dorfman disease are positive for S100 and contrast to histiocytic sarcoma, which is negative for S100. There is nuclear and cytoplasmic staining usually[8] (Figure 9.84).

CD1a and Langerin: They are both markers specific for Langerhans cells. CD1a is additionally positive in T lymphoblastic lymphoma and also stains the amastigotes of Leishmania.[9]

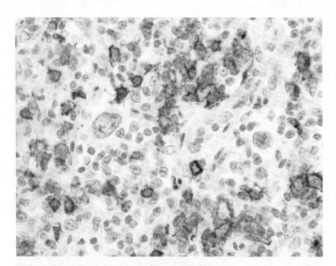

Figure 9.70. CD20 highlights numerous background small B-cells, but the Hodgkin-like cells are negative for CD20.

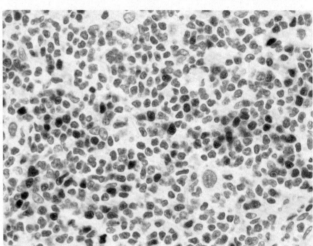

Figure 9.71. There is weak PAX 5 expression on these Hodgkin-like cells with background small B-cells demonstrating strong PAX 5 expression.

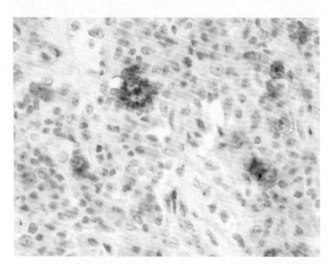

Figure 9.72. The Hodgkin-like cells are strongly positive for CD30.

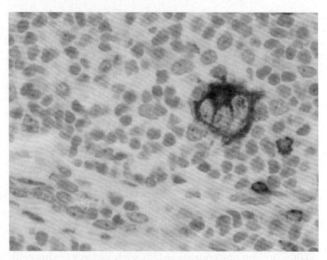

Figure 9.73. The Hodgkin-like cells are additionally positive for CD15. Note the presence of scattered small strongly positive neutrophils in the same field to the bottom right.

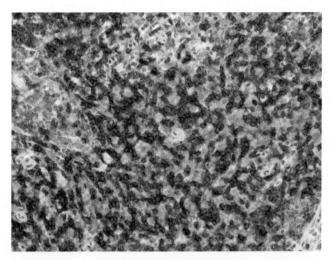

Figure 9.74. There is strong CD4 expression in the background lymphoid cells.

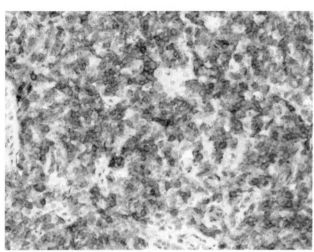

Figure 9.75. The cells are also positive for the follicular helper T-cell marker, PD-1.

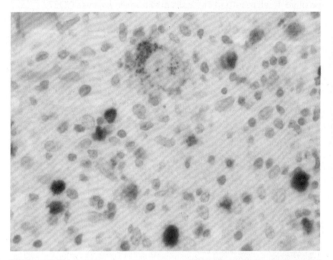

Figure 9.76. CD15 immunostain in classical Hodgkin lymphoma demonstrating granular cytoplasmic expression in the single cells seen at the top of the field. Several neutrophils are seen to demonstrate variable moderate to strong expression. Monocytes express weak CD15 and can serve as low positive internal controls.

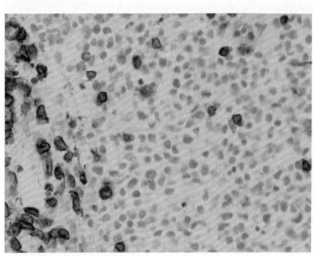

Figure 9.77. T-cell receptor (TCR) beta immunohistochemistry demonstrating nodal peripheral T-cell lymphoma with a cytotoxic phenotype demonstrating diffuse loss of surface TCR beta expression while background T-cells are strongly positive.

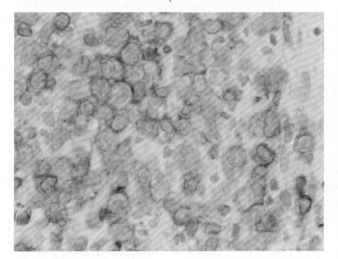

Figure 9.78. Mycosis fungoides at transformation demonstrating dual expression of T-cell receptor (TCR) beta (shown here) and TCR gamma.

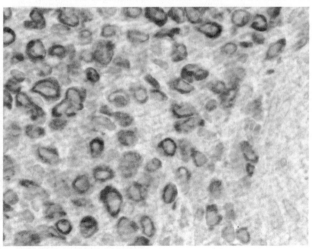

Figure 9.79. T-cell receptor–delta immunohistochemistry in the case above (mycosis fungoides) expressing TCR delta in the transformed neoplastic cells in conjunction with strong, T-cell receptor beta. Different functional T-cell receptor rearrangements may occur in neoplastic T-cells on the different alleles explaining the simultaneous coexpression of both TCR delta and TCR beta.

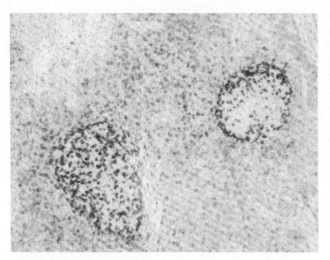

Figure 9.80. Reactive follicular hyperplasia demonstrating rim of strongly PD1-positive normal follicular helper T-cells within the germinal center abutting the mantle zones. Note the week positive lymphoid cells outside the context of germinal centers within the paracortex.

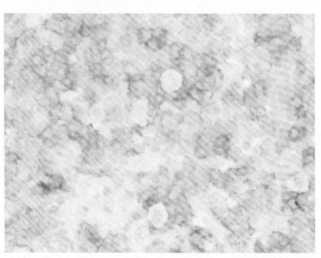

Figure 9.81. Nodular lymphocyte predominant Hodgkin lymphoma demonstrating scattered popcorn cells surrounded by PD1-positive T-cell rosettes. The cells additionally express CD57.

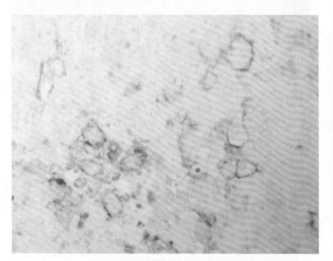

Figure 9.82. A case of nodal double hit high-grade B-cell lymphoma demonstrating scattered macrophages with strong PD-L1 expression, but lymphoma cells are negative in the background.

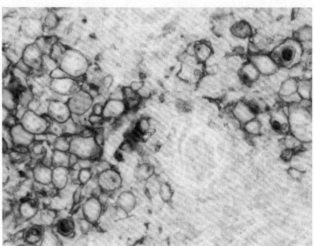

Figure 9.83. A case of classical Hodgkin lymphoma with high content of Hodgkin cells expressing strong membranous PD-L1 in the neoplastic cells. A significant proportion of classical Hodgkin lymphoma contain amplifications of the PD–L1 with near universal expression by immunohistochemistry. Although there are several companion diagnostic antibody clones packaged for PD–L1 for several solid tumors, at this time, there is no mandate for utilization of any specific companion diagnostic antibody for lymphoma for current clinical trials.

STAINS RELATED TO MICROORGANISMS

Epstein-Barr virus early RNA (EBER): EBER is an RNA in situ hybridization for EBV RNA and is expressed in all latency phases and hence is a very sensitive marker for detection of EBV. RNA in situ hybridization must be performed with an additional RNA control probe (U6) which is directed against the poly-A tail of RNA in the tissue of interest. This probe ensures that the tissue of interest has viable RNA that can be detected by the EBER probe. Hence EBER staining requires three unstained slides, one for negative control, one for RNA control, and one for EBV-specific probes.

HHV8/LANA: Staining is typically nuclear and stippled in infected cells. Typical positive control use is one from Kaposi sarcoma, which is always positive for HHV8 (Figure 9.88).

Checklist of Best Practices While Examining and Reporting IHCs in Cases With Inside and Outside Stains

☐ Separate out control slides.

☐ Arrange stains in the tray in order in a logical order depending on the diagnosis starting with CD20 and CD3.

☐ Make a note of stains positive in neoplastic controls with note on nonworking stains based on comparison with internal controls (for example, cyclin D1 is suboptimal with absent stain in endothelial cells or histiocytes).

☐ List background stains after neoplastic compartment.

☐ Quantify extent of staining in reports when possible.

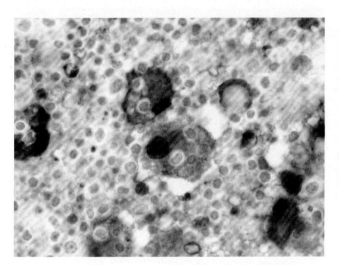

Figure 9.84. S100 immunostain in Rosai-Dorfman disease demonstrating staining within histiocytes showing emperipolesis.

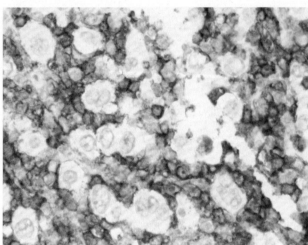

Figure 9.85. Classical Hodgkin lymphoma demonstrates absent staining in the Hodgkin/Reed-Sternberg cells, while surrounding lymphocytes demonstrate strong staining. Often, interpretation of CD45 status on large neoplastic cells is hampered by presence of numerous surrounding lymphocytes and when in doubt, it is good to look for clusters of abnormal cells abutting each other and determine membrane staining in between two abnormal cells.

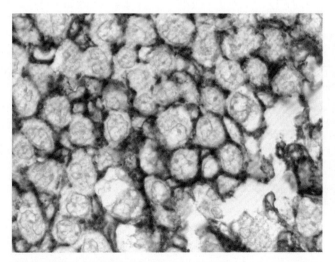

Figure 9.86. Mediastinal gray zone lymphoma demonstrating sheets of neoplastic Hodgkin-like cells demonstrating strong membrane staining for CD45.

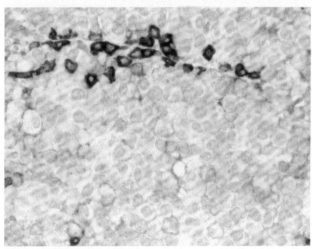

Figure 9.87. Plasmablastic lymphoma demonstrating largely negative CD45 expression with scattered perivascular lymphocytes demonstrating strong CD45 positivity. Comparison with internal control cells is important in most stains in hematopathology.

NEAR MISS

CASE: EXTRACAVITARY PRIMARY EFFUSION LYMPHOMA

This is a 73-year-old male with well-controlled HIV with scattered enlarged lymph nodes that were biopsied. Morphologically these were thought to be reactive but sent for second opinion due to persistent lymphadenopathy (Figures 9.89-9.94).

Herpes simplex virus 1/2: This antibody is usually a cocktail of primary antibody directed against HSV1 and HSV2. Careful review of the necrotic areas and lymph nodes is essential to be able to recognize the purpose pattern of necrosis with nuclear changes characteristic of HSV. Necrosis in lymph nodes of patients with CLL/SLL must raise suspicion for infection by HSV and tested appropriately (Figures 9.95 and 9.96).

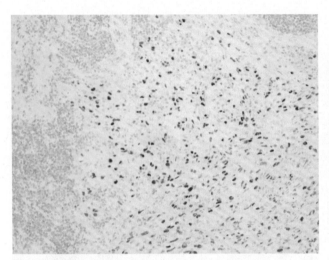

Figure 9.88. Kaposi sarcoma involving the lymph node demonstrating strong nuclear HHV8/LANA staining with a stable pattern in the spindly neoplastic cells.

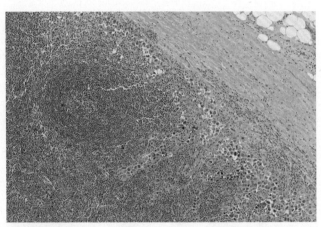

Figure 9.89. H&E image at low power demonstrates prominent capsular fibrosis with scattered atypical cells within the subcapsular and trabecular sinus associated with regressed lymphoid follicles.

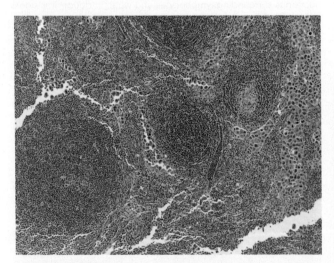

Figure 9.90. H&E image of the deeper parts of this lymph node demonstrating several scattered reactive regressed Castleman-like follicles associated with several linear intrasinusoidal clusters of large plasmablastic cells. The cells were distributed patchily.

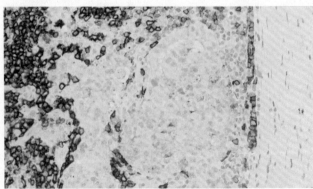

Figure 9.91. CD20 is negative in the large atypical cells while background normal small B-cells are identified.

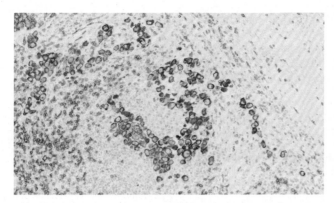

Figure 9.92. CD3 is, however, strongly positive in these large cells with surrounding background reactive T-cells. Her T-cell lymphoma was considered in view of this abnormal CD3 positivity.

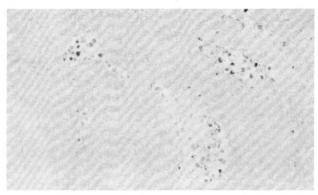

Figure 9.93. EBV in situ hybridization demonstrates that these large cells are infected by EBV raising the possibility of extranodal NK/T-cell lymphoma based on CD3/EBV coexpression.

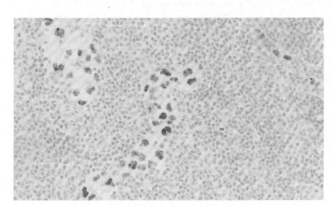

Figure 9.94. However, HHV8 immunostain is also coexpressed indicating coinfection by EBV and HHV8 in the cells. The combination of stains supporting the diagnosis of extracavitary primary effusion lymphoma. Similar atypical lymphoid proliferations restricted to the germinal centers may be observed outside the context of HIV and are termed as germinal tropic lymphoproliferative disorder.

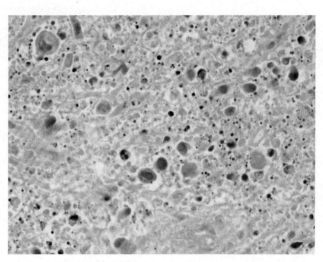

Figure 9.95. H&E image of necrotic areas of the lymph node in a patient with small lymphocytic lymphoma and suspected transformation. Note scattered virally transformed cellular nuclei with smudging typical of Cowdry type A inclusions of herpes simplex virus.

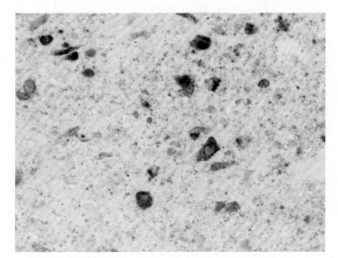

Figure 9.96. Additional staining with antibody for HSV 1/2 demonstrates staining within the cells confirming the infection.

KEY FEATURES Diagnostic of Certain Lymphoma Entities Based on CD20, CD21, and EBER

Stain	Entity	Pattern	Figure number
CD20			
	Nodular lymphocyte predominant Hodgkin lymphoma (NLPHL)	Scattered large CD20+ B-cells with nodules of small B-cells	Figure 9.97
	T-cell/histiocyte-rich large B-cell lymphoma	Scattered large CD20+ B-cells without small B-cells	Figure 9.98
	Diffuse large B-cell lymphoma (DLBCL)	Sheets of strong large B-cells	Figure 9.99
	Classical Hodgkin lymphoma	Scattered CD20-negative	Figure 9.100
	EBV + DLBCL, NOS	Variable size, strong CD20+	Figure 9.101
	Plasmablastic lymphoma	Sheets of large dim-negative CD20+	Figure 9.102
	Small lymphocytic lymphoma	Small dim CD20+ cells	Figure 9.103
	Angioimmunoblastic T-cell lymphoma	Subcapsular CD20+ small cells and large CD20+ immunoblasts	Figure 9.104
CD21			
	NLPHL and FL	Expanded and disrupted	Figure 9.105
	AITL	Extrafollicular dendritic meshworks	Figure 9.106
	FL	Areas of missing FDC meshworks-transformation	Figure 9.107
	NLPHL vs T/HRBCL	Retained vs absent meshworks	Figure 9.108
	MCL and FL	Lymphoma cells expressing CD21	Figure 9.109
	Progressive transformation of germinal center	Expanded meshworks	Figure 9.110
	Castleman disease	Regressed meshworks	Figure 9.111
EBER			
	EBV reactivation	Scattered small and large cells	Figure 9.112
	Classical Hodgkin lymphoma	Scattered large cells only	Figure 9.113
	EBV + DLBCL and polymorphic B-cell lymphoma	Mixed and small large and Hodgkin-like cells	Figure 9.114
	Plasmablastic lymphoma	Diffuse positive	Figure 9.115
	Germinotropic LPD	Isolated EBV in follicles only	Figure 9.116

Checklist of Triaging and IHC Ordering Practices for Cases—Algorithm First

☐ Touch preparation at lymphoma work-up with sheets of large cells (likely DLBCL, no flow).

☐ Cases with concurrent flow: restrict ordering corresponds IHCs if flow is positive.

☐ Other IHC practices

　o Small lymphoid processes: CD20, CD3, CD5, CD10, cyclin D1, and CD21 (kappa/lambda if plasmacytic differentiation)

　　■ Large sheetlike lymphoid processes (DLBCL panel with CD20, CD3, CD5, CD10, BCL6, MUM1, MYC, BCL2, CD30, EBER, and PD-L1)

　　■ Hodgkin-like processes: CD20, CD3, CD30, CD15, PAX5, and EBER

　　■ Large morphologically reactive nodal processes. No need for all stains or flow upfront.

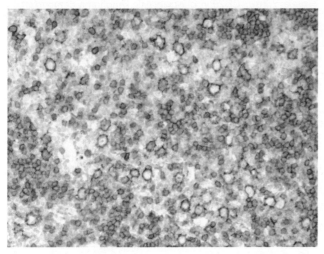

Figure 9.97. CD20 in nodular lymphocyte predominant Hodgkin lymphoma (NLPHL) demonstrating singly scattered large cells present in the background of small B-cells within the nodules. The nodular architecture and small B-cells start diminishing with progression toward variant pattern NLPHL through overt T-cell/histiocyte-rich large B-cell lymphoma.

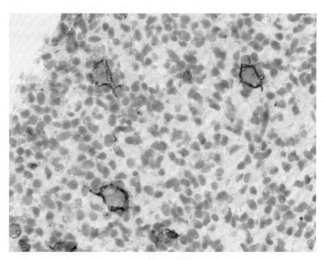

Figure 9.98. CD20 in T-cell/histiocyte-rich large B-cell lymphoma demonstrating three scattered large B-cells with rare small B-cells seen in the top of the field. Note the lack of any nodular architecture or any small B-cells in the background.

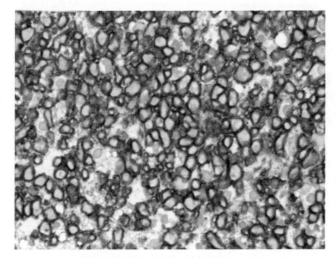

Figure 9.99. CD20 in diffuse large B-cell lymphoma demonstrating sheets of large B-cells with strong staining.

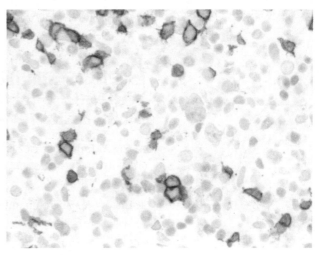

Figure 9.100. CD20 in classical Hodgkin lymphoma showing CD20-negative Hodgkin cells with surrounding reactive small B-cells. Variable weak to negative CD20 is typical of classical Hodgkin lymphoma. In cases like this, if there is uniform strong staining for CD20, EBV + large B-cell lymphoma must be entertained and additional EBV staining should be done.

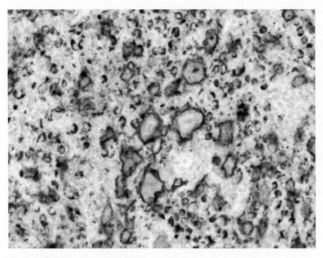

Figure 9.101. CD20 in EBV + large B-cell lymphoma demonstrating pleomorphic small medium and Hodgkin-like large B-cells with uniform strong staining for CD20. This case was additionally strongly positive for EBV by in situ hybridization.

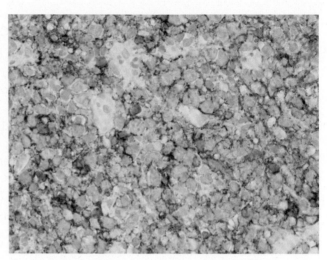

Figure 9.102. CD20 in plasmablastic lymphoma demonstrating weak to negative CD20 on the large plasmablastic cells. Some cases can be uniformly negative for CD20 and CD45 and hence additional MUM1 and EBER confirm the diagnosis in many instances.

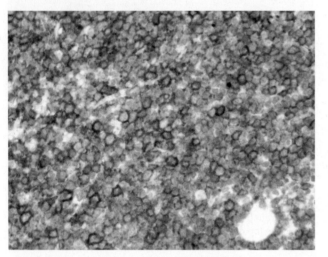

Figure 9.103. CD20 in small lymphocytic lymphoma (SLL) demonstrating weak to moderate staining in the SLL cells. Occasional prolymphocytes demonstrate stronger CD20 immunostaining. Flow cytometry is often better at demonstrating dim CD20 expression in SLL.

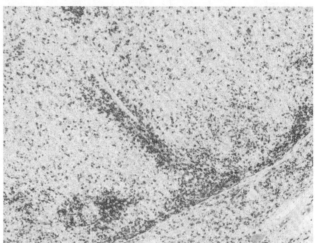

Figure 9.104. CD20 immunostain pattern in angioimmunoblastic T-cell lymphoma demonstrating collections of subcapsular small B-cells with increased numbers of larger immunoblasts in the deeper areas. Careful attention must be paid to CD20 in the situation since large B-cell lymphomas can arise within angioimmunoblastic T-cell lymphoma. In this case, however, there is no evidence of such progression.

EXERCISE IN INTERPRETATION, SAMPLE WRITE-UPS IN ONE SINGLE CASE, AND BEST PRACTICES IN WRITE-UPS

ALCL–ALK-negative case.

Write-up in case as above. Note the following key aspects of the write-up below that ties in several aspects:

1. History of patient up until now
2. Diagnosis that takes into account prior treatment with CD30 status at this time relevant for patients with PTCL
3. Note that expression of aberrant CD20 that does not connote B-cell lymphoma
4. Separation of submitted stains and new stains in the right order
5. Final explanation that ties the morphologic clues and explains rationale for the chosen diagnosis
6. Correlation of the morphology and IHC data with possible molecular data that might impact outcome

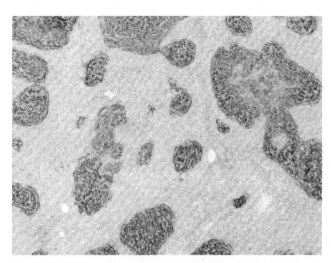

Figure 9.105. CD21 immunostain in follicular lymphoma demonstrating expanded and serpiginous follicular dendritic cell meshworks.

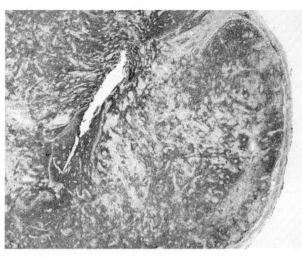

Figure 9.106. CD21 immunostain in angioimmunoblastic T-cell lymphoma with numerous CD21 follicular dendritic cell meshworks coursing throughout the lymph node. This pattern is highly atypical since follicular dendritic cell meshworks should be restricted only to lymphoid follicles.

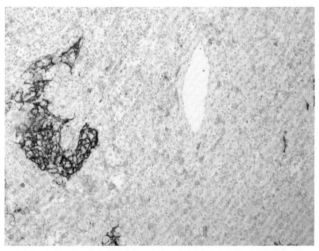

Figure 9.107. CD21 immunostain in transformed follicular lymphoma demonstrating attenuated and disrupted meshworks in a single follicular structure to the left with absent meshworks in the area to the right demonstrating increased numbers of large cells expressing weak CD21 consistent with a transformed component.

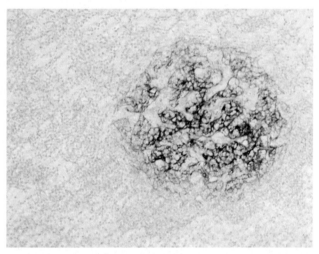

Figure 9.108. CD21 immunostain in nodular lymphocyte predominant Hodgkin lymphoma demonstrating expanded dendritic cell meshworks.

Clinical history: The patient is a 69-year-old male with history of peripheral T-cell lymphoma, NOS undergoing liver biopsy. He was diagnosed to have PTCL nos in early 2017 and given CHOP x 6 and BV with CR and then autotransplant with BEAM conditioning with recent relapse in November 2018. The initial biopsy is not available for review.

Liver; core needle biopsies:

• Relapsed T-cell lymphoma best subclassified as ALCL, ALK-negative, CD30+ (100%) with aberrant partial CD20 expression, and diffuse P63 expression, see microscopic description.

Microscopic description: There are several core needle sections of the liver, one of which shows complete effacement of liver parenchyma by diffuse sheetlike infiltrate of intermediate to large pleomorphic lymphoid cells with irregular nuclear membranes, prominent nucleoli, and scant basophilic cytoplasm. Scattered hallmark cells and donut cells (cells with intranuclear cytoplasmic inclusions) are noted in addition to frequent single cell

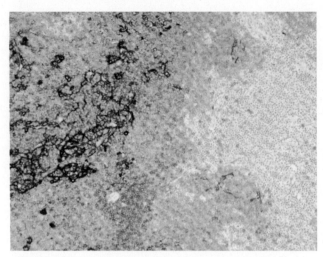

Figure 9.109. CD21 immunostain in mantle cell lymphoma (MCL) demonstrating disrupted follicular dendritic cell meshworks within the central areas in addition to moderate CD21 expression by the MCL cells. Frequently, lymphoma cells including follicular lymphoma may express CD21. CD23 is also often positive in normal mantle zone cells. This must be kept in mind as one evaluates both these stains.

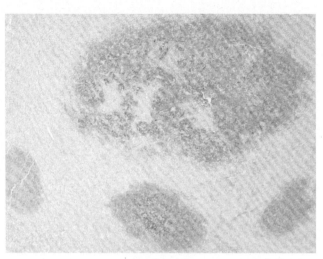

Figure 9.110. CD21 immunostain in progressive transformation of germinal centers demonstrating three normal follicles at the bottom with a markedly expanded follicular structure, consistent with progressively transformed germinal center demonstrating expanded and disrupted follicular dendritic cell meshworks with additional staining for CD21 in some of the mantle zone lymphocytes.

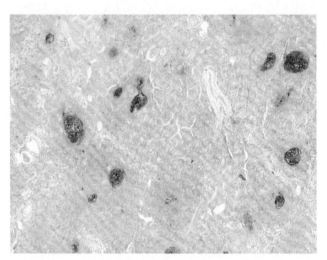

Figure 9.111. CD21 immunostain demonstrating small regressed follicular structures in a patient with idiopathic multicentric Castleman disease. Regressed lymphoid follicles may be seen in a variety of situations and not only in hyaline vascular Castleman disease.

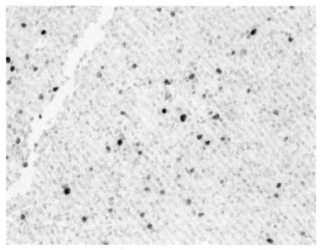

Figure 9.112. EBV-ISH in a patient with EBV reactivation demonstrating predominantly small and occasional medium-sized EBV + lymphoid cells.

apoptosis and mitotic figures. There is a patchy sprinkling of eosinophils amidst the tumor cells. The other fragments of liver show multifocal portal-centric lymphoma infiltrates with sparing of the sinusoidal spaces.

Provided immunohistochemical stains include CD3, CD20, CD5, CD4, CD8, and CD7 and additional stains performed at UOC (CD30, EBER, TIA-1, granzyme B, perforin, P63, TCRB, CD15, ALK, and PAX5) are also examined. The large neoplastic cells are positive for CD3 (dim-moderate), CD4, TCRB, P63 (strong), and CD30 (strong and uniform, 100% of cells) with aberrant weak CD20 (significant subset). They are negative for PAX5, CD15, CD8, and ALK, as well all three cytotoxic markers. They have complete loss of CD5 and CD7.

The overall findings (cohesive sheets of large pleomorphic cells, donut, and hallmark cells) coupled with strong CD30 and CD4 support designation as ALCL rather than PTCL, nos. Lack of cytotoxic markers is not infrequent in ALCL. Cases with DUSP22-IRF4 rearrangement are reported to exhibit more hallmark cells and donut cells with monomorphic

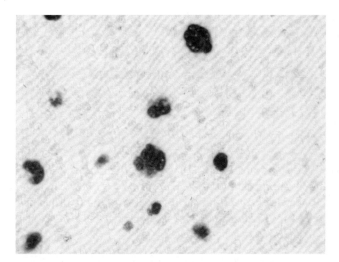

Figure 9.113. EBV–ISH in a patient with classical Hodgkin lymphoma demonstrating isolated staining of the Hodgkin cells with EBV. This is the typical pattern in immunocompetent patients with classical Hodgkin lymphoma that is EBV+. Background small EBV + lymphoid cells are typically not seen in such patients.

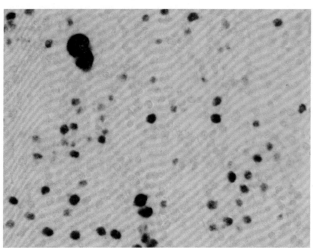

Figure 9.114. EBV–ISH pattern in polymorphic post-transplant lymphoproliferative disorder demonstrating small to medium and Hodgkin-like EBV + lymphoid cells. Identical patterns are typically seen in patients with EBV + large B-cell lymphoma outside the setting of transplant.

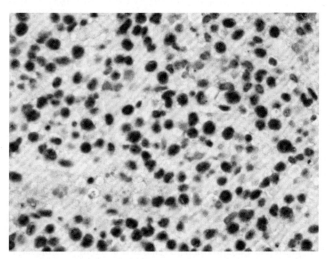

Figure 9.115. EBV–ISH pattern in EBV + plasmablastic lymphoma demonstrating sheets of large EBV + lymphoid cells.

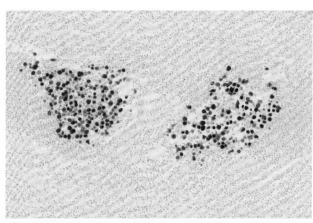

Figure 9.116. EBV–ISH pattern demonstrating large EBV + lymphoid cells restricted only to germinal centers in a case of germinotropic lymphoproliferative disorder. (Case courtesy, Dr. Christos Masaoutis, Evangelismos General Hospital, Athens, Greece.)

cytomorphology and often lack cytotoxic markers more frequently compared to DUSP–non-rearranged ALCLs as noted here. However, there is rather striking pleomorphism in most areas with diffuse P63 expression and hence possible TP63-rearranged or triple negative (ALK, DUSP22, and TP63) disease is favored based on morphologic features. Additional TP63 and IRF4 FISH will both be performed (send out) and reported separately in a week or so.

Review of the treatment naïve biopsy in early 2017, which reportedly showed small CD4+/CD30 (variable) lymphoma cells, would be informative, and additional polymerase chain reaction studies might be helpful in knowing if the two processes are clonally related. Although evolution/progression of previously diagnosed PTCL is a possibility, based on the current morphologic features, the above diagnosis of ALCL is favored at this time. Expression of CD20 has been reported in PTCLs although not in ALCL.

References:

Rahemtullah, et al. CD20+ T-cell lymphoma: clinicopathologic analysis of 9 cases and a review of the literature. *Am J Surg Pathol.* 2008;32(11):1593-1607.

King RL, Parrilla Castellar E, Feldman AL, coworkers. Morphologic features of ALK-negative anaplastic large cell lymphomas with DUSP22 rearrangements. *Am J Surg Pathol.* 2016;40(1):36-43.

SAMPLE OF BAD AND GOOD WRITE-UPS WITH FOCUS ON IMMUNOHISTOCHEMISTRY IN A CASE OF ANGIOIMMUNOBLASTIC T-CELL LYMPHOMA WHERE STAINS ARE PERFORMED IN-HOUSE AND AT ORIGINATING INSTITUTION

Bad Write-up:

Immunostains reveal numerous T-cells with a mixture of CD4 and CD8 T-cells along with CD5- and CD7-positive cells. Scattered B-cells are also noted with occasional large CD20+ B-cells. CD21 shows several scattered dendritic cell meshworks and scattered EBV+ cells are present. In addition, scattered CD30+, BCL6+, PD1, and Mum1+ cells are also present. Kappa and lambda are non-contributory while CD10, keratin, and HHV8 are both negative.

Why this write-up is bad:

1. This does not give the relative proportion of B-cells and T-cells. Also, the CD4:CD8 ratio is not clarified. Expression of CD4 in excess will support the diagnosis.
2. Furthermore, loss of CD5 or CD7 is not stated. Presence of some loss would corroborate T-cell lymphoma.
3. The location of B-cells and follicular dendritic cell meshworks is not indicated. In this lymphoma, follicular dendritic cell meshworks are often present outside of follicular structures in the perisinusoidal areas.
4. Size of the CD30+ cells is not indicated. Immunoblasts are typically large and express CD20 (variable) and CD30.
5. It is unclear what the BCL6+ cells are and if they correspond to the numbers of CD4 and PD1 or CD10. Follicular helper T-cells (cell of origin for angioimmunoblastic T-cell lymphoma) coexpress CD4, BCL 6, CD10, and PD1.
6. Noncontributory does not clarify if the stain did not work or there was no positive finding.

Good Write-Up in the Case Above:

Submitted immunostains (CD20, CD3, CD4, CD8, keratin, HHV8) and additional stains performed in-house (CD5, CD7, CD21, CD30, CD10, BCL6, PD1, MUM1, kappa, and lambda) as well as in situ hybridization for EBV are examined. The stains reveal numerous diffuse infiltrate of small- to medium-sized CD3+ T-cells with lesser numbers of CD5 and CD7. CD4 T-cells markedly outnumber CD8 T-cells. In addition, numerous PD-1+ lymphoid cells corresponding with the numbers of CD4 are present. Lesser numbers of scattered BCL6+ are noted outside of follicular structures, likely corresponding to CD4/PD1+ follicular helper T-cells are noted. Several scattered large CD30+ lymphoid cells expressing variable CD20 are noted, likely corresponding to background immunoblasts. In addition, numerous small B-cells are seen within scattered residual nodular structures corresponding to lymphoid follicles. CD21 highlights numerous expanded extra-follicular perisinusoidal follicular dendritic cell meshworks. Kappa and lambda immunostains highlight rich background of polytypic plasma cells. Moderate numbers of small- to medium-sized EBV+ lymphoid cells are present. Keratin and HHV8 immunostain (controls appropriate) are both negative. CD10 is also negative but stain is suboptimal since there is no staining in background neutrophils.

Why this write-up is good:

1. Separates out stains performed in-house from submitted stains.
2. Addresses the CD4:CD8 ratio as well as loss of T-cell antigens.
3. Makes good correlation between markers likely coexpressed on the same cells based on numbers of cells, size, and spatial location.
4. Addresses the spatial location of important immunostains (follicular vs extra-follicular).
5. Addresses the size of some of the cells as well as speculations on lineage based on markers expressed (CD20, EBVISH, and CD21).
6. Negative stains versus nonworking stains are also addressed (CD10) with reference to internal controls, which are usually present in most stains.

ACKNOWLEDGMENTS

Anirudh V Girish for helping with citations.

References

1. Vyberg M, Nielsen S. Proficiency testing in immunohistochemistry--experiences from Nordic immunohistochemical quality control (NordiQC). *Virchows Arch*. 2016;468:19-29.

2. NordiQC https://www.nordiqc.org/.

3. Swerdlow SH, Campo E, Harris NL, et al. eds. *WHO Classification of Tumours of Haematopoietic and Lymphoid Tissues*. Revised 4th ed. Lyons: IARC; 2017.

4. Prakash S, Fountaine T, Raffeld M, Jaffe ES, Pittaluga S. IgD positive L&H cells identify a unique subset of nodular lymphocyte predominant Hodgkin lymphoma. *Am J Surg Pathol*. 2006;30:585-592.

5. Adam P, Baumann R, Schmidt J, et al. The BCL2 E17 and SP66 antibodies discriminate 2 immunophenotypically and genetically distinct subgroups of conventionally BCL2-"negative" grade 1/2 follicular lymphomas. *Hum Pathol*. 2013;44:1817-1826.

6. Xu J, Wang L, Li J, et al. SOX11-negative mantle cell lymphoma: clinicopathologic and prognostic features of 75 patients. *Am J Surg Pathol*. 2019;43:710-716.

7. Quintanilla-Martinez L, Fend F, Moguel LR, et al. Peripheral T-cell lymphoma with Reed-Sternberg-like cells of B-cell phenotype and genotype associated with Epstein-Barr virus infection. *Am J Surg Pathol*. 1999;23:1233-1240.

8. Ioachim HL. *Lymph Node Biopsy*. Philadelphia, PA: Lippincott; 1982.

9. Sundharkrishnan L, North JP. Histopathologic features of cutaneous leishmaniasis and use of CD1a staining for amastigotes in Old World and New World leishmaniasis. *J Cutan Pathol*. 2017;44:1005-1011.

10. Attygalle AD, Kyriakou C, Dupuis J, et al. Histologic evolution of angioimmunoblastic T-cell lymphoma in consecutive biopsies: clinical correlation and insights into natural history and disease progression. *Am J Surg Pathol*. 2007;31:1077-1088.

11. Hart M, Thakral B, Yohe S, et al. EBV-positive mucocutaneous ulcer in organ transplant recipients: a localized indolent posttransplant lymphoproliferative disorder. *Am J Surg Pathol*. 2014;38:1522-1529.

12. Barry TS, Jaffe ES, Sorbara L, Raffeld M, Pittaluga S. Peripheral T-cell lymphomas expressing CD30 and CD15. *Am J Surg Pathol*. 2003;27:1513-1522.

CHAPTER 1 INTRODUCTION

1-1. Which of the following is true for the structure in the center of this image (Figure 1A.1)?

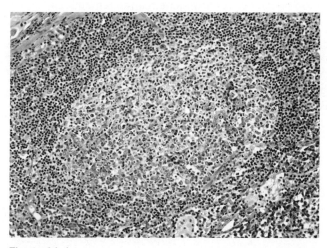

Figure 1A.1.

    A. It has a low Ki-67 proliferation index
    B. It is entirely composed of B-cells
    C. Most of the cells are BCL-2-positive
    D. Most of the cells are CD10-positive
    E. Most of the cells are CD23-positive

1-2. Which part of the normal lymph node is rich in plasma cells, as seen in Figure 1A.2?

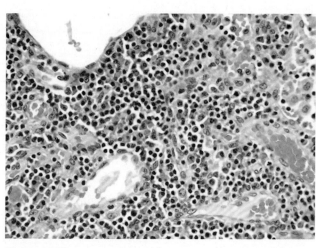

    A. Capsule
    B. Sinuses
    C. Cortex
    D. Paracortex
    E. Medullary cords

Figure 1A.2.

1-3. **Which panel is most appropriate for the initial workup of a core biopsy of a lymph node with no morphologic involvement by metastatic disease?**

    A. AE1/AE3, Cam5.2, CK903

    B. AE1/AE3, S100, CD45

    C. CD45, CD43, MUM-1, CD30

    D. CD3, CD20, Ki-67, CD30

    E. AFB, GMS, Brown-Hopps, Wright-Giemsa, Warthin-Starry

1-4. **Which of the following ancillary tests requires fresh tissue and cannot be performed on formalin-fixed and paraffin-embedded tissue?**

    A. Fluorescence in situ hybridization for t(14;18) (IGH/BCL2)

    B. PCR studies for immunoglobulin heavy chain gene rearrangements

    C. PCR studies for immunoglobulin light chain gene rearrangements

    D. Flow cytometry

    E. PCR studies for T-cell receptor gene rearrangement studies

1-5. **Which of the following cells are not present in the interfollicular area in Figure 1A.3 that is rich in CD3+ T-cells (Figure 1A.4)?**

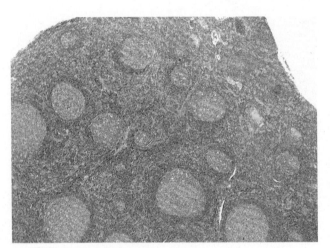

Figure 1A.3.

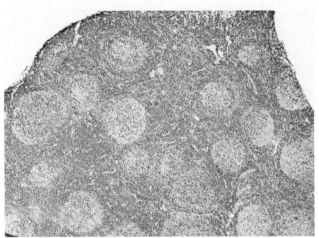

Figure 1A.4.

    A. Endothelial cells

    B. Germinal center B-cells

    C. Activated B- and T-lymphocytes (immunoblasts)

    D. Interdigitating dendritic cells

    E. Histiocytes

1-6. **The diagnosis of hematolymphoid disorders is facilitated by which of the following procedures?**

    A. Overnight fixation of the tissue

    B. Submitting the entire specimen for frozen section analysis

    C. Rushing the specimen with minimal fixation

    D. Submitting the entire specimen for fixation/embedding

    E. Flow cytometric analysis and morphologic evaluation of an aspirate without a concomitant core biopsy

CHAPTER 2 CAPSULE

2-1. **Which lymphoma often shows a predilection for continuation into the perinodal soft tissue, leaving a largely patent subcapsular sinus?**

    A. Angioimmunoblastic lymphoma

    B. Anaplastic large cell lymphoma

    C. Classical Hodgkin lymphoma

    D. Burkitt lymphoma

    E. B-lymphoblastic lymphoma

2-2. **The atypical vascular proliferation that involves the lymph node capsule seen in Figure 2A.1 is associated with which of the following disorders?**

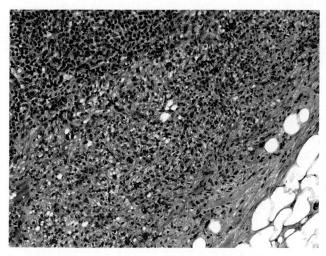

    A. Herpes lymphadenitis

    B. Syphilitic lymphadenitis

    C. Diffuse large B-cell lymphoma

    D. Kaposi sarcoma

    E. Nodular sclerosing classical Hodgkin lymphoma

Figure 2A.1.

2-3. **Capsular fibrosis is often associated with the entity in Figures 2A.2 and 2A.3. What is the most likely diagnosis?**

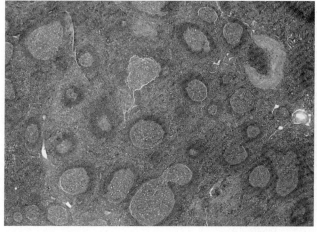
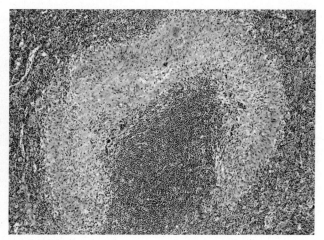

Figure 2A.2.

Figure 2A.3.

    A. Inflammatory liposarcoma

    B. Burkitt lymphoma

    C. IgG4-associated lymphadenopathy

    D. Mixed cellularity variant of classical Hodgkin lymphoma

    E. Lymphocyte-rich variant of classical Hodgkin lymphoma

2-4. Which of the following is true of these inclusions (Figure 2A.4) seen in a pelvic lymph node in a 35-year-old woman?

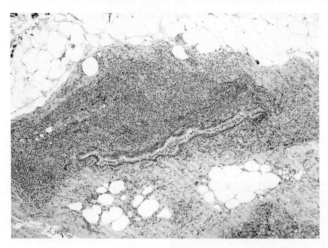

Figure 2A.4.

A. The inclusions may represent foci of endosalpingiosis, and careful cytomorphologic evaluation is warranted

B. The inclusions are diagnostic for endosalpingiosis involving the lymph node capsule, and careful cytomorphologic evaluation is not necessary

C. The inclusions are diagnostic for metastatic carcinoma

D. The inclusions are positive for S100

E. The inclusions are positive for CD45

2-5. The cells associated with the capsule in this image (Figure A2.5) will likely show which of the following staining patterns?

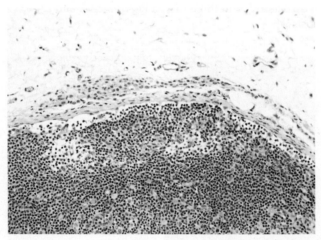

Figure 2A.5.

A. S100+, Melan-A/MART-1+, HMB-45+

B. S100+, Melan-A/MART-1+, HMB-45−

C. S100+, Melan-A/MART-1−, HMB-45−

D. S100−, Melan-A/MART-1−, HMB-45−

E. S100−, Melan-A/MART-1+, HMB-45+

2-6. Which of the following is NOT a typical feature of Kimura lymphadenopathy?

A. Increased eosinophils

B. Thickened capsule

C. Occasional Warthin-Finkeldey-type cells

D. Involvement of cervical lymph nodes, often near the ear

E. A peripheral monocytosis

CHAPTER 3 SINUS

3-1. A useful marker for distinguishing lymph nodes from spleniculi is

A. CD34

B. CD8

C. CD163

D. CD207

3-2. Which of the following sentences best describes vascular transformation of sinuses?

A. Neoplastic transformation of nodal sinus endothelium with potential for metastasis

B. Condition associated with congenital vascular malformations

C. Reactive changes often associated with neoplastic conditions in draining territory of lymph nodes.

D. Precursor lesion preceding development of Kaposi sarcoma

3-3. All the following malignancies can be seen in sinuses except

A. Metastatic breast cancer

B. Anaplastic large cell lymphoma

C. Extracavitary primary effusion lymphoma

D. Classical Hodgkin lymphoma

3-4. A 14-year-old boy had extensive bilateral neck lymphadenopathy with an excisional biopsy demonstrating effacement of the lymphoid architecture by marked expansion of the sinuses. Numerous large polygonal histiocytes were observed within the sinuses without cytologic atypia (Figure 3A.1). In addition, numerous background plasma cells and small lymphoid cells were also noted. He had normal LDH with localized disease. The most useful set stains to order in this clinical and pathologic setting is

A. CD20, CD10, MYC, and BCL2

B. S100, IgG4, CD68

C. CD30, CD15, PAX5

D. S100, CD1a, CD207

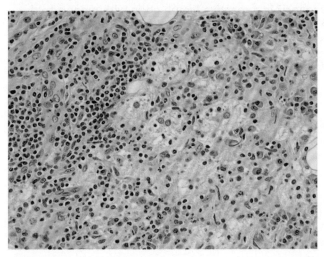

Figure 3A.1.

3-5. A reactive-appearing lymph node showed perisinusoidal clusters of mononuclear cells with irregular centrocyte-like nuclei and scant to moderate amount of clear cytoplasm. Few admixed neutrophils were also seen within these clusters. This description is most compatible with

    A. Monocytoid B-cells

    B. Plasmacytoid dendritic cells

    C. Germinal center B-cells

    D. Lymphoblasts

CHAPTER 4 CORTEX

4-1. Reactive immunoblasts are usually located in the

    A. Germinal center dark zone

    B. Mantle zone

    C. Subcapsular region

    D. Perifollicular region

4-2. Secondary lymphoid follicle germinal centers exhibit which of following phenotype?

    A. CD10+/BCL2+/IGD+

    B. CD10–/BCL2+/IGD+

    C. CD10+/BCL2–/IGD–

    D. CD10–/BCL2–/IGD–

4-3. Hyperplastic follicles may be seen rarely in this lymphoma:

    A. Follicular lymphoma

    B. Angioimmunoblastic T-cell lymphoma

    C. Anaplastic large cell lymphoma

    D. Plasmablastic lymphoma

4-4. Useful set of stains to diagnose progressive transformation of germinal centers are:

    A. CD20, MYC, and BCL2

    B. CD20, IGD, and BCL2

    C. CD20, MYC, and KI67

    D. CD3, CD20, and BCL6

4-5. The most plausible diagnosis in a reactive lymph node with monocytoid B-cell clusters and clusters of epithelioid histiocytes within the mantle zones is

    A. EBV lymphadenitis

    B. Cat scratch disease

    C. Toxoplasma

    D. HIV

CHAPTER 5 PARACORTEX

5-1. Which infectious lymphadenitis shows nuclear changes characterized by a ground glass appearance with margination of the chromatin (Figure 5A.1)?

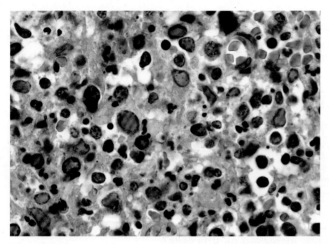

Figure 5A.1.

    A. Epstein-Barr virus (EBV)

    B. Herpes simplex virus (HSV)

    C. Cytomegalovirus (CMV)

    D. HIV

    E. HHV-8

5-2. Markedly enlarged tonsils with follicular hyperplasia and numerous EBV-positive cells in a 7-year-old boy 6 months after a renal transplant are best classified as which of the following entities?

    A. Infectious mononucleosis

    B. Reactive lymph node with follicular hyperplasia

    C. Posttransplant lymphoproliferative disorder (PTLD), polymorphous type

    D. Posttransplant lymphoproliferative disorder (PTLD), monomorphic type (EBV+ diffuse large B-cell lymphoma)

    E. Posttransplant lymphoproliferative disorder (PTLD), infectious mononucleosis type

5-3. Which class of medications is most frequently associated with drug-associated lymphadenopathy?

    A. Antihypertensive agents

    B. Antihistamines

    C. Anticonvulsants

    D. Statins

    E. Selective serotonin reuptake inhibitors

5-4. Which of the following cases of lymphadenopathy is NOT associated with increased histiocytes within the paracortex?

    A. Toxoplasma lymphadenopathy

    B. Kikuchi lymphadenitis

    C. Chronic lymphocytic leukemia/small lymphocytic lymphoma (CLL/SLL)

    D. Sarcoidosis

    E. Atypical mycobacterial infection

5-5. Which of the following findings is often true of light chain deposition disease?

    A. Amorphous eosinophilic deposits that stain salmon pink with a Congo red stain and show apple green birefringence under polarized light

    B. A brisk foreign-body giant cell reaction

    C. More frequently associated with lambda light chain than with kappa light chain

    D. Spares the vessel walls

    E. Associated with localized deposition, and systemic disease is not seen

5-6. Which of the following causes of lymphadenopathy are NOT characteristically associated with relatively increased plasma cells?

    A. Rheumatoid lymphadenopathy

    B. Drug-associated lymphadenopathy

    C. HIV-associated lymphadenopathy

    D. Kaposi sarcoma

    E. Castleman lymphadenopathy, plasma cell variant

5-7. How can an indolent T-lymphoblastic proliferation be distinguished from T-lymphoblastic lymphoma?

    A. PCR studies for T-cell receptor gene rearrangements

    B. Ki-67 proliferation index

    C. CD4/CD8 double positive T-cells

    D. Bright expression of CD7

    E. Expression of TdT

5-8. Which of the following markers is not expressed by normal mast cells?

    A. CD45

    B. CD117

    C. Mast cell tryptase

    D. Calretinin

    E. CD25

CHAPTER 6 OBLITERATED NODAL PATTERN

6-1. All the following entities frequently demonstrate obliterated pattern of nodular architecture except

    A. Nodular lymphocyte-predominant Hodgkin lymphoma

    B. Hyaline vascular Castleman disease

    C. Follicular T-cell lymphoma

    D. Marginal zone lymphoma

6-2. **Useful panel of stains in nodular lymphocyte-predominant Hodgkin lymphoma include**

    A. CD20, CD3, IgD, OCT2
    B. CD30, CD15, PAX5
    C. CD20, CD10, MYC
    D. CD163, PU.1, and S100

6-3. **In the context of neoplasms of follicular helper T-cell derivation, identification of follicular helper T-cell phenotype can be aided by**

    A. PU.1 and BCL6
    B. PD-1 and ICOS
    C. CD10 and BCL6
    D. MUM1 and CD4

6-4. **All the following cells are seen within follicular structures except these cells which normally express CD30 (Figure 6A.1)**

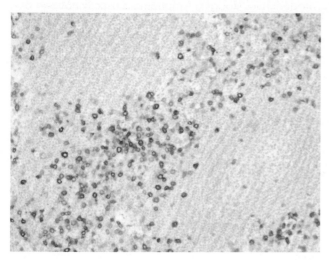

    A. Follicular dendritic cells
    B. Centrocytes
    C. Immunoblasts
    D. Tingible body macrophages

Figure 6A.1.

6-5. **Abnormal large atypical cells are seen in the context of these nodular proliferations except**

    A. Nodular lymphocyte-predominant Hodgkin lymphoma
    B. Lymphocyte-rich classical Hodgkin lymphoma
    C. Follicular variant of peripheral T-cell lymphoma
    D. Mantle cell lymphoma

CHAPTER 7 DIFFUSE

7-1. **Proliferation centers in small lymphocytic lymphoma usually**

    A. Have a low proliferation index seen with Ki-67
    B. Have a MYC rearrangement seen by FISH analysis
    C. May be positive for MYC and cyclin D1 by IHC
    D. Express BCL6 by IHC

7-2. **Cyclin D1-negative mantle cell lymphomas**

    A. Are mostly negative for SOX11

    B. Have a similar gene expression profiling as cyclin D1-positive mantle cell lymphoma

    C. Tend to be more aggressive and have a blastoid morphology

    D. Has a cryptic translocation of CCND1

7-3. **Plasma cell myelomas**

    A. May be indistinguishable from plasmablastic lymphoma especially if they have plasmablastic morphology

    B. Usually present in the skin as a mass-like lesion

    C. Never have a MYC translocation

    D. Can sometimes have less than 10% plasma cells in the bone marrow

7-4. **When evaluating a case of T-cell/histiocyte-rich large B-cell lymphoma (THRLBL):**

    A. Nodular lymphocyte-predominant Hodgkin lymphoma is usually not part of the differential

    B. CD30 is a helpful marker as it is usually positive in the large atypical cells

    C. One can encounter many small B-cells admixed with the large atypical cells

    D. The CD20 immunostain helps with identifying the large cells as they are usually scattered and singly distributed

7-5. **The EBV-positive large cells seen in some cases of peripheral T-cell lymphoma (PTCL) are**

    A. Usually T-cells

    B. Usually histiocytes

    C. May coexpress CD30 by IHC

    D. Usually seen with the PTCL with cytotoxic phenotype

7-6. **Cutaneous T-cell lymphomas that involve the lymph node can mimic classical Hodgkin lymphoma because**

    A. They morphologically mimic classical Hodgkin lymphoma and have an inflammatory background with eosinophils

    B. The abnormal T-cells usually express B-cell markers such as CD20 and CD79a

    C. Usually they are positive for immunoglobulin gene rearrangement studies

    D. Present with B symptoms and mediastinal mass

CHAPTER 8 NECROSIS

8-1. **CD20 immunostain is a helpful stain in cases with diffuse large B-cell lymphoma and necrosis because**

    A. If the B-cells are nonviable or necrotic, they will still stain with CD20

    B. It can be used in conjunction with EBER-ISH in the necrotic cells

    C. Plasma cells are mostly positive for CD20, and you can identify plasmacytic differentiation

    D. You can distinguish which cells are viable or nonviable by CD20

8-2. **EBV-positive mucocutaneous ulcer is**

A. Only seen in elderly patients

B. Usually does not benefit from withdrawal of immunosuppressive therapy

C. Has a limited growth potential

D. Characterized by large atypical cells forming sheets

8-3. **Which of the following statements is true?**

A. The two main groups of posttransplant lymphoproliferative disorder (PTLD) are aggressive and nonaggressive

B. The two main groups of PTLD are destructive and nondestructive

C. T-cell PTLD are more common than B-cell PTLD

D. Nearly all PTLD cases are positive for EBV

8-4. **Which of the following statement is true regarding anaplastic large cell lymphoma (ALCL)?**

A. *DUSP22* rearrangement is seen in ALK-positive ALCL and associated with a good prognosis

B. Some cases of ALCL have variable CD30 expression and are commonly seen with ALK-negative ALCL

C. Cases of ALCL involving the lymph node may be focal and involve the sub-capsular spaces and sinuses

D. Most cases of ALCL have intact T-cell makers such as CD3, CD2, CD5, and CD7

8-5. **All of the following are true except**

A. Kikuchi-Fujimoto lymphadenitis (KFL) usually affects women of Asian descent

B. Neutrophils are commonly seen and are highlighted by the myeloperoxidase stain

C. KFL can be misdiagnosed as a T-cell lymphoma, because the T-cells can have cytologic atypia

D. T-cell gene rearrangement studies are usually negative in KFL which is helpful in distinguishing from a lymphoma

CHAPTER 9 IMMUNOHISTOCHEMISTRY

9-1. **Figure 9.49 IHC chapter**

This immunostain image depicts scattered spindly cells with nuclear staining in addition to scattered mononuclear cells demonstrating nuclear staining, both of which serve as internal controls. Based on the staining pattern, this immunostain is most likely to represent

A. ERG

B. CD20

C. Cyclin D1

D. CD33

9-2. **Figure 9.116**

This 34-year-old male with no evidence of HIV infection demonstrated lymphadenopathy which was biopsied. Numerous EBV-positive cells were located within the follicular structures as noted in this image. Which additional immunostains are most likely to be diagnostic in this lymphoid neoplasm?

A. CD20, MUM1, and HHV8

B. CD30, ALK1

C. Mammaglobin and ER

D. S100 and SOX10

9-3. CD30 is useful in all the following entities except

    A. Angioimmunoblastic T-cell lymphoma

    B. Extramedullary myeloid tumor

    C. Classical Hodgkin lymphoma

    D. Primary mediastinal (thymic) large B-cell lymphoma

9-4. BCL-2 is expressed in all the following cells except

    A. Normal T-cells

    B. Mantle zone B-cells

    C. Follicular lymphoma

    D. Burkitt lymphoma cells

9-5. CD123 is a useful marker for identification of

    A. Follicular dendritic cells

    B. Plasmacytoid dendritic cells

    C. Monocytoid B-cells

    D. Interfollicular immunoblasts

SELF-ASSESSMENT ANSWERS

CHAPTER 1 INTRODUCTION

1-1. Answer – D. This is a normal germinal center. Germinal center B-cells are CD10 and BCL-6-positive but are negative for BCL-2. Germinal centers have a high Ki-67 proliferation index and have a few admixed follicular helper T-cells and tingible body macrophages. The follicular helper T-cells in the germinal centers are also CD10-positive (bright). CD23 marks the follicular dendritic cell meshworks that underlie the follicles.

1-2. Answer – E. The medullary sinuses are near the center of the lymph node and are surrounded by an area rich in lymphocytes, plasmacytoid lymphocytes, and plasma cells. This area, known as the medullary cords, is the area in which plasma cells proliferate and produce antibodies.

1-3. Answer – D. Panel D will determine the distribution of T-cells (CD3) and B-cells (CD20), evaluate the proliferation index of various parts of the node (Ki-67), and identify possible Hodgkin/Reed-Sternberg cells or immunoblasts (CD30). Panel A (AE1/AE3, Cam5.2, CK903) includes cytokeratins; one or more of these stains would typically highlight a possible metastatic carcinoma. Panel B (AE1/AE3, S100, CD45) is appropriate for the initial workup of atypical cells of uncertain etiology in order to determine whether they represent carcinoma (AE1/AE3), melanoma (S100) or a hematolymphoid (CD45) neoplasm. Panel C (CD45, CD43, MUM-1, CD30) is useful for ruling in or ruling out the possibility of a hematolymphoid neoplasm, as nearly all hematolymphoid neoplasms are positive for at least one of these markers. Panel E (AFB, GMS, Brown-Hopps, Wright-Giemsa, Warthin-Starry) is appropriate for the workup of a possible infectious lymphadenitis.

1-4. Answer – D. Flow cytometry requires fresh tissue and cannot be performed on fixed tissue. Thus, it is important to submit (or hold) a portion of the fresh tissue for flow cytometry when grossing a specimen with possible or suspected involvement by a hematolymphoid neoplasm. Selected fluorescence in situ hybridization (FISH) studies and PCR studies for clonal gene rearrangements (IGH, IGK, TCR) can be performed on formalin-fixed and paraffin-embedded tissue.

1-5. Answer – B. The paracortex comprises the area between follicles and the medullary cords and is composed of a mixture of lymphocytes, small vessels, and scattered activated lymphocytes known as immunoblasts. Most of the lymphocytes in the paracortex are CD3-positive T-cells. The paracortex also contains antigen presenting cells, including Langerhans cells, interdigitating dendritic cells, and histiocytes. Germinal center B-cells are present in reactive follicles, which are part of the cortex rather than the paracortex.

1-6. Answer – A. Adequate fixation is crucial for evaluation of the overall lymph node architecture and cytomorphology. "Rushing" the specimen may lead to inadequate fixation. When the tissue is frozen or poorly fixed, the cells become distorted, making it difficult to assess both the overall architecture of the node and the cytomorphology of the lymphocytes. A portion of the node should be submitted (or held) for flow cytometric analysis at the time of grossing, because flow cytometry requires fresh tissue. Flow cytometry is able to readily detect clonal B-cells or abnormal T-cell populations that can be difficult to identify on tissue sections. Fine-needle aspirates with concomitant flow cytometric analysis may be diagnostic in some instances; however, if a core biopsy is not submitted for evaluation then hematolymphoid neoplasms that are not readily detected by flow cytometric analysis or seen on smears (such as classical Hodgkin lymphoma) may be missed.

CHAPTER 2 CAPSULE

2-1. Answer – A. So-called skip lesions are often seen in angioimmunoblastic lymphoma, though they can occasionally be seen in other lymphomas as well. Anaplastic large cell lymphoma may show a sinusoidal distribution. The nodular sclerosing variant of classical Hodgkin lymphoma is typically associated with a thickened capsule. Nodal involvement by Burkitt and B-lymphoblastic lymphoma do not characteristically show this growth pattern.

2-2. Answer – D. Early Kaposi sarcoma lesions involve the lymph node capsule. These lesions are comprised of a proliferation of endothelial cells in the capsule that result in poorly formed slitlike vascular spaces, often with extravasated red blood cells and admixed hemosiderin-laden macrophages. Syphilitic lymphadenitis and nodular sclerosing classical Hodgkin lymphoma often exhibit thickening of the lymph node capsule. Syphilitic lymphadenitis has a characteristic lymphoplasmacytic infiltrate around vessels within the capsule but does not show a marked vascular proliferation. Neither herpes lymphadenitis nor Burkitt lymphoma is associated with specific abnormalities of the lymph node capsule.

2-3. Answer – C. IgG4-associated lymphadenopathy does not have a single characteristic morphologic appearance, but capsular thickening and reactive changes are often seen in involved lymph nodes. This node also contains granulomas that curve around reactive germinal centers, which can be seen in IgG4-associated lymphadenopathy. The nodular sclerosing variant of classical Hodgkin lymphoma is characteristically associated with capsular fibrosis; however, the other three variants of classical Hodgkin lymphoma (mixed cellularity, lymphocyte-rich, and lymphocyte-depleted) do not typically show marked capsular fibrosis. Liposarcomas with a dense associated lymphoid infiltrate can mimic atypical lymphoid infiltrates but are not lymph nodes and do not have a lymph node capsule. Burkitt lymphoma is an aggressive and rapidly growing neoplasm and is not associated with capsular thickening.

2-4. Answer – A. One of the most common inclusions in pelvic lymph nodes is endosalpingiosis. Foci of endosalpingiosis may be subtle. They are highlighted with a cytokeratin immunohistochemical stain but are not positive for either S100 or CD45. Occasionally these benign structures can mimic carcinoma; however, unlike carcinoma, capsular endosalpingiosis is cytologically bland, and cilia can often be identified on a subset of the cells.

2-5. Answer – B. Capsular nevi may be seen in peripheral lymph nodes that drain the skin. The cells are cytologically bland. They typically express S100 and Melan A (MART-1) but are negative for HMB-45. Capsular nevi also have a low Ki-67 proliferation index. In contrast, metastatic melanoma is more likely to be positive for S100, Melan-A/MART-1, and HMB-45 and typically has a high Ki-67 proliferation index.

2-6. Answer – E. The enlarged nodes in Kimura lymphadenopathy are characteristically found in the cervical area or near the ears. The lymph node architecture is intact, displaying follicular hyperplasia and vascular proliferation. Multinucleated cells that resemble Warthin-Finkeldey cells are often readily identified in Kimura lymphadenopathy. The capsule is typically thickened and there may be bands of fibrosis, and as the disease progresses, the lymph nodes may become matted together. Both the peripheral blood and lymph node are notable for an eosinophilia.

CHAPTER 3 SINUS

3.1. Answer – B. The splenic littoral endothelium expresses strong CD8, whereas the lymph node sinus endothelium is negative for CD8 and allows the distinction of lymph node from spleniculi. CD34 is positive on both whereas CD163 stains histiocytes, and CD207 (Langerin) stains only Langerhans cells.

3-2. Answer – C. Vascular transformation of sinuses is a benign condition often associated with extensive endothelialization and vascularization of sinuses of lymph nodes often seen in the context of other solid tumor malignancies such as renal cell carcinoma. Sometimes, it may be confused with metastatic vascular tumors, specifically Kaposi sarcoma. Careful examination for possible hyaline globules and positivity for HHV 8 is typical of Kaposi sarcoma and allows its distinction.

3-3. Answer – D. Most metastatic malignancies including breast cancer as well as melanoma typically involve subcapsular sinus and trabecular sinuses. Likewise, anaplastic large cell lymphoma frequently involves lymphatics including cases of extracavitary primary effusion lymphoma which is often seen in the sinusoidal location. It is very unusual to see classical Hodgkin lymphoma localized to the sinuses.

3-4. Answer – B. The overall clinical and histologic picture is suggestive of a benign histiocytic process most consistent with Rosai-Dorfman disease. All histiocytic cells are positive for CD68 while only Rosai-Dorfman histiocytes coexpress S100. Frequently increased numbers of IgG4+ plasmacytic cells are increased in the background of Rosai-Dorfman lesions. Choice A would be appropriate in a case of Burkitt lymphoma which can occur in the child, although localized disease and the histologic description is not compatible with this diagnosis. Likewise, choice C is appropriate in the context of classical Hodgkin lymphoma which can occur in children. However, the histologic description is not compatible with this possibility. Choice D would be appropriate when Langerhans cell histiocytosis is a consideration. However, the clinical presentation and histologic description is not compatible with Langerhans cells which often contain elongated and grooved nuclei with scant to moderate amount of cytoplasm.

3-5. Answer – A. The morphology is compatible with monocytoid B-cells, which typically occurs in the perisinusoidal location and can be confirmed with CD20. Plasmacytoid dendritic cells often contain apoptotic structures (see Figure 3.71) with round nuclei and clumped but dispersed chromatin. Although germinal center centrocytes exhibit identical nuclei, the cells have very scant cytoplasm and are restricted topographically to germinal centers and are not seen in the perisinusoidal location outside the confines of the lymphoid follicle. Lymphoblasts typically involve the paracortex and exhibit finely dispersed chromatin with scant cytoplasm.

CHAPTER 4 CORTEX

4-1. Answer – D. Reactive immunoblasts are typically formed from antigens selected germinal center B-cells. The cells developed either into memory B-cells or progress to develop into reactive immunoblasts which in turn mature into plasma cells filled with intracytoplasmic immunoglobulin. Germinal center dark zone (choice A) typically contains centroblasts, while mantle zone (choice B) contains naïve B-cells, and subcapsular region (choice C) contains histiocytes and dendritic cells.

4-2. Answer – C. Reactive secondary germinal centers typically expressed germinal center B-cell marker CD10 and are negative for IgD and BCL-2. Coexpression of CD10 and BCL-2 (choice A) is typical of follicular lymphoma. Choice B corresponds to mantle zone naïve B-cells which coexpress IgD and BCL-2. Primary follicles exhibit identical immunophenotype as mantle zone–naïve B-cells of secondary lymphoid follicles.

4-3. Answer – B. Reactive hyperplastic follicles may often be seen in the context of early angioimmunoblastic T-cell lymphoma which may often show perifollicular accumulations of CD4+/PD–1+ follicular helper T-cells corresponding to the cell of origin for this lymphoma. Although lymph nodes partially involved by follicular lymphoma may show scattered reactive follicles, most of the time, there is diffuse effacement of the lymphoid architecture in follicular lymphoma as well as anaplastic large cell lymphoma and plasmablastic lymphoma which typically overrun the entire lymph node.

4-4. Answer – B. CD20 confirms B-cell origin while coexpression of IgD and BCL-2 supports mantle zone phenotype. Progressive transformation of germinal centers is defined by the ingression of naïve mantle zone B-cells into the germinal centers with resulting expansion of the follicular structure with disruption of germinal center B-cell reaction. MYC is not expressed in mantle zone B-cells and BCL6 stains germinal center B-cells.

4-5: Answer – C. Toxoplasma involvement of lymph node is characterized by the combination of monocytoid B-cell clusters and tight epithelioid cell clusters in the mantle zones. While monocytoid B-cell expansion may be seen in EBV lymphadenitis, frequently there is extensive paracortical expansion, immunoblastic reaction, and variable amount of interfollicular increase in histiocytes. Numerous stellate abscesses containing neutrophils are typical of cat scratch disease, while in HIV lymphadenitis, there is prominent follicular hyperplasia or follicular lysis in the stages of primary generalized lymphadenopathy.

CHAPTER 5 PARACORTEX

5-1. Answer – B. HSV lymphadenitis shows nonspecific morphologic findings similar to those in EBV and CMV lymphadenitis; however, cells infected with HSV exhibit characteristic nuclear changes, including a ground glass appearance with margination of the chromatin. HSV lymphadenitis is rare in immunocompetent individuals and can also be seen in association with chronic lymphocytic leukemia/small lymphocytic lymphoma (CLL/SLL). EBV lymphadenitis is associated with scattered atypical cells that resemble Hodgkin/Reed-Sternberg cells, CMV lymphadenitis exhibits immunoblasts containing large eosinophilic intranuclear inclusions surrounded by a clear halo, and HIV lymphadenopathy can show scattered Warthin-Finkeldey-type cells. HHV-8 infection is associated with various neoplasms, including the plasma cell variant of Castleman disease, large B-cell lymphoma, and Kaposi sarcoma.

5-2. Answer – E. As this patient is status-post transplant, the findings in this lymph node are best classified as a posttransplant lymphoproliferative disorder (PTLD). There is no destruction of the tissue architecture; thus, it is a nondestructive subtype of PTLD. The three nondestructive subtypes of PTLD include infectious mononucleosis, follicular hyperplasia, and plasmacytic hyperplasia. As there are numerous EBV+ cells, the infectious mononucleosis subtype of PTLD is the best classification. The infectious mononucleosis subtype of PTLD is typically seen in patients who were previously EBV- but received an organ from an EBV+ donor. It is most frequently seen in younger patients.

5-3. Answer – C. While many other drugs have been implicated in drug-associated lymphadenopathy, the anticonvulsants (ie, phenytoin and phenobarbital) are most frequently reported causative agents. The nodes show follicular and paracortical hyperplasia, and eosinophils may also be increased. The lymph node findings in drug-associated lymphadenopathy are nonspecific, and clinical correlation is needed to make the diagnosis.

5-4. Answer – C. CLL/SLL is not typically associated with increased histiocytes within involved lymph nodes. However, increased histiocytes can be seen in nodal marginal zone lymphoma, and singly scattered epithelioid histiocytes are often seen in lymph nodes involved by mantle cell lymphoma. Toxoplasma lymphadenopathy is characterized by a triad of findings, including follicular hyperplasia, areas of monocytoid B-cells, and clusters of epithelioid histiocytes that encroach on germinal centers. Kikuchi lymphadenitis exhibits patchy aneutrophilic necrosis with abundant admixed histiocytes, immunoblasts, and plasmacytoid dendritic cells. Of note, systemic lupus lymphadenitis and Kikuchi lymphadenopathy are difficult to distinguish from one another based on morphologic and immunophenotypic findings. Sarcoid lymphadenopathy is characterized by closely packed and well-demarcated noncaseating granulomas. Atypical mycobacterial infections in immunocompromised patients can result in spindle cell pseudotumor, in which lymph nodes are partially or completely replaced by spindled histiocytes that contain mycobacterial organisms.

5-5. Answer – B. Both amyloidosis and light chain deposition can show either localized or systemic involvement, and both may involve vessel walls. While amyloid is readily identified by its characteristic salmon pink staining with a Congo red special stain and apple green birefringence under polarized light, light chain deposits are not highlighted by a Congo red stain. Amyloidosis is often, but not always, associated with lambda light chain-positive neoplasms, whereas light chain deposition disease is more strongly correlated with kappa light chain expression by the associated neoplasm. The light chains deposited within tissue can incite a vigorous foreign-body giant cell response.

5-6. Answer – B. Drug-associated lymphadenopathy demonstrates follicular and paracortical hyperplasia and may also show eosinophilia. It is not characteristically associated with increased plasma cells. The lymph nodes in long-standing HIV lymphadenopathy have atretic and fibrosed follicles, but the paracortex remains expanded with abundant plasma cells and prominent vasculature. Early Kaposi sarcoma lesions involve the lymph node capsule, and the remainder of the lymph node typically shows reactive changes, including follicular hyperplasia and a polytypic plasmacytosis. As the name suggests, increased plasma cells are characteristic of the plasma cell variant of Castleman lymphadenopathy.

5-7. Answer – A. Molecular studies are of value in distinguishing iT-LBP from T-ALL because iT-LBP exhibits a polyclonal pattern on T-cell receptor gene rearrangement studies. In contrast, CD4+/CD8+ T-lymphoblastic lymphoma is typically clonal. The T-lymphoblasts in iT-LBP are CD4/CD8 double-positive cells, which can also be seen in T-ALL with a cortical thymocyte-like phenotype. Both iT-LBP and T-ALL usually coexpress TdT and bright CD7, and both have a high Ki-67 proliferation index.

5-8. Answer – E. Normal mast cells express CD45, CD117 (bright), mast cell tryptase, and calretinin; however, abnormal mast cells typically show immunophenotypic abnormalities. The abnormalities may include aberrant expression of CD2, CD25, and/or CD30; loss of mast cell tryptase expression; and variation in the intensity of CD117 and CD45 expression.

CHAPTER 6 OBLITERATED NODAL PATTERN

6-1. Answer – D. Marginal zone lymphoma occurring in lymph nodes is an interfollicular proliferation that may occasionally demonstrate disruption of the follicles but is primarily interfollicular. All the other entities demonstrate varying degrees of expansile or regressed nodular follicular structures. In rare instances, nodal marginal zone lymphoma with follicular colonization may demonstrate nodular motheaten pattern.

6-2. Answer – A. The neoplastic cells of nodular lymphocyte-predominant Hodgkin lymphoma, ie, LP cells, express CD20 and OCT2. Additionally, both stains will highlight background small B-cells within the nodular structures which may occasionally be T-cell rich on CD3. IgD typically highlights the nodular small B-cells within the nodules in the background. In rare instances, LP cells may express IgD in younger patients in the cervical location.

6-3. Answer – B. Both PD-1 and ICOS are sensitive and specific markers for follicular helper T-cell phenotype. Although CD10, BCL6, and MUM1 are expressed in follicular helper T-cells to a varying degree, consistent expression on neoplastic follicular helper T-cells is not observed in these markers. CD4, however, is sensitive but is not specific to follicular helper phenotype, because regulatory T-cells and other T-cell subsets may also be positive for CD4.

6-4. Answer – C. Immunoblasts are typically located in the perifollicular regions while all the other cells noted here occur within the lymphoid follicles. CD30 is a useful stain to identify perifollicular immunoblasts in reactive follicular hyperplasia.

6-5. Answer – D. The cells of mantle cell lymphoma are usually pretty uniform with either classical, blastoid, or pleomorphic cytomorphology. Scattered benign macrophages are noted, but Hodgkin-like cells are not present. Both nodular lymphocyte-predominant Hodgkin lymphoma and lymphocyte-rich classical Hodgkin lymphoma consistently contain abnormal large atypical neoplastic cells, whereas scattered reactive Hodgkin-like B-cells may be seen in follicular variant of peripheral T-cell lymphoma.

CHAPTER 7 DIFFUSE

7-1. Answer – C. Proliferation centers in SLL can be positive for MYC and cyclin D1 by immunohistochemistry but lack translocations for MYC and CCND1. The proliferation index in the proliferation centers is usually high by Ki-67. They are pseudofollicles and not true germinal centers, so they are negative for BCL6 by IHC.

7-2. Answer – B. Cyclin D1-negative mantle cell lymphomas (MCL) are usually positive for SOX11 by IHC. They are not usually more aggressive than typical MCL. These cases have a gene expression profiling similar to conventional MCL, and some cases have increased expression with CCND2 and CCND3.

7-3. Answer – A. Plasmablastic lymphoma (PBL) may have the same immunophenotype as plasma cell myeloma especially if you are dealing with a PBL that is EBV negative. Plasma cell myeloma does not usually present in the skin but more commonly in the respiratory tract or soft tissue. Plasma cell myeloma can also have an MYC translocation just like PBL, and a diagnosis of plasma cell myeloma requires greater than 10% plasma cells in the bone marrow.

7-4. Answer – D. Sometimes the large atypical cells are subtle because of the extensive T-cell and histiocyte infiltrate; therefore, CD20 is helpful in highlighting these large cells. Some cases of nodular lymphocyte-predominant Hodgkin lymphoma (NLPHL) can be seen concurrently with THRLBL, and CD21 immunostaining may be helpful in identifying these nodular structures associated with the NLPHL. CD30 is positive in a subset of large cells in THRLBL, and one should not encounter very many small B-cells.

7-5. Answer – C. In cases of PTCL, especially in PTCL with a TFH-phenotype, the EBV-positive large cells have Hodgkin-like morphology and can express CD30. These are usually B-cells and not T-cells or histiocytes.

7-6. Answer – A. Cutaneous T-cell lymphoma (CTCL) involving the lymph node can mimic Hodgkin lymphoma, because there can be large atypical cells characteristic of Hodgkin cells with CD30 expression. These cells are usually negative for PAX5 and are positive for T-cell gene rearrangements when there are a lot of tumor cells or if enriched by microdissection. CTCL does not usually present with B symptoms or a mediastinal mass.

CHAPTER 8 NECROSIS

8-1. Answer – A. There are cases of DLBCL with necrosis where the CD20 is helpful in that it will still stain the nonviable cells and showing their outline, "ghost cells." In situ hybridization for EBER, however, would be negative in nonviable or necrotic areas due to the degradation of RNA. Plasma cells can aberrantly express CD20, but this is not the norm.

8-2. Answer – C. EBV-positive mucocutaneous ulcer (MCU) can be seen mainly in elder patients but can also be seen in younger patients, especially if immuno-compromised. Usually the initial step is to withdraw or lower immunosuppressive therapy to see if the lesions will regress on their own. The large atypical cells are usually scattered or can form small clusters but are not usually forming sheets of large cells as you would see in diffuse large B-cell lymphoma.

8-3. Answer – B. PTLD is differentiated by whether there is destruction of the normal architecture. Destructive PTLD (eg, monomorphic PTLD) are typically clonal, and B-cell type is more common compared with T-cell type (eg, Hepatosplenic T-cell lymphoma). PTLD are not always positive for EBV, and some PTLD that develop years after the transplant may be negative for EBV.

8-4. Answer – C. *DUSP22* rearrangements are usually seen in ALK-negative ALCL and not ALK-positive and are associated with an improved prognosis compared with typical ALK-negative ALCL. CD30 is strong and uniform by IHC in ALCL. Variable staining for CD30 is more typical of PTCL, NOS. Loss of T-cell markers is common in ALCL, and some cases may be considered "null cell" lacking the majority of pan T-cell markers.

8-5. Answer – B. Neutrophils are not usually seen in KFL, but the histiocytes usually have myeloperoxidase staining by IHC. KLF is common in women of Asian de-scent, and the cytologic atypia in the T-cells can be concerning for a T-cell lym-phoma. However, T-cell gene rearrangements are usually negative in KFL which is helpful in making that distinction from lymphoma.

CHAPTER 9 IMMUNOHISTOCHEMISTRY

9-1. Answer – C. Both endothelial cells and histiocytes serve as internal control cells for cyclin D1 which demonstrates nuclear staining in both compartments. While ERG marks endothelial cells with nuclear pattern, staining in histiocytes would be incompatible with ERG. Likewise, CD20 stains background small lymphoid cells including B-cells while CD33 stains scattered histiocytes, in the cytoplasm, and membrane, but nuclear staining for CD33 in endothelial cells is incompatible.

9-2. Answer – A. This characteristic immunostaining pattern for large cells restricted to lymphoid follicles on EBER is typical of germinotropic lymphoproliferative dis-order which typically occurs in immunocompetent individuals. The cells exhibit plasmablastic phenotype and are negative for CD20 but positive for MUM1 as well as HHV8. The second choice (choice B) is useful in cases of anaplastic large cell lymphoma, although isolated location within the follicles and EBV expression is not compatible with this diagnosis. Metastatic breast cancer and metastatic melanoma are positive for choices C and D, respectively, but again, restriction within lymphoid follicles and EBV expression as noted here is not compatible with both diagnosis.

9-3. Answer – B. Extramedullary myeloid tumor is typically positive for myeloid markers, and CD30 is not useful in the diagnosis or prognostication of this entity. However, scattered immunoblasts of angioimmunoblastic T-cell lymphoma are positive for CD30 while the neoplastic cells of classical Hodgkin lymphoma are positive for CD30 while moderate diffuse staining for CD30 is also present in pri-mary mediastinal (thymic) large B-cell lymphoma.

9-4. Answer – D. BCL-2 is normally expressed in all mantle zone B-cells and normal T-cells. Although germinal center B-cells are negative, follicular lymphoma is pos-itive for BCL-2, while Burkitt lymphoma is characteristically negative for BCL-2 despite origin from germinal center B-cells.

9-5. Answer – B. CD123 is a specific marker for plasmacytoid dendritic cells and ad-ditionally stains basophils and bone marrows. None of the other cells stain with CD123.

Note: Page numbers followed by "*f*" indicate figures and "*b*" indicate boxes.